Table of Contents

W9-AWB-047

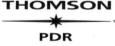

SECTION I
CLINICAL STRATEGIES

STRATEGIES FOR THE MANAGEMENT OF PATIENTS WITH COLORECTAL CANCER

Al B. Benson III, MD, FACP
Professor of Medicine
Associate Director for Clinical Investigations
Robert H. Lurie Comprehensive Cancer Center of Northwestern University
Chicago, IL

INTRODUCTION

Our knowledge of colorectal cancer (CRC) and how to prevent and treat it has been enhanced in the last few years, uncovering new truths and dispelling commonly held myths. For example, a recent meta-analysis of 13 prospective cohort studies involving 725,628 adults followed for six to 20 years concluded that high dietary fiber is not associated with a reduced risk of colorectal cancer, thereby confusing a populace that has been indoctrinated to include more dietary roughage to ensure a healthy colon.[1]

The drugs available to treat the disease are changing, as well. Aimed at molecular targets such as epidermal growth factors, agents are becoming more widely researched both as monotherapy and in combination with traditional therapies. Pharmaceutical protectants like the 3-hydroxy-3-methylglutaryl coenzyme A (HMG-CoA) reductase inhibitors, or "statins," are also being assessed as means to protect one against CRC. Some say they work.[2] Others disagree with this approach.[3,4]

Another issue: Should adjuvant chemotherapy be offered to patients with stage II CRC? Not unless the patients are part of a clinical trial, according to a 1990 National Institutes of Health Consensus Panel.[5] On the other hand, in 2004 the American Society of Clinical Oncology recommended against the routine use of adjuvant therapy. However, for high-risk subsets of stage III patients, adjuvant therapy could be considered after thorough discussion with the patient about risks vs benefits.[6]

This article will review the current treatment options for CRC, including the advantages and disadvantages of adjuvant therapy in early stage CRC, as well as some of the newer molecules under consideration, and other issues that can impact therapeutic success.

EPIDEMIOLOGY: THE BURDEN OF GENDER AND HERITAGE

Colorectal cancer is the third most common cancer and the second leading cause of cancer death in the United States, with approximately

145,290 new cases and 56,290 deaths from CRC estimated to have occurred in 2005.[7] Although the lifetime probability (magnitude of absolute risk) for the development of CRC in the United States is about 6%, the incidence and mortality of colorectal cancer increase with age. Over 90% of newly diagnosed cases and 94% of deaths from CRC occur in people over age 50.[7] The incidence rate of CRC is almost 60 times higher in men and 48 times higher among women aged 60 to 79 years than in those under the age of 39.[8] CRC incidence and mortality rates are more than 35% higher in men than in women.[7]

Racial disparities in the disease exist, as well. The incidence and mortality of CRC are highest in African Americans, with rates of incidence about 15% higher compared with non-Hispanic whites and mortality rates about 40% higher than for whites

(**Table 1**). Before 1987, the incidence rates for CRC were higher for non-Hispanic white males than for their African American counterparts. The current reversal of that trend may reflect historical underdiagnosis of CRC in African Americans, with some studies showing that members of this group were more likely to be diagnosed after the disease has metastasized and were less likely than white patients to receive surgical treatment and recommended adjuvant therapy.[9,10] Considerable variation exists across Asian/Pacific Islander and Hispanic white subgroups (**Table 2**). A study of American subgroups revealed that compared with non-Hispanic whites, African Americans, American Indians, Chinese, Filipinos, Koreans, Hawaiians, Mexicans, South/Central Americans, and Puerto Ricans were 10% to 60% more likely to be diagnosed with Stage III or

Table 1. Colorectal Cancer Incidence and Mortality Rates* According to Heritage and Gender, 1997-2001[12]

Heritage	Incidence		Mortality	
	Male	*Female*	*Male*	*Female*
African Americans	72.9	56.5	34.3	24.5
Asian Americans/Pacific Islanders	56.3	38.6	15.8	10.8
Hispanics/Latinos	49.6	32.5	18.0	11.6
American Indians/Alaskan Natives	38.3	32.7	17.1	11.7
Non-Hispanic Whites	63.1	45.9	24.8	17.1
All heritages	*63.4*	*46.4*	*25.3*	*17.7*
*Per 100,000, age-adjusted to the 2000 U.S. Standard Population.				

Table 2. Stage Distribution of Colorectal Cancer Diagnosed in 5 Heritage Populations, 1992-2000[12]

Heritage	Stage distribution (%)			
	Local	Regional	Distant	Unstaged
African Americans	34.5	34.7	23.8	7.0
Asian Americans/Pacific Islanders	38.7	39.5	17.2	4.6
Hispanics/Latinos	34.9	38.4	21.4	5.3
American Indians/Alaskan Natives	34.8	38.7	23.3	3.2
Non-Hispanic whites	38.1	37.8	19.0	5.2

IV CRC.[11] Conversely, Japanese-Americans had a 20% lower risk of advanced-stage CRC. In addition to African Americans and American Indians, Hawaiians and Mexicans had a 20% to 30% greater risk of mortality, while Chinese, Japanese, and Indians/Pakistanis had a 10% to 40% lower risk. Although the etiology of these disparities was multifactorial, developing screening and treatment programs that target racial/ethnic populations with elevated risks of poor CRC outcomes may be an important means of reducing these disparities.

There is good news, however. In the United States, the overall incidence of CRC declined by 2.4% a year from 1998 through 2001.[8] Statistics also show that from the mid 1970s until the 1995-2000 period, the survival rate for CRC increased from 52% to 63% in women and from 50% to 64% in men, principally because of the introduction and use of 5-fluorouracil adjuvant therapy for resectable stage III CRC, which reduced mortality by as much as 30%.[12]

PATHOGENESIS: THE POLYP AS PRECURSOR TO DISEASE

Most colorectal cancers begin with preexisting adenomatous polyps, or adenomas. While other types of polyps such as hamartomas and inflammatory polyps are present in the colon, only adenomas are believed to progress to CRC. The risk of subsequent CRC appears to depend on the histologic type, size, and number of adenomas found at the time of initial examination.[13]

From a histologic standpoint, early CRC and its precursor lesions are displayed as grossly visible elevated polyps or non-polypoid flat lesions. Macroscopically, precursor lesions are characterized by intraepithelial neoplasia and present as either pedunculated adenomas (attached by a narrow base and long stalk) or sessile (serrated) adenomas (attached by a long, flat base with no stalk).[14] In recent years, evidence has grown to identify the sessile adenomas as the probable precursor lesion for some cases of microsatellite unstable CRC.[15] They have a significant malignant potential; in an analysis of the clinicopathologic characteristics of 110 colorectal mixed hyperplastic adenomatous polyps, 11% contained foci of early carcinoma.[16] Approximately 55% to 66% of CRC arises from adenomatous polyps, while 10% to 30% originate from sessile adenomas.[17]

Autopsy studies have shown that adenomas are common and exist in more than 30% of persons over age 50 years, with their prevalence increasing with age.[18] However, only a fraction (2% at five years; 3% at 10 years) of adenomatous polyps ever becomes malignant.[19] After an adenomatous polyp is detected, the entire large bowel should be visualized endoscopically due to polyp recurrence. A study that assessed polyp recurrence among older, increased-risk patients who have been diagnosed and excised of colorectal polyps found that polyp recurrence rates for one, three, and five years were 11%, 38%, and 53%, respectively.[20] Males and younger patients were more likely to undergo surveillance and showed higher polyp recurrence rates.

The average time from onset of a polyp to onset of carcinoma, termed the "dwell time," is 10 to 20 years. However, dwell time appears to vary with the location of the cancer. This period is longer in the distal colon than in the proximal colon, and shortest in the rectosigmoid segment.[21] Although rectosigmoid cancer develops more rapidly, its clinical manifestation is earlier because of associated stool changes and hematochezia. This explains the lower mortality rate for rectosigmoid cancers compared with colon cancers.

A polyp's potential for malignancy is based on its size. Relatively small polyps—5 mm or less in diameter—have a negligible malignant potential.[17] Polyps with a diameter of 5 mm to 10 mm are considered small. Very large lesions are considered to be greater than 20 mm in diameter with a prevalence of 0.8 to 5.2% in patients undergoing colonoscopy.[22] The prevalence of malignancy in these lesions is 5% to 22.1%.

Approximately one third of polyps and one half of colorectal cancers occur proximal to the splenic flexure.[17] Proximal lesions carry a poorer prognosis than distal cancers, partly because of delayed diagnosis secondary to the later development of hematochezia or obstruction. The rate of carcinomatous degeneration of polyps is low—about 2.5 cases per 1,000 polyps annually.[17]

PREDISPOSITION TO DISEASE—GENETIC, SITUATIONAL, AND ENVIRONMENTAL

The development of CRC is often a complex intertwining of environmental and genetic factors, as well as situational circumstances, such as ulcerative colitis. The majority of CRC is acquired sporadically. Almost one in four patients diagnosed with CRC has a family history of the disease, suggesting the involvement of a genetic factor. Two major forms of CRC predisposition are known to exist and both show autosomal dominant inheritance. They are familial adenomatous polyposis (FAP), which accounts for approximately 1% of cases of colon cancer annually, and the more common hereditary nonpolyposis colorectal cancer (HNPCC), which accounts for 5% to 10% of cases.[23]

Familial Adenomatous Polyposis (FAP)

FAP is characterized by the presence of multiple adenomas—hundreds or even thousands—in the colon starting in the second and third decades. FAP patients have an almost 100% risk of developing CRC by their 60s.[24]

FAP is associated with a deletion of chromosome 5q21, known as the adenomatous polyposis coli (APC) gene in neoplastic cells (somatic mutation) and normal cells (germline mutation); this deletion apparently leads to abnormal proliferative patterns in the colonic mucosa.[25] The different mutation sites in the gene are associated with varying severities of the disease. For instance, mutations at the 5' end and the 3' distal end and occasional specific mutations in other areas of the APC gene result in an attenuated form of FAP characterized by fewer adenomas, a proximal colonic distribution of polyps, a slightly delayed development of adenomas and cancer, and a decreased CRC risk.[26] Individuals with the same germline mutation may show different disease manifestations, suggesting that other factors, both genetic and/or environmental, may act as modifiers. Prophylactic surgery is offered to affected individuals, usually in their teens. Restorative proctocolectomy (RPC) eliminates the risk of colorectal adenocarcinoma in FAP patients, but desmoid tumors, duodenal adenomas, and ileal adenomas can still develop.[27] Close upper GI surveillance may help prevent duodenal malignancy. Once CRC is prevented, mesenteric desmoid tumors are the principal cause of mortality, and the main reason for worsening functional results.

Genetic testing is now the standard of care for FAP, although this is an evolving field. One small study showed that fecal DNA testing for APC gene mutations has a sensitivity of 57% and a specificity of 100%.[28] If the test result is positive or the test is not available, flexible sigmoidoscopy is performed at 10 to 12 years of age. During the procedure, mucosal biopsy specimens are taken to identify subtle adenomatous changes. Colonoscopy with mucosal biopsies is advisable at 18 to 20 years of age. If adenomas are detected, surgical prophylaxis should be considered. Routine gastroduodenoscopic surveillance is also recommended for patients with FAP, because these patients are at high risk for potentially precancerous gastric and duodenal adenomas.[29]

Hereditary Non-Polyposis Colorectal Cancer (HNPCC)

HNPCC is caused by a fault in a DNA mismatch repair (MMR) gene; faults in the MMR genes account for over 90% of detectable mutations.[30]

The mean age at which adenomatous malignancies appear in HNPCC is age 45 years, which is 10 to 15 years younger than the median age at which they appear in the general non-HNPCC population.[31] Unlike FAP, HNPCC is associated with a very high frequency of neoplasms in the proximal large bowel. Also, families with HNPCC often include persons with multiple primary cancers; in women, an association between colorectal cancer and either endometrial or ovarian carcinoma is especially prominent.

Genetic testing for predisposing mutations in people with a strong family history of these cancers enables screening and prevention to be targeted at those individuals at highest risk. For those with a documented mutation, especially young patients with a family history of HNPCC, prophylactic surgery may be advisable. Pilot studies in CRC patients under 30 years old have shown that 41% have MMR gene mutations.[32] The risk for developing CRC by age 70 years in people with these mutations has been shown to be 91% for men and 69% for women.[33]

Apart from FAP and HNPCC, other conditions that predispose to CRC include rare polyposis autosomal dominant conditions such as Peutz-Jeghers syndrome and familial juvenile polyposis.[34]

APC Mutations

Despite the genetic predisposition of CRC in some people, the majority of persons who are diagnosed with CRC develop it as a result of environmental or other disease states. CRC occurs in conjunction with the accumulation of multiple mutations within a cell in the bowel lining, allowing it to escape the normal growth control mechanisms. The step-wise accumulation of mutations drives the histological transition from normal tissue to adenoma to carcinoma.[34] The most common genetic alterations in sporadic bowel cancers are activating mutations in the oncogene KRAS and mutation or loss of the tumor suppressor genes APC, SMAD4 and TP53. Evidence points to the strong likelihood that somatic mutations of the APC gene are associated with development of a great majority of colorectal tumors and that the occurrence of such APC mutations represents an initial step in CRC.[35,36] In an analysis of APC gene mutations in 63

colorectal tumors that developed in FAP and non-FAP patients, over 80% of tumors (14 adenomas and 39 carcinomas) had at least one APC gene mutation, of which more than 60% (nine adenomas and 23 carcinomas) had two mutations.[35] The APC protein has many vital functions including control of the Wnt developmental signalling pathway, cell adhesion, migration, apoptosis, and chromosomal segregation. Loss of APC causes stabilization of beta catenin which binds the TCF/LEF family of transcription factors, activating gene expression.[37] CRC arises through a gradual series of histological changes, each of which is accompanied by a specific genetic alteration. In general, an intestinal cell needs to comply with two essential requirements to develop into a malignancy: the acquisition of selective advantage to allow for its initial clonal expansion, and genetic instability to permit multiple hits in other genes that are responsible for tumor progression and malignant transformation. Inactivation of APC might fulfill both requirements.

Inflammatory Bowel Disease

Other conditions linked to an increased risk include the inflammatory bowel diseases, ulcerative colitis (UC) and Crohn's disease, estimated to be responsible for around 1% to 2% of CRC cases.[38] However, CRC is considered a serious complication of these bowel diseases and accounts for approximately 15% of all deaths in inflammatory bowel disease (IBD) patients. Statistical analyses suggest that the risk of CRC for people with IBD increases by 0.5% to 1.0% yearly in the eight to 10 years after diagnosis.[38] The magnitude of CRC risk increases with early age at IBD diagnosis, longer duration of symptoms, and extent of the disease.

The morphological development of UC-related CRC differs from that of its sporadic counterpart. Recent research suggests that environmental factors related to long-term inflammation of the bowel may contribute more to the increased cancer risk in UC than inherited susceptibility.[39] UC-related CRC is likely a result of chronic inflammation, a mechanism that is still elusive.[40] Similarly, detailed molecular analyses have indicated that whereas many of the genetic alterations observed in sporadic colon cancers also occur in UC-associated malignancies, the timing and frequency of those changes in the UC arena are different. These histological and molecular signatures may very well be reflective of an inflammation-driven carcinogenesis process in UC patients. Studies in animal models of UC have partly unraveled the mechanisms of inflammation-driven CRC. The available evidence implies that DNA damage caused by oxidative stress in the characteristic damage-regeneration cycle is a major factor in the development of CRC in UC patients.

Environmental and Situational Factors

Specific factors that increase the CRC risk have been identified, as have factors that reduce risk (**Table 3**). Recent findings have sought to clarify clinical issues or to announce paradigm shifts in our present knowledge of CRC.

Fiber is Not Protective for CRC

An analysis of 13 prospective cohort studies newly published by the Harvard School of Public Health and involving 725,628 adults revealed that high dietary fiber intake was not associated with a reduced risk of CRC.[1] The study population was followed for six to 20 years. These findings are discordant

Table 3. Risk Factors for Colorectal Cancer[12]

Increased risk	• Age >50 yrs • Male gender • African American heritage • Family history of CRC, colorectal polyps, or chronic inflammatory disease • Inherited genetic abnormalities, such as familial adenomatous polyposis, or hereditary nonpolyposis CRC • Sedentary lifestyle • Obesity • Diet that includes high amount of red and/or processed meat • Smoking • Alcohol consumption (>4 drinks per week)
Decreased risk	• Hormonal replacement therapy • Moderate to vigorous physical activity most days per week • Diet that includes low-fat dairy products, fish, poultry • Diet rich in fruits and vegetables • Use of aspirin, non-steroidal anti-inflammatory drugs

with previously published studies that tout the benefits of high-fiber diets. Even in this study, dietary fiber intake was inversely associated with risk of CRC until other dietary risk factors were considered. The researchers of the present study contend that persons who eat high-fiber diets also eat less red meat, take folate-rich multivitamins, and have otherwise healthier lifestyles. Even if fiber does not have a major impact on CRC, convincing evidence exists to show that dietary fiber helps to prevent heart disease, type 2 diabetes, diverticulitis, and other several chronic conditions.

Dietary Acrylamide Does Not Increase CRC in Women

Acrylamide is classified as a probable human carcinogen, and animal studies have shown an increased incidence of tumors in rats exposed to very high levels. The substance is found in coffee, fried potato products, pretzels, popcorn, and crisp bread. The first prospective study of acrylamide in food and CRC risk, done through Harvard Medical School, has shown that intake of food items associated with elevated levels of acrylamide was not associated with CRC risk.[41] The researchers comment that in light of the null findings of this study, an important question is why the epidemiologic data on dietary acrylamide thus far appear to contradict data from animal experiments and risk assessment models.

Exercise Impacts CRC Survival

While sedentary lifestyle and obesity increase the risk of CRC, new evidence shows that these risk factors also impact survival after CRC diagnosis.[42] A prospective cohort study of 526 Australians who had CRC showed that after adjusting for age, sex, and tumor stage, patients who reported regular exercise before their CRC were 31% less likely to die from the disease than were non-exercisers. In fact, 73% of exercisers survived at least five years, versus 61% of non-exercisers. Increasing percent body fat resulted in an increase in disease-specific deaths, (hazard ratio 1.33 per 10 kg [22 pounds]). Similarly, increasing waist circumference reduced disease-specific survival (hazard ratio 1.20 per 10 cm [four inches]).

Chicken vs Processed Meats: Risk of Adenoma Recurrence

Specific meats may have different effects in adenoma recurrence, a Dartmouth Medical School study has revealed.[43] Researchers found that among 1,520 adults with a history of colon polyps, those who ate a diet heavy in processed meats had a higher risk of polyp recurrence than those with the lowest intake. Conversely, patients who favored chicken had a lesser risk of new polyps than those who ate the least. Patients in the quartile with the highest intake of processed meat were 75% more likely to develop an advanced adenoma compared with the quartile that ingested the lowest amount of processed meat. In contrast, those with the highest chicken intake were 39% less likely than those who ate the least to develop an advanced polyp.

Do Statins Prevent CRC?

The 3-hydroxy-3-methylglutaryl coenzyme A reductase inhibitors, otherwise known as statins, are effective lipid-lowering agents. They can inhibit the growth of colon cancer cell lines, and secondary analyses of some, but not all, clinical trials suggest that they reduce CRC risk. In 2005, the Molecular Epidemiology of Colorectal Cancer study, a population-based case-control study of 1,953 patients with CRC and 2,015 controls, compared the use of statins for at least five years versus the nonuse of statins, and concluded that statin use was associated with a 47% relative reduction in CRC risk after adjustment for other known risk factors.[2] In 2006, two more studies with conflicting results were published. One study, conducted by the American Cancer Society, examined the association between use of statins and CRC incidence among 132,136 men and women in the Cancer Prevention Study II Nutrition Cohort, and found that current use of such drugs for five years or more was only associated with a weak impact on CRC incidence (multivariable adjusted relative risk = 1.09).[4] The investigators did concede, however, that the small reduction in risk could be associated with only specific types or doses of statins. The other study looked at 27 trials of statins involving 86,936 patients and showed an even weaker association with a reduction in cancer incidence (overall risk [OR], 1.01) or in cancer mortality (OR, 1.01).[3] They concluded that no type of cancer was affected by statin use and no subtype of statin affected cancer risk. Undoubtedly, more studies will follow.

TREATMENT OPTIONS

Surgery

The greatest potential for cure in patients with CRC is curative resection.[44] Patients considered for such surgery are often elderly and should be evaluated preoperatively for metastatic disease by thorough physical examination, biochemical studies, and imaging of the chest and pelvis. The identification of metastases does not constitute an absolute contraindication to surgery in patients experiencing tumor-induced gastrointestinal bleeding or obstruction, but evidence of metastasization often warrants a more conservative operative procedure designed primarily to relieve symptoms. Before surgery, the carcinoembryonic antigen (CEA) titer should be determined and, if possible, the entire bowel mucosa should be visualized by colonoscopy to detect synchronous polyps or neoplasms.[44]

The principles of surgery in treating CRC

Lymphadenectomy. If lymphadenectomy is to be preformed, lymph nodes at the origin of the feeding vessels should be identified for pathologic exam.[44] Lymph nodes outside the field of resection considered suspicious should be biopsied or removed. Residual positive nodes indicate an incomplete (R2) resection. The new 2006 NCCN guidelines encourage surgeons to remove a minimum of 12 lymph nodes for examination to clearly establish stage II (T 3-4, N0) colon cancer.[44] Even for stage III disease, the number of lymph nodes correlates with overall survival, as demonstrated by a secondary survey of Intergroup trial INT-0089, which showed that the number of lymph nodes analyzed for staging colon cancers is, itself, a prognostic variable on outcome.[45]

Laparoscopic-assisted colectomy. A multi-institutional study conducted by the Clinical Outcomes of Surgical

Therapy Study Group showed the rates of recurrent cancer were similar after minimally invasive laparoscopically assisted colectomy and open colectomy, suggesting that the laparoscopic approach is an acceptable alternative to open surgery for colon cancer.[46] Laparoscopic-assisted colectomy may be considered if the surgeon has experience performing laparoscopically assisted colorectal operations.[47,48] Following that, additional criteria include no disease in rectum or prohibitive abdominal adhesions, and no advanced local or metastatic disease. The procedure is not indicated for acute bowel obstruction or perforation from cancer, and a thorough abdominal exploration is required. The surgeon may consider preoperative marking of small lesions.

Principles for resectability of metastases

Liver. Hepatic resection effectively controls hepatic tumor in a substantial number of patients.[49,50] Based on that finding, complete resection must be feasible based on anatomic grounds and the extent of disease; maintenance of normal hepatic function is required. There should be no unresectable extrahepatic sites of disease. Fong and colleagues used a five-criterion preoperative scoring system to produce a score that was highly predictive of outcome ($P<.0001$):[50]

1. node-positive primary ($P=.02$)
2. disease-free interval from primary to metastases less than 12 months ($P=.03$)
3. number of hepatic tumors more than one ($P=.0004$)
4. largest hepatic tumor greater than 5 cm ($P=.01$)
5. CEA level greater than 200 ng/mL ($P=.01$)

A scoring system by Nordlinger and colleagues that included the most relevant disease characteristics was developed using data from 1,568 patients with resected liver metastases from CRC carcinoma.[50a] The prognostic value of different factors was studied through uni- and multivariate analyses. They found that two- and five-year survival rates were 64% and 28%, respectively, and were affected by age, size of largest metastasis or CEA level, stage of the primary tumor, disease free-interval, number of liver nodules, and resection margin. Giving one point to each factor, the population was divided into three risk groups with different two-year survival rates: 0-2 (79%), 3-4 (60%), or 5-7 (43%).

According to a study by Fujita et al,[50b] synchronous liver metastases should be resected with the primary lesion if the patient can tolerate the procedure. The only true prognostic factor is the number of regional lymph node metastases. When six or more distinct metastatic lymph nodes are detected during resection of the primary cancer, synchronous liver resection should be postponed. In such cases, resection of the liver tumors should be considered only when no new lesions and no recurrences are detected several months after the primary resection.

Re-evaluation for resection can be considered in otherwise unresectable patients after neoadjuvant therapy.[51] Hepatic resection is the treatment of choice for resectable liver metastases from CRC; radiofrequency ablation (RFA) alone or in combination with resection for unresectable patients does not provide survival comparable to resection, and only slightly superior to nonsurgical treatment.[52]

Lung. Complete resection of the lung is based on the anatomic location and extent of disease with maintenance of adequate function required. A Japanese study showed that the median interval between colorectal resection and lung resection was 33 months.[53] Overall, five-year survival was 48%; five-year survival was 51% for patients with solitary metastasis, 47% for patients with ipsilateral multiple metastases, and 50% for patients with bilateral metastases. Resectable extrapulmonary metastases do not preclude resection.[54] Re-resection can be considered in selected patients.

Radiotherapy

Radiotherapy is advantageous to patients with stage II or III rectal tumors. Approximately 40% of these patients experience tumor recurrence following complete resection, compared with 7% for patients who receive postoperative radiotherapy.[55] This unusually high frequency of recurrence in non-radiation-treated patients is presumably the result of two factors: the loss of integrity of the serosa of the large bowel as it enters the pelvis facilitates the infiltration of tumor, and the rich lymphatic supply of the pelvic side wall immediately adjacent to the rectum enhances the early spread of malignant cells into surgically inaccessible tissue. Therefore, adjuvant radiation therapy was introduced to remove tumor cells from perirectal tissue and to boost the potential of cure.

The use of adjuvant radiation therapy to decrease pelvic recurrence appears rational, but controversy has existed as to whether such treatment should be administered prior to or after surgery. Patients with large, potentially unresectable rectal cancers may need preoperative irradiation to shrink the tumor sufficiently to allow its resection. Survival is prolonged when adjuvant radiation therapy is combined with concomitant chemotherapy. Preoperative chemoradiation has now emerged as the treatment of choice for many stage II and stage III rectal cancer patients.

Radiation therapy fields should include the tumor bed, which should be defined by preoperative radiological imaging and/or surgical clips.[44] Radiation doses should be 45-50 Gy in 25 to 28 fractions; small bowel doses should be limited to 45 Gy. Chemotherapy based on 5-FU should be delivered concurrently with radiation. Intraoperative radiotherapy (IORT), if available, should be considered for patients with T4 or recurrent cancers as an additional boost. Preoperative radiation is preferred for these patients to aid resectability.

Chemotherapy

After virtually having only one drug, 5-fluorouracil, to use against CRC for decades, the arrival of new and more effective agents has changed the approach to chemotherapy for the treatment of CRC. Although 5-FU remains the backbone of most regimens, the new agents—irinotecan, capecitabine, oxaliplatin, bevacizumab, and cetuximab—are being incorporated into frontline therapies for advanced CRC.

5-Fluorouracil

Synthesized in 1952 and approved by the FDA in 1962, 5-FU remains an important drug in the treatment of advanced CRC. At one time, it was given as a bolus injection, but today permanent venous access devices and portable infusion pumps allow the continuous infusion of 5-FU on an outpatient basis. Such uninterrupted infusion increases the likelihood that 5-FU will be present during the S phase of the tumor cell cycle, when this agent is most effective.

5-FU is modulated by leucovorin, which raises the level of 5,10-methylenetetrahydrofolate and results in the formation of a stable ternary complex of the folate coenzyme thymidylate synthase with 5-FU in the form of its principal metabolite, fluorodeoxyuridine. The use of 5-FU with leucovorin has resulted in a higher response rate than with 5-FU alone. The NCCN guidelines recommend several 5-FU regimens, including a continuous infusion administered 24 hours a day for a protracted time (10 weeks or more).[44,56] Administration of 5-FU as a continuous infusion for protracted periods improves the therapeutic index for this agent in patients with advanced CRC with respect to response rate and reduced toxicity. The schedule appears workable in the community setting and yields response rates similar to those reported for 5-FU with high-dose leucovorin, but without the gastrointestinal toxicity profile of the latter combination. Other recommended regimens include bolus 5-FU given one hour after leucovorin and repeated weekly for six cycles, and 5-FU and leucovorin given daily for five days every four or five weeks .[44]

Irinotecan

Irinotecan is a novel topoisomerase inhibitor that has significant therapeutic activity in metastatic CRC. It is indicated for patients with metastatic CRC and for patients whose disease recurred or progressed following initial 5-FU-based therapy. The drug is used as first-line therapy in combination with 5-FU/leucovorin and considered standard chemotherapy for CRC.[44] In a phase 3 trial, irinotecan with an infusion 5-FU/leucovorin regimen increased median survival by 35% vs 22% (P<.005) and improved overall survival (17.4 months vs 14 months; P>0.03)[57] In an intent-to-treat analysis, treatment with irinotecan, bolus 5-FU and leucovorin produced a significantly longer median progression-free survival (7.0 vs 4.3 months; P=.004), compared with bolus 5-FU/leucovorin treatment.[58] The incidence of grade 4 diarrhea was similar in both groups (<8%).[58] However, grade 4 neutropenia and grade 3 and grade 4 mucositis were less common in the triple drug regimen.

Capecitabine

Capecitabine is an oral fluoropyrimidine—specifically a prodrug of 5-FU—and appears to mimic continuous-infusion 5-FU. The drug is indicated for adjuvant treatment in patients with Dukes' C colon cancer who have undergone complete resection of the primary tumor. It is also approved as first-line treatment in patients with metastatic CRC. In two studies that compared capecitabine with bolus 5-FU/leucovorin in patients with advanced disease, capecitabine therapy was associated with an improved response rate (18.9% vs 15%; and 24.8% vs 15%; P=0.005), but there was not a significant benefit in survival (12.9 months vs 12.8 months).[59-61]

Oxaliplatin

Although a platinum-based molecule, oxaliplatin differs in its preclinical activity profile from cisplatin and also has a distinct toxicity profile. In most patients, it causes no renal toxicity and minimal hematologic toxicity, but it is associated with both a reversible, acute, cold-related dysesthesia and a dose-limiting, cumulative, peripheral sensory neuropathy.

In 2004, the FDA approved oxaliplatin injection in combination with infusional 5-fluorouracil (5-FU) and leucovorin for the treatment of patients with stage III CRC who have undergone complete resection of the primary tumor, as well as for the first-line treatment of advanced carcinoma of the colon or rectum. The combination including oxaliplatin was shown to shrink tumors in some patients and delay tumor growth. The approval was based on the efforts to find the best first-line regimen in advanced CRC in which the National Cancer Institute GI intergroup designed a six-arm study that compared various combinations of 5-FU, leucovorin, irinotecan, and oxaliplatin.[62] Data suggest that the combination of oxaliplatin and 5-FU infusion is superior to the combination of irinotecan and bolus 5-FU (response rate, 45% vs 31%; time to disease progression, 8.7 months vs 6.9 months; and overall survival, 19.5 months vs 15 months).[62]

Bevacizumab and cetuximab

Bevacizumab and cetuximab are monoclonal antibodies that work by preventing angiogenesis. Both agents were approved by the FDA in 2004 for the treatment of advanced CRC. A pivotal study showed that bevacizumab (5 mg/kg), when combined with irinotecan, 5-FU/leucovorin, produced a significantly higher response rate (45% vs 35%, P=0.004), progression-free survival (10.6 months vs 6.2 months; P<0.001), and median duration of survival (20.3 months vs 15.6 months; P<0.001).[63-65] A pivotal phase 2 trial investigated the safety and efficacy of two doses of bevacizumab—5 mg/kg and 10 mg/kg every two weeks—plus 5-FU/LV vs 5-FU/LV alone in 104 treatment-naïve patients with metastatic CRC.[66] Compared with the 5-FU/LV control arm, treatment with bevacizumab (at both dose levels) plus FU/LV resulted in higher response rates (control arm, 17%; low-dose arm, 40%; high-dose arm, 24%), longer median time to disease progression (control arm, 5.2 months; low-dose arm, 9.0 months; high-dose arm, 7.2 months), and longer median survival (control arm, 13.8 months; low-dose arm, 21.5 months; high-dose arm, 16.1 months). Thrombosis was the most significant adverse event and was fatal in one patient.

A large randomized phase 2 trial, which became known as the BOND trial, compared cetuximab alone with cetuximab plus irinotecan in patients with irinotecan-refractory CRC.[67] While the response rates favored the combination over monotherapy in terms of response rate (23% vs 11%; P=.007), disease control (56% vs 32%; P=.0001), and median time to progression (4.1 vs 1.5 months; P<.0001), the study was not designed or powered to address the survival advantage of cetuximab. Toxic effects were more frequent in the combination-therapy group, an observation that was attributed to the intrinsic toxicity of irinotecan.

[See Appendix for a review of relevant mechanisms of action.]

Table 4. Estimates of 5-Year Disease-Free Survival (%) with Surgery Versus Surgery Plus Adjuvant Therapy[68]

Nodal status	T Stage	Low Grade		High Grade	
		S	+AT	S	+AT
0 nodes	T3	79	81	72	76
	T4	70	74	62	66
1-4 nodes	T1-T2	69	78	60	72
	T3	58	70	48	62
	T4	45	59	34	49
>5 nodes	T1-T2	44	59	33	49
	T3	31	47	20	36
	T4	18	33	10	22

S=surgery; AT=adjuvant therapy
Note: Referent age is 60-69 years.

TREATMENTS BY DISEASE STAGE

Changes in Staging Classifications

Staging systems are changing so that treatment options can be more precisely targeted to the patient's disease risk status. The sixth edition of the American Joint Committee on Cancer Staging Manual includes several modifications to the colon and rectum TNM staging system, which have been incorporated into the NCCN treatment guidelines.[44,69] In the latest revision of the staging system, smooth metastatic nodules in the pericolic or perirectal fat are considered lymph node metastases and should be included in N staging. Irregularly contoured metastatic nodules in the peritumoral fat are considered vascular invasion.

Stage II is now subdivided into IIA (T3N0M0, if the primary tumor is T3) and IIB (T4N0M0 for T4 lesions).

Stage III is subdivided into IIIA (T1 to T2, N1, M0), IIIB (T3 to T4, N1, M0), and IIIC (any T, N2, M0). The number of nodes separates N1 and N2 disease: N1 lesions have one to three positive regional lymph nodes, whereas N2 tumors have four or more positive regional nodes. Understanding the significant differences in survival among diagnostic subsets is important when assessing individual patient treatment options and design of clinical trials.

For example, the difference in five-year disease-free survival (DFS) is substantial: stage IIIA is 59.8%, stage IIIB is 42.0%, and stage IIIC is 27.3%.[69] DFS decreases with higher T stage, greater extent of nodal involvement and high grade of tumor. Gill and colleagues have generated estimates suggesting that the addition of adjuvant chemotherapy to surgery can improve rates of DFS in all groups (**Table 4**).[68]

Treatment goals for CRC are based on the stage of disease at presentation.

Stages I, II, and III disease are considered potentially curable, and are best managed with the intent of eradicating known and micrometastatic sites to achieve remission and avoid recurrence. Because stage IV is considered incurable in most cases, efforts are directed to reducing symptoms and prolonging survival.

The latest version of NCCN's colon cancer guidelines includes several major changes to recommended courses of treatment based on recent relevant clinical studies and changing practice patterns. One significant change is the recommendation that all first-line therapy for advanced or metastatic disease should include bevacizumab in the treatment regimen. The panel also added a new regimen, capecitabine and oxaliplatin (a combination known as CAPOX) as a treatment option in first-line therapy (Category 2B).[44]

In addition to changing treatment recommendations in advanced or metastatic disease, there are also new options in the adjuvant setting. The panel added new treatment regimens for Stage IIA patients, including capecitabine, 5-FU/leucovorin or 5-FU/leucovorin/oxaliplatin (Category 2B) and the election of this regimen would be based on risk assessment discussions between physician and patient.

Stage I

Because of its localized nature, stage I colon cancer has a high cure rate. The treatment of stage I colon cancer is usually wide surgical resection and anastomosis.[44] The treatment of early stage rectal cancer includes transabdominal resection or transanal excision.[66]

Stage II

The treatment of stage II colon cancer is usually wide surgical resection and anastomosis. Following surgery, patients should be considered for entry into controlled clinical trials evaluating the use of systemic or regional chemotherapy, radiation therapy, biologic therapy, or observation without post-operative therapy. (Information about ongoing clinical trials is available from the NCI website at www.cancer.gov/clinicaltrials.)

About 55% of all cases of colon cancer presently diagnosed are either stage II or stage III disease, and therefore eligible for adjuvant chemotherapy.[71,72] However, adjuvant therapy is not indicated for most stage II colon cancer patients unless they are entered into a clinical trial. The principles of risk assessment for stage II colon cancer include asking the patient how much information he or she would like to know regarding prognosis. Following that, a patient/physician discussion should ensue regarding the potential risks of therapy compared with potential benefits. This should include discussion of evidence supporting treatment, assumptions of benefit from indirect evidence, morbidity associated with treatment, high-risk prognostic characteristics, and patient preferences.

When determining whether adjuvant therapy will offer clinical benefits, the following points should be considered: the number of lymph nodes analyzed after surgery; poor prognostic features (eg, T4 lesion, perforation, peritumoral lymphovascular involvement, poorly differentiated histology); assessment of other comorbidities; anticipated life expectancy.

The potential value of adjuvant therapy for patients with stage II colon cancer remains controversial.

Although subgroups of patients with stage II colon cancer (including those with anatomic features such as tumor adherence to adjacent structures, perforation, complete obstruction, emergency presentation, a primary tumor site in the left colon, pT3 tumors with a depth of invasion of greater than 15 mm beyond the outer border of the muscularis propria, and pT4 lesions[73]) may be at relatively increased risk for recurrence, the evidence is conflicting as to whether adjuvant chemotherapy based on 5-FU is associated with an overall improved survival compared to surgery alone. Investigators from the National Surgical Adjuvant Breast and Bowel Project (NSABP) have indicated that the reduction in risk of recurrence by adjuvant therapy in patients with stage II disease is of similar magnitude to the benefit seen in patients with stage III disease treated with adjuvant therapy.[74] The Intergroup 0035 Trial, which randomized stage II patients to either follow-up only or 5-FU plus levamisole, showed no survival advantage to postoperative adjuvant chemotherapy in that patient population.[75] In its meta-analysis of 1,000 stage II patients, the International Multicentre Pooled Analysis of B2 Colon Cancer Trials (IMPACT B2) found a 2% advantage in overall survival at five years when adjuvant patients were treated with 5-FU/leucovorin, compared with untreated controls.[76]

The SEER Medicare Cohort study of 3,151 cases of resected stage II colon cancer distinguishes between the great majority of patients (92%) who have T3N0 disease and "usual" risk and a small number (8%) at high risk (T4N0 disease, obstruction or perforation).[77] Among the "usual" risk group, 27% received chemotherapy; 33%

high-risk patients were treated. Treatment was started at a median of 5.5 weeks from surgery. Of those patients who consulted with a medical oncologist, 54% received adjuvant therapy. Survival curves between treated and untreated patients in this SEER cohort are identical until three years from surgery, when the curve for chemotherapy-treated patients starts to diverge. However, the absolute difference in survival at five years among this non-randomized population is only around 3%.

A panel convened by the American Society of Clinical Oncology (ASCO), in partnership with the Cancer Care Ontario Program in Evidence-Based Care Gastrointestinal Cancer Disease Site Group, made recommendations on adjuvant therapy for stage II colon cancer patients based on a literature meta-analysis that included 37 trials, 11 meta-analyses, and 20,317 patients.[6,78] The panel concluded that while a 5% to 10% improvement in the DFS was observed with adjuvant treatment, no significant improvement was seen in overall survival. Thus, the panel did not recommend the routine administration of adjuvant chemotherapy for stage II colon cancer patients. The panel did emphasize the importance of a discussion outlining the risks vs benefits of adjuvant therapy to help guide the decision process. Patients with stage II colon cancer remain candidates for clinical trials in which surgery alone represents standard therapy.

The efficacy of postoperative radiation and 5-FU-based chemotherapy for stage II and III rectal cancer was established by a series of prospective, randomized clinical trials (the Gastrointestinal Tumor Study Group (GITSG) Protocol 7175, the Mayo/North Central Cancer

Treatment Group (NCCTG) Protocol 79-47-51, and the National Surgical Adjuvant Breast and Bowel Project (NSABP) R-01.[79-81] These studies showed an increase in both disease-free interval and overall survival when radiotherapy is combined with chemotherapy following surgical resection.

A recent randomized trial from the German Rectal Cancer Study Group included 823 stage II and stage III rectal cancer patients randomized to receive either preoperative chemoradiotherapy or postoperative chemoradiation. The study demonstrated comparable overall five-year survival (76% vs 74%, respectively). However, local relapse rate favored preoperative chemoradiotherapy (6% vs 13%; $P=0.006$), with less acute (27% vs 40%; $P=.001$) and long-term toxicity (14% vs 24%; $P=0.01$).[82]

Stage III

The treatment options for colon cancer include wide surgical resection and anastomosis as well as chemotherapy and radiation. The results of the MOSAIC trial demonstrated the benefit of adding oxaliplatin to 5-FU and leucovorin (FOLFOX) in adjuvant therapy for stage II and III disease.[83]

Some of the newer regimens in phase 3 trials presented at the 2005 ASCO meeting included:

• A phase 3 trial in which XELOX was compared with bolus 5-FU/LV (the standard regimen at the start of the study) as adjuvant therapy for stage III colon cancer.[84] Patients with resected stage III colon cancer received XELOX (capecitabine 1000mg/m^2 bid d1-14 + oxaliplatin 130mg/m^2 d1, q3w x8) or IV bolus 5-FU/LV (Mayo Clinic, LV 20mg/m^2 + 5-FU 425mg/m^2 d1-5, q4w x6; or Roswell Park [RP], LV 500mg/m^2 + 5-FU 500mg/m^2 d1, w1-6

in 8w cycles x4). Early safety data from the largest population of patients treated with XELOX indicate that XELOX causes less myelosuppression (neutropenia – XELOX 5.3% vs 5-FU/LV 10.9%) and stomatitis (0.6% vs 7.9%), but more skin (hand-foot syndrome (3.6% vs 0.2%) and neurosensory toxicity (8.1% vs 0%) than 5-FU/LV, and compares favorably with FOLFOX4. XELOX has now been incorporated in the three-arm AVANT adjuvant trial (FOLFOX4 vs FOLFOX4 + bevacizumab vs XELOX + bevacizumab).

The NSABP recently reported three-year disease-free survival results from a randomized trial comparing bolus 5-FU and leucovorin with 5-FU and oxaliplatin (FLOX) in patients with stage II and stage III colon cancer. Results favored the FLOX regimen and were comparable to data from the MOSAIC trial.[85]

Various adjuvant regimens are now recommended by the NCCN.[44] These include 5-FU/leucovorin given in various cycles[86,87] (without the use of levamisole, which had been included in 5-FU/leucovorin in the past[88]). Also, capecitabine used as monotherapy, and mFOLFOX6, which adds oxaliplatin to a 5-FU/leucovorin regimen are also proposed as standard adjuvant therapy.[85,89]

Based on results from the MOSAIC trial presented at the American Society of Clinical Oncology meeting in 2005, adjuvant FOLFOX4 demonstrated prolonged four-year survival over 5-FU/leucovorin (69.7% vs 61.0% translating into a relative risk reduction of 25% in the subset of stage III patients).[90] FOLFOX4 is now considered a standard treatment for patients with stage III CRC.

Stage IV

- Stage IV CRC represents distant metastatic disease. Treatment of recurrent CRC depends on the sites of recurrent disease demonstrable by physical examination and/or radiographic studies.[44]

Treatment options include:
- Surgical resection of locally recurrent cancer.
- Surgical resection/anastomosis or bypass of obstructing or bleeding primary lesions in selected metastatic cases.
- Resection of liver metastases or ablation in selected metastatic patients.
- Resection of isolated ovarian or pulmonary metastases in selected patients.
- Palliative radiotherapy and/or chemotherapy.
- Clinical trials evaluating new drugs, biological therapy, or comparisons of different chemotherapy regimens which may include biologic agents

In stage IV and recurrent colon cancer, chemotherapy has been used for palliation. For patients who can tolerate intensive therapy, recommended first-line regimens for advanced or metastatic CRC include:[44]
- FOLFOX (5-FU, leucovorin, oxaliplatin) plus bevacizumab.
- FOLFIRI (5-FU, leucovorin, irinotecan) plus bevacizumab.
- IFL (or Saltz regimen irinotecan, 5-FU, leucovorin) plus bevacizumab.
- 5-FU/leucovorin plus bevacizumab.
- CAPOX (capecitabine, oxaliplatin) plus bevacizumab.

For patients who cannot tolerate intensive therapy, recommended first-line regimens for advanced or metastatic CRC are:
- Capecitabine.
- Bolus 5-FU/leucovorin with or without bevacizumab.
- Infusional 5-FU with or without leucovorin and/or bevacizumab.
- Protracted 5-FU with or without leucovorin.

Table 5. Selected Prognostic Factors and 5-Year Relapse-Free Survival[45,94,100]

Prognostic factors*	Stage	5-yr relapse-free survival (%)
T3N0 (11-20 nodes analyzed) Stage IIa	IIA	79
T3N0 low grade	IIA	73
T3N0 (≤10 nodes analyzed)	IIA	72
T3N0 high grade	IIA	65
T4N0 low grade Stage IIb	IIB	60
T4N0 high grade	IIB	51
T3N1	IIIB	49
T3N2	IIIC	15

*All stages in this table are M0. Results derived from *www.mayoclinic.com/calcs* using a referent age of 60-69 years old.

It should be emphasized that the overall survival of patients with metastatic colorectal cancer represents a continuum of care and correlates with the availability of all active agents over the course of a patient's illness.[91]

Tournigand and colleagues compared irinotecan-based and oxaliplatin-based chemotherapy in patients with newly diagnosed advanced CRC.[92] In this study, patients were crossed over from one regimen to the other at the time of progression. These two first-line treatments for metastatic and advanced CRC demonstrated similar response rates and acceptable toxic effects profiles with no differences in median time to first progression (eight months vs 8.5 months; $P=.26$) or overall survival (20.6 months vs 21.5 months; $P=.99$) for FOLFOX6 followed by FOLFIRI regimen versus FOLFIRI followed by FOLFOX regimen, respectively. However, the toxicity profiles were different. In first-line therapy, National Cancer Institute Common Toxicity Criteria grade 3/4 mucositis, nausea/vomiting, and grade 2 alopecia were more frequent with FOLFIRI, and grade 3/4 neutropenia and neurosensory toxicity were more frequent with FOLFOX6.

Cetuximab plus FOLFOX4 (oxaliplatin, leucovorin, 5-FU) was recently evaluated in patients with metastatic EGFR-positive CRC who had progressed on prior first-line irinotecan therapy with an ECOG performance status ≤2.[92] Response rates and progression-free survival showed a trend toward improvement with the combination of FOLFOX4 and cetuximab in irinotecan-refractory patients with advanced CRC. Another study presented at the 2005 ASCO meeting assessed irinotecan versus

FOLFOX4 in 5-FU-experienced patients.[93] In patients failing prior 5-FU, overall survival was not significantly different based on whether second-line therapy began with either irinotecan or FOLFOX4 (HR=1.04, 95% CI 0.9-1.3). However, second-line FOLFOX4 produced a higher response rate than irinotecan (27% vs 15%; $P<.01$) and a trend toward longer time to progression.

SURVEILLANCE

Surveillance after curative treatment of CRC commonly includes periodic history taking and physical examinations; some combination of laboratory tests (eg, CEA tests, liver-function tests, complete blood counts, and fecal occult-blood tests); diagnostic imaging studies (eg, chest radiography, ultrasonography, computed tomography, magnetic resonance imaging, and barium enema); and endoscopic procedures (eg, sigmoidoscopy and colonoscopy).[94] Is such an exhaustive list the standard of care and does intensive follow-up improve survival and preserve quality of life?

The ASCO Expert Panel published a 2005 surveillance guideline update based on results from three independently reported meta-analyses of randomized controlled trials.[95] These trials compared low-intensity and high-intensity programs of colorectal cancer surveillance with recent analyses of data from major clinical trials in colon and rectal cancer.[78,96,97] The Panel recommended the following:

• Annual computed tomography (CT) of the chest and abdomen for three years after primary therapy for patients who are at higher risk of recurrence and who could be candi-

dates for curative-intent surgery.
- Pelvic CT scan for rectal cancer surveillance, especially for patients with several poor prognostic factors, including those who have not been treated with radiation.
- Colonoscopy at three years after operative treatment, and, if results are normal, every five years thereafter.
- Flexible proctosigmoidoscopy every six months for five years for rectal cancer patients who have not been treated with pelvic radiation.
- History and physical examination every three to six months for the first three years, every six months during years 4 and 5, and subsequently at the discretion of the physician.
- CEA every three months postoperatively for at least three years after diagnosis, if the patient is a candidate for surgery or systemic therapy.
- Chest x-rays, CBCs, and liver function tests are not recommended, and molecular or cellular markers should not influence the surveillance strategy based on available evidence.

For individuals with familial or inherited risk, ASCO recommends the following based on a report by Winawer and colleagues:[98]
- Colonoscopy every five years for a person with two or more first-degree relatives with CRC, or a single first-degree relative with CRC or adenomatous polyps at age <60 years.
- Annual sigmoidoscopy beginning at age 10-12 years for a gene carrier of (or at risk for) FAP.
- Colonoscopy every one to two years, beginning at age 20-25 years or 10 years younger than the first diagnosis in the family, whichever comes first, for a gene carrier of (or at risk for) HNPCC.

PATIENT INVOLVEMENT

An ongoing working relationship between patient and oncologist is essential for survival. An analysis of patient data from 15 large adjuvant CRC trials showed that 85% of CRC recurrences are diagnosed within the first three years following initial treatment.[99] Based on that, the 2005 ASCO Surveillance Guidelines recommend seeing the patient every three to six months for the first three years after treatment, with longer intervals possible during the fourth and fifth years, to determine symptoms and to offer counseling.[95]

Risk assessment should also be reviewed with the patient, using the latest TMN classifications as mentioned above. This is especially important for stage II and III patients in whom the subsets within these stages have varying relapse-free survival rates (**Table 5**) based on Internet-based predictive tools such as those found at *www.mayoclinic.com/calcs* and *www.adjuvantonline.com*.[100,101]

Stage II patients who opt for adjuvant treatment must understand that the magnitude of benefit is less than 5% in overall survival at five years. Treatment decision-making with all stage II patients should include an assessment of comorbid conditions and life expectancy. When life expectancy is limited, then adjuvant treatment offers less benefit.[6]

Other than stage and stage subsets, no single pathological feature or statistical model exists in CRC to build a surveillance strategy with the patient. Likewise, no predictive markers exist in CRC that can show who is most likely to benefit from therapy.[95] Yet, risk assessment should be part of the patient discussion to prepare a surveillance strategy for that patient.

CONCLUSIONS

While the treatment of CRC is advancing as research continues to forge ahead, fulfilling specific needs should be the focus of our efforts. This includes designing individualized treatment strategies and developing molecular CRC classification subtypes, as well as creating and assessing new molecules that can prevent and treat CRC, particularly the use of molecularly targeted agents and combinations of drugs and/or treatment modalities. Also, diagnostic accuracy should be enhanced using the newest imaging technology to identify precancerous and cancerous lesions as well as to noninvasively assess treatment effects. In the future, functional imaging might detect molecular activity in cells and their surroundings and could, potentially, signal the interaction of a treatment agent with its intended molecular target.

Finally, methods are needed to subtype tumors on the basis of genetic and molecular alterations to help define the biologic characteristics of normal, premalignant, and malignant lesions that indicate the likelihood of neoplastic transformation, recurrence after initial treatment, and positive response to a particular treatment.

DISCLOSURE

Dr. Benson discloses that he has received grant/research support from and been retained as a consultant by Bristol-Myers Squibb Company, Genentech, Inc., ImClone Systems Incorporated, Pfizer Inc, Roche Laboratories Inc., and sanofi-aventis.

REFERENCES

1. Park Y, Hunter DJ, Spiegelman D, et al. Dietary fiber intake and risk of colorectal cancer: a pooled analysis of prospective cohort studies. JAMA. 2005;294:2849-2857.
2. Poynter JN, Gruber SB, Higgins PD, et al. Statins and the risk of colorectal cancer. N Engl J Med. 2005;352:2184-2192.
3. Dale KM, Coleman CI, Henyan NN, et al. Statins and cancer risk: a meta-analysis. JAMA. 2006;295:74-80.
4. Jacobs EJ, Rodriguez C, Brady KA, et al. Cholesterol-lowering drugs and colorectal cancer incidence in a large United States cohort. J Natl Cancer Inst. 2006;98:69-72.
5. NIH consensus conference. Adjuvant therapy for patients with colon and rectal cancer. JAMA. 1990;264:1444-1450.
6. Benson AB 3rd, Schrag D, Somerfield MR, et al. American Society of Clinical Oncology recommendations on adjuvant chemotherapy for stage II colon cancer. J Clin Oncol. 2004;22:3408-3419.
7. American Cancer Society. Cancer Facts & Figures 2005. Available at: http://www.cancer.org. Accessed January 17, 2006.
8. Jemal A, Murray T, Ward E, et al. Cancer statistics, 2005. CA Cancer J Clin. 2005;55:10-30.
9. Cooper GS, Yuan Z, Landefeld CS, et al. Surgery for colorectal cancer: Race-related differences in rates and survival among Medicare beneficiaries. Am J Public Health. 1996;86:582-586.
10. Potosky AL, Harlan LC, Kaplan RS, et al. Age, sex, and racial differences in the use of standard adjuvant therapy for colorectal cancer. J Clin Oncol. 2002;20:1192-1202.
11. Chien C, Morimoto LM, Tom J, et al. Differences in colorectal carcinoma stage and survival by race and ethnicity. Cancer. 2005;104:629-639.
12. American Cancer Society. Colorectal Cancer Facts & Figures 2005. Available at: http://www.cancer.org/downloads/STT/CAFF2005CR4PWSecured.pdf. Accessed January 17, 2006.
13. Atkin WS, Morson BC, Cuzick J. Long-term risk of colorectal cancer after excision of rectosigmoid adenomas. N Engl J Med. 1992;326:658-662.
14. Geboes K, Ectors N, Geboes KP. Pathology of early lower GI cancer. Best Pract Res Clin Gastroenterol. 2005;19:963-978.
15. Wynter CVA, Walsh MD, Higuchi T, et al. Methylation patterns define two types of hyperplastic polyp associated with colorectal cancer. Gut. 2004;53:573-580.
16. Longacre TA, Fenoglio-Preiser CM. Mixed hyperplastic adenomatous polyps/serrated adenomas. A distinct form of colorectal neoplasia. Am J Surg Pathol. 1990; 14:524-537.
17. Winawer SJ, Fletcher RH, Miller L, et al. Colorectal cancer screening: clinical guidelines and rationale. Gastroenterology. 1997;112:594-642.
18. Rickert RR, Auerbach O, Garfinkel L, et al. Adenomatous lesions of the large bowel: an autopsy survey. Cancer. 1979;43:1847-1857.
19. Levi F, Randimbison L, La Vecchia C. Incidence of colorectal cancer following adenomatous polyps of the large intestine. Int J Cancer. 1993;55:415-418.
20. Amonkar MM, Hunt TL, Zhou Z, et al.. Surveillance patterns and polyp recurrence following diagnosis and excision of colorectal polyps in a Medicare population. Cancer Epidemiol Biomarkers Prev. 2005;14:417-421.
21. Launoy G, Smith TC, Duffy SW, et al. Colorectal cancer mass-screening: estimation of faecal occult blood test sensitivity, taking into account cancer mean sojourn time. Int J Cancer. 1997;73:220-224.
22. Fukami N, Lee JH. Endoscopic treatment of large sessile and flat colorectal lesions. Curr Opin Gastroenterol. 2006; 22:54-59.
23. Rustgi AK. Hereditary gastrointestinal polyposis and nonpolyposis syndromes. N Engl J Med. 1994;331:1694-1702.
24. Ionescu DN, Papachristou G, Schoen RE, et al. Attenuated familial adenomatous polyposis: a case report with mixed features and review of genotype-phenotype correlation. Arch Pathol Lab Med. 2005;129:1401-1404.
25. Cottrell S, Bicknell D, Kaklamanis L, et al. Molecular analysis of APC mutations in familial adenomatous polyposis and sporadic colon carcinomas. Lancet. 1992;340: 626-630.

26. Soravia C, Berk T, Maklensky L, et al. Genotype phenotype correlations in attenuated adenomatous polyposis coli. *Am J Hum Genet.* 1998;62:1290-1301.

27. Parc Y, Piquard A, Dozois RR, et al. Long-term outcome of familial adenomatous polyposis patients after restorative coloproctectomy. *Ann Surg.* 2004;239:378-382.

28. Traverso G, Shuber A, Levin B, et al. Detection of APC mutations in fecal DNA from patients with colorectal tumors. *N Engl J Med.* 2002;346:311-320.

29. Sarre RG, Frost AG, Jagelman DG, et al. Gastric and duodenal polyps in familial adenomatous polyposis: a prospective study of the nature and prevalence of upper gastrointestinal polyps. *Gut.* 1987;28:306-314.

30. Liu B, Parsons R, Papadopoulos N, et al. Analysis of mismatch repair genes in hereditary non-polyposis colorectal cancer patients. *Nat Med.* 1996;2:169-174.

31. Vasen HF, Watson P, Mecklin JP, et al. New clinical criteria for hereditary nonpolyposis colorectal cancer (HNPCC, Lynch syndrome) proposed by the International Collaborative Group on HNPCC. *Gastroenterology.* 1999; 116:1453-1456.

32. Farrington SM, Lin-Goerke J, Ling J, et al. Systematic analysis of hMSH2 and hMLH1 in young colon cancer patients and controls. *Am J Hum Genet.* 1998;63:749-759.

33. Dunlop MG, Farrington SM, Carothers AD, et al. Cancer risk associated with germline DNA mismatch repair gene mutations. *Hum Mol Genet.* 1997;6:105-110.

34. Fearnhead NS, Wilding JL, Bodmer WF. Genetics of colorectal cancer: hereditary aspects and overview of colorectal tumorigenesis. *Br Med Bull.* 2002; 64:27-43.

35. Miyoshi Y, Nagase H, Ando H, et al. Somatic mutations of the APC gene in colorectal tumors: mutation cluster region in the APC gene. *Hum Mol Genet.* 1992;1:229-233.

36. Powell SM, Zilz N, Beazer-Barclay Y, et al. APC mutations occur early during colorectal tumorigenesis. *Nature.* 1992;359:235-237.

37. Fodde RR, Smits R, Clevers H. APC, signal transduction and genetic instability in colorectal cancer. *Nat Rev Cancer.* 2001;1:55-67.

38. Munkholm P. Review article: the incidence and prevalence of colorectal cancer in inflammatory bowel disease. *Aliment Pharmacol Ther.* 2003;18(Suppl 2):1-5.

39. Wong NA, Harrison DJ. Colorectal neoplasia in ulcerative colitis-related advances. *Histopathology.* 2001;39:221-234.

40. Seril DN, Liao J, Yang GY, et al. Oxidative stress and ulcerative colitis-associated carcinogenesis: studies in humans and animal models. *Carcinogenesis.* 2003;24:353-362.

41. Mucci LA, Adami HO, Wolk A. Prospective study of dietary acrylamide and risk of colorectal cancer among women. *Int J Cancer.* 2006;18:169-173.

42. Haydon AM, Macinnis RJ, English DR, et al. Effect of physical activity and body size on survival after diagnosis with colorectal cancer. *Gut.* 2006;55:62-67.

43. Robertson DJ, Sandler RS, Haile R, et al. Fat, fiber, meat and the risk of colorectal adenomas. *Am J Gastroenterol.* 2005;100:2789-2795.

44. National Comprehensive Cancer Network (NCCN). Clinical Practical Guidelines in Oncology – v.2.2006. *Colon Cancer.* Version 2.2006. *http://www.nccn.org/professionals/physician_gls/PDF/colon.pdf.* Accessed February 22, 2006.

45. Le Voyer TE, Sigurdson ER, Hanlon AL, et al. Colon cancer survival is associated with increasing number of lymph nodes analyzed: a secondary survey of intergroup trial INT-0089. *J Clin Oncol.* 2003;21:2912-2919.

46. Clinical Outcomes of Surgical therapy Study Group. A comparison of laparoscopically assisted and open colectomy for colon cancer. *N Engl J Med.* 2004;350:2050-2059.

47. Wishner JD, Baker JW, Jr., Hoffman GC, et al. Laparoscopic-assisted colectomy. The learning curve. *Surg Endosc.* 1995;9:1179-1183.

48. Nelson H, Weeks JC, Wieand HS. Proposed phase III trial comparing laparoscopic-assisted colectomy versus open colectomy for colon cancer. *J Natl Cancer Inst Monogr.* 1995:51-56.

49. Hughes KS, Simon R, Songhorabodi S, et al. Resection of the liver for colorectal carcinoma metastases: a multi-institutional study of patterns of recurrence. *Surgery.* 1986;100:278-284.

50. Fong Y, Fortner J, Sun RL, et al. Clinical score for predicting recurrence after hepatic resection for metastatic colorectal cancer: analysis of 1001 consecutive cases. *Ann Surg.* 1999;230:309-318.

50a. Nordlinger B, Guiguet M, Vaillant JC, et al. Surgical resection of colorectal carcinoma metastases to the liver. A prognostic scoring system to improve case selection, based on 1568 patients. Association Francaise de Chirurgie. *Cancer.* 1996;77:1254-1262.

50b. Fujita S, Akasu T, Moriya Y. Resection of synchronous liver metastases from colorectal cancer. *Jpn J Clin Oncol.* 2000;30:7-11.

51. Rivoire M, De Cian F, Meeus P, et al. Combination of neoadjuvant chemotherapy with cryotherapy and surgical resection for the treatment of unresectable liver metastases from colorectal carcinoma. *Cancer.* 2002;95:2283-2292.

52. Abdalla EK, Vauthey JN, Ellis LM, et al. Recurrence and outcomes following hepatic resection, radiofrequency ablation, and combined resection/ablation for colorectal liver metastases. *Ann Surg.* 2004;239:818-825.

53. Sakamoto T, Tsubota N, Iwanaga K, et al. Pulmonary resection for metastases from colorectal cancer. *Chest.* 2001;119:1069-1072.

54. Mohiuddin M, Marks G. Adjuvant radiation therapy for colon and rectal cancer. *Semin Oncol.* 1991;18:411-420.

55. Rena O, Casadio C, Viano F, et al. Pulmonary resection for metastases from colorectal cancer: factors influencing prognosis. Twenty-year experience. *Eur J Cardiothorac Surg.* 2002;21:906-912.

56. Lokich JJ, Ahlgren JD, Gullo JJ, et al. A prospective randomized comparison of continuous infusion fluorouracil with a conventional bolus schedule in metastatic colorectal carcinoma: a Mid-Atlantic Oncology Program Study. *J Clin Oncol.* 1989;7:425-432.

57. Douillard JY, Cunningham D, Roth AD, et al. Irinotecan combined with fluorouracil compared with fluorouracil alone as first-line treatment for metastatic colorectal cancer: a multicentre randomized trial. *Lancet.* 2000;355:1041-1047.

58. Saltz LB, Blanke JV, Rosen C, et al. Irinotecan plus fluorouracil and leucovorin for metastatic colorectal cancer. *N Engl J Med.* 2000;343:905-914.

59. Van Cutsem E, Twelves C, Cassidy J, et al. Oral capecitabine compared with intravenous fluorouracil plus leucovorin in patients with metastatic colorectal cancer: Results of a large phase III study. *J Clin Oncol.* 2001;19:4097-4106.

60. Van Cutsem E, Hoff PM, Harper P, et al. Oral capecitabine vs intravenous 5-fluorouracil and leucovorin: Integrated efficacy data and novel analyses from two large, randomised, phase III trials. *Br J Cancer.* 2004;90:1190-1197.

61. Hoff PM, Ansari R, Batist G. Comparison of oral capecitabine versus intravenous fluorouracil plus leucovorin as first-line treatment in 605 patients with metastatic colorectal cancer: Results of a randomized phase III study. *J Clin Oncol.* 2001;19:2282-2292.

62. Goldberg RM, Sargent DJ, Morton RF. A randomized controlled trial of fluorouracil plus leucovorin, irinotecan, and oxaliplatin combinations in patients with previously untreated metastatic colorectal cancer. *J Clin Oncol.* 2004;22:23-30.

63. Kabbinavar FF, Hambleton J, Mass RD, et al. Combined analysis of efficacy: the addition of bevacizumab to fluorouracil/leucovorin improves survival for patients with metastatic colorectal cancer. *J Clin Oncol.* 2005;23:3706-3712.

64. Hurwitz HI, Fehrenbacher L, Hainsworth JD, et al. Bevacizumab in combination with fluorouracil and leucovorin: an active regimen for first-line metastatic colorectal cancer. *J Clin Oncol.* 2005;23:3502-3508.

65. Hurwitz H, Fehrenbacher L, Novotny W, et al. Bevacizumab plus irinotecan, fluorouracil, and leucovorin for metastatic colorectal cancer. *N Engl J Med.* 2004;350:2335-2342.

66. Kabbinavar F, Hurwitz HI, Fehrenbacher L, et al. Phase II, randomized trial comparing bevacizumab plus fluorouracil (FU)/leucovorin (LV) with FU/LV alone in patients with metastatic colorectal cancer. *J Clin Oncol.* 2003;21:60-65.

67. Cunningham D, Humblet Y, Siena S, et al. Cetuximab monotherapy and cetuximab plus irinotecan in irinotecan-refractory metastatic colorectal cancer. *N Engl J Med.* 2004;351:337-345.

68. Gill S, Loprinzi CL, Sargent DJ, et al. Pooled analysis of fluorouracil-based adjuvant therapy for stage II and III colon cancer: who benefits and by how much? *J Clin Oncol.* 2004;22:1797-1806.

69. Greene FL, Stewart AK, Norton HJ. A new TNM staging strategy for node-positive (stage III) colon cancer 2002. An analysis of 50,042 patients. *Am Surg.* 2002;236:416-442.

70. National Comprehensive Cancer Network (NCCN). Clinical Practical Guidelines in Oncology – v.2.2006. *Rectal Cancer.* Version 2.2006. *http://www.nccn.org/professionals/physician_gls/PDF/rectal.*pdf. Accessed February 22, 2006.

71. Hobday TJ. An overview of approaches to adjuvant therapy for colorectal cancer in the United States. *Clin Colorectal Cancer.* 2005; 5(Suppl 1): S11-S18.

72. Mattar M, Frankel P, David D, et al. Clinicopathologic significance of synchronous and metachronous adenomas in colorectal cancer. *Clin Colorectal Cancer.* 2005;5:274-278.

73. Merkel S, Wein A, Günther K, et al. High-risk groups of patients with Stage II colon carcinoma. *Cancer.* 2001;92: 1435-1443.

74. Mamounas E, Wieand S, Wolmark N, et al. Comparative efficacy of adjuvant chemotherapy in patients with Dukes' B versus Dukes' C colon cancer: results from four National Surgical Adjuvant Breast and Bowel Project adjuvant studies (C-01, C-02, C-03, and C-04) *J Clin Oncol.* 1999;17:1349-1355.

75. Moertel CG, Fleming TR, Macdonald JS, et al. Intergroup study of fluorouracil plus levamisole as adjuvant therapy for stage II/Dukes' B2 colon cancer. *J Clin Oncol.* 1995; 13:2936-2943.

76. International Multicentre Pooled Analysis of B2 Colon Cancer Trials (IMPACT B2) Investigators. Efficacy of adjuvant fluorouracil and folinic acid in B2 colon cancer. *J Clin Oncol.* 1999;17:1356-1363.

77. Schrag D, Rifas-Shiman S, Saltz L, et al. Adjuvant chemotherapy use for Medicare beneficiaries with stage II colon cancer. *J Clin Oncol.* 2002;20:3999-4005.

78. Figueredo A, Charette ML, Maroun J, et al. Adjuvant therapy for stage II colon cancer: a systematic review from the Cancer Care Ontario Program in evidence-based care's gastrointestinal cancer disease site group. *J Clin Oncol.* 2004;22:3395-3407.

79. Thomas PR, Lindblad AS. Adjuvant postoperative radiotherapy and chemotherapy in rectal carcinoma: a review of the Gastrointestinal Tumor Study Group experience. *Radiother Oncol.* 1988;13:245-52.

80. Krook JE, Moertel CG, Gunderson LL, et al. Effective surgical adjuvant therapy for high-risk rectal carcinoma. *N Engl J Med.*1991;324:709-715.

81. Fisher B, Wolmark N, Rockette H, et al. Postoperative adjuvant chemotherapy or radiation therapy for rectal cancer: results from NSABP protocol R-01. *J Natl Cancer Inst.* 1988;80:21-9.

82. Sauer R, Becker H, Hohenberger W, et al. Preoperative versus postoperative chemoradiotherapy for rectal cancer. *N Engl J Med.* 2004;351:1731-1740.

83. Andre T, Boni C, Mounedji-Boudiaf L, et al. Oxaliplatin, fluorouracil, and leucovorin as adjuvant treatment for colon cancer. *N Engl J Med.* 2004;350:2343-2351.

84. Sastre J, Massuti B, Tabernero JM, et al. Preliminary results of a randomized phase III trial of the TTD Group comparing Capecitabine and Oxaliplatin (CapeOx) vs Oxaliplatin and 5-Fluorouracil in continuous infusion (5-FU CI) as first line treatment in advanced or metastatic colorectal cancer (CRC) [abstract 3524]. Presented at the 41st Annual Meeting American Society of Clinical Oncology; May 13-17, 2005; Orlando, Florida.

85. Wolmark N, Wieand HS, Kuebler JP, et al. A phase III trial comparing FULV to FULV + oxaliplatin in stage II or III carcinoma of the colon: Results of NSABP Protocol C-07 [abstract 3500]. Presented at the 41st Annual Meeting American Society of Clinical Oncology; May 13-17, 2005; Orlando, Florida.

86. O'Connell MJ, Mailliard JA, Kahn MJ, et al. Controlled trial of fluorouracil and low-dose leucovorin given for 6 months as postoperative adjuvant therapy for colon cancer. *J Clin Oncol.* 1997;15:246-250.

87. International multicentre pooled analysis of colon cancer trials (IMPACT) investigators. Efficacy of adjuvant fluorouracil and folinic acid in colon cancer. *Lancet.* 1995; 345:939-944.

88. Haller DG, Catalano PJ, Macdonald JS, et al. Phase III study of fluorouracil, leucovorin, and levamisole in high-risk stage II and III colon cancer: final report of Intergroup 0089. *J Clin Oncol.* 2005;23:8671-8678.

89. Twelves C, Wong A, Nowacki MP, et al. Capecitabine as adjuvant treatment for stage III colon cancer. *N Engl J Med.* 2005;352:2696-2704.

90. de Gramont A, Boni C, Navarro M, et al. Oxaliplatin/5FU/LV in the adjuvant treatment of stage II and stage III colon cancer: Efficacy results with a median follow-up of 4 years [abstract 3501]. Presented at the 41st Annual Meeting American Society of Clinical Oncology; May 13-17, 2005; Orlando, Florida.

91. Grothey A, Sargent D, Goldberg RM, et al. Survival of patients with advanced colorectal cancer improves with the availability of fluorouracil-leucovorin, irinotecan, and oxaliplatin in the course of treatment. *J Clin Oncol.* 2004;22:1209-1214.

92. Tournigand C, André T, Achille E, et al. FOLFIRI followed by FOLFOX6 or the reverse sequence in advanced colorectal cancer: a randomized GERCOR study. *J Clin Oncol.* 2004;22:229-237.

93. Jennis A, Polikoff J, Mitchell E, et al. Erbitux (Cetuximab) plus FOLFOX for colorectal cancer (EXPLORE): Preliminary efficacy analysis of a randomized phase III trial [abstract 3574]. Presented at the 41st Annual Meeting American Society of Clinical Oncology; May 13-17, 2005; Orlando, Florida.

94. Pfister DG, Benson AB 3rd, Somerfield MR. Clinical practice. Surveillance strategies after curative treatment of colorectal cancer. *N Engl J Med.* 2004;350:2375-2382

95. Desch CE, Benson AB 3rd, Somerfield MR, et al. American Society of Clinical Oncology. Colorectal cancer surveillance: 2005 update of an American Society of Clinical Oncology practice guideline. *J Clin Oncol.* 2005;23:8512-8519.

96. Renehan AG, Egger M, Saunders MP, et al. Impact on survival of intensive follow up after curative resection for colorectal cancer: Systematic review and meta-analysis of randomised trials. *BMJ.* 2002;324:813.

97. Jeffery GM, Hickey BE, Hider P. Follow-up strategies for patients treated for non-metastatic colorectal cancer *Cochrane Database Syst Rev.* 2002;(1):CD002200.

98. Winawer S, Fletcher R, Rex D, et al. Colorectal cancer screening and surveillance: Clinical guidelines and rationale–Update based on new evidence. *Gastroenterology.* 2003;124:544-560.

99. Sargent DJ, Wieand S, Benedetti J, et al. Disease-free survival (DFS) vs overall survival (OS) as a primary endpoint for adjuvant colon cancer studies: Individual patient data from 12,915 patients on 15 randomized trials [abstract 3502]. Presented at the 40th Annual Meeting of the American Society of Clinical Oncology; June 5-8, 2004; New Orleans, La.

100. Adjuvant systemic therapy tools; 2005. *www.mayoclinic.com/calcs.* Accessed January 23, 2006.

101. Adjuvantonline.com; 2005. *www.adjuvantonline.com.* Accessed January 23, 2006.

Appendix. Mechanisms of Action of Agents Currently Used in Colorectal Cancer

Drug	Mechanism of Action
Bevacizumab	• Humanized MAb. • Binds to VEGF. • Reduces the ability of the VEGF ligand for its receptor and thus prevents receptor activation.[a]
Capecitabine	• In the liver, drug is hydrolyzed to 5-FU.[59] • Both normal and tumor cells metabolize 5-FU to 5-fluoro-2'-deoxyuridine monophosphate (FdUMP) and 5-fluorouridine triphosphate (FUTP). • This causes cell injury by forming a complex with thymidylate synthase, which inhibits the formation of thymidylate, the necessary precursor of thymidine triphosphate (TT), and essential for DNA synthesis. • TT deficiency inhibits cell division. • Also, nuclear transcriptional enzymes can mistakenly incorporate FUTP in place of uridine triphosphate during the synthesis of RNA. • This metabolic error can interfere with RNA processing and protein synthesis.
Cetuximab	• When the external binding domain of EGFR, a transmembrane glycoprotein, binds to specific ligands, such as EGF, receptor dimerization occurs, which in turn stimulates phosphorylation of the tyrosine kinases.[b] • This initiates a signaling cascade that regulates cell proliferation and survival. • Cetuximab, a chimeric immunoglobulin G_1 MAb, recognizes the bind to the extracellular domain of EGFR.[c] • This results in a steric interference with the ligand binding site and prevents ligand activation of the receptor.
5-Fluorouracil	• Incorporated into DNA during DNA synthesis. • This promutagenic DNA lesion is excised by the base excision repair enzyme uracil DNA glycosylase (UDG). • 5-FU, as the free base, specifically binds in vivo to the UDG in noncycling human cells, thereby inhibiting its activity.[d]
Irinotecan	• Semi-synthetic, water-soluble derivative of camptothecin, a cytotoxic alkaloid extracted from plants such as Camptotheca acuminate.[e] • Along with its active metabolite, SN-38, they inhibit the action of topoisomerase I, an enzyme that produces reversible single-strand breaks in DNA during DNA replication. • These single-strand breaks relieve torsional strain and allow DNA replication to proceed. Irinotecan and SN-38 bind to the topoisomerase I-DNA complex and prevent relegation of the DNA strand, resulting in double-strand DNA breakage and cell death. • Cell cycle phase-specific (S-phase).[f]
Oxaliplatin	• A platinum-based chemotherapeutic agent with a 1,2-diaminocyclohexane (DACH) carrier ligand.[g] • Retention of the bulky DACH ring by activated oxaliplatin is thought to result in the formation of platinum-DNA adducts, which appear to be more effective at blocking DNA replication and are more cytotoxic than adducts formed from cisplatin.

EGF, endothelial growth factor; EGFR, endothelial growth factor receptor; MAb, monoclonal antibody; UDG, uracil DNA glycosylase; VEGF, vascular endothelial growth factor.

REFERENCES

a. Ferrara N. Vascular endothelial growth factor: basic science and clinical progress. *Endocr Rev.* 2004;25:581-611.

b. Ciardiello F, Tortora G. A novel approach in the treatment of cancer: targeting the epidermal growth factor receptor. *Clin Cancer Res.* 2001;7:2958-2970.

c. Thomas SM, Grandis JR. Pharmacokinetic and pharmacodynamic properties of EGFR inhibitors under clinical investigation. *Cancer Treat Rev.* 2004;30:255-268.

d. Wurzer JC, Tallarida RJ, Sirover MA. New mechanism of action of the cancer chemotherapeutic agent 5-fluorouracil in human cells. *J Pharmacol Exp Ther.* 1994;269:39-43.

e. Camptosar [prescribing information]. New York, NY: Pfizer, Inc.; 2005.

f. Rothenberg ML, Kuhn JG, Schaaf LJ, et al. Alternative dosing schedules for irinotecan. *Oncology* (Huntington). 1998;12(8 Suppl 6):68-71.

g. Raymond E, Faivre S, Woynarowski JM, Chaney SG. Oxaliplatin: mechanism of action and antineoplastic activity. *Semin Oncol.* 1998;25(2 Suppl 5):4-12.

SECTION II
GUIDELINES

COLON CANCER (PDQ®): TREATMENT HEALTH PROFESSIONAL VERSION

GENERAL INFORMATION

[Note: Separate PDQ summaries on *Screening for Colorectal Cancer, Prevention of Colorectal Cancer,* and *Genetics of Colorectal Cancer* are also available. Information about colon cancer in children is available in the PDQ summary on *Unusual Cancers of Childhood: Treatment.*
Note: Estimated new cases and deaths from colon cancer in the United States in 2005:[1]

- New cases: 104,950.
- Deaths (colon and rectal cancers combined): 56,290.

Note: Some citations in the text of this section are followed by a level of evidence. The PDQ editorial boards use a formal ranking system to help the reader judge the strength of evidence linked to the reported results of a therapeutic strategy. (Refer to the PDQ summary on *Levels of Evidence* for more information.)]
(Table 1.)

Cancer of the colon is a highly treatable and often curable disease when localized to the bowel. Surgery is the primary form of treatment and results in cure in approximately 50% of patients. Recurrence following surgery is a major problem and is often the ultimate cause of death.

Table 1. PDQ Levels of Evidence

Level of evidence 1iiA
Randomized, controlled, nonblinded clinical trial with total mortality as an endpoint.

Level of evidence 1iiB
Randomized, controlled, nonblinded clinical trial with cause-specific mortality as an endpoint.

Level of evidence 1iiC
Randomized, controlled, nonblinded clinical trial with carefully assessed quality of life as an endpoint.

Level of evidence 1iiDiii
Randomized, controlled, nonblinded clinical trial with tumor response rate as an endpoint.

Level of evidence 3iiiA
Nonconsecutive case series with total mortality as an endpoint.

Level of evidence 3iiiDi
Nonconsecutive case series with total disease-free survival as an endpoint.

Prognostic Factors

The prognosis of patients with colon cancer is clearly related to the degree of penetration of the tumor through the bowel wall, the presence or absence of nodal involvement, and the presence or absence of distant metastases. These three characteristics form the basis for all staging systems developed for this disease. Bowel obstruction and bowel perforation are indicators of poor prognosis.[2] Elevated pretreatment serum levels of carcinoembryonic antigen (CEA) have a negative prognostic significance.[3] The American Joint Committee on Cancer and a National Cancer Institute-sponsored panel recommended that at least 12 lymph nodes be examined in patients with colon and rectal cancer to confirm the absence of nodal involvement by tumor.[4-6] This recommendation takes into consideration that the number of lymph nodes examined is a reflection of the aggressiveness of lymphovascular mesenteric dissection at the time of surgical resection and the pathologic identification of nodes in the specimen. Retrospective studies demonstrated that the number of lymph nodes examined in colon and rectal surgery may be associated with patient outcome.[7-10]

Many other prognostic markers have been evaluated retrospectively for patients with colon cancer, though most, including allelic loss of chromosome 18q or thymidylate synthase expression, have not been prospectively validated.[11-20] Microsatellite instability, also associated with hereditary nonpolyposis colon cancer (HNPCC), has been associated with improved survival independent of tumor stage in a population-based series of 607 patients younger than 50 years with colorectal cancer.[21] Treatment decisions depend on factors such as physician and patient preferences and the stage of the disease rather than the age of the patient.[22-24] Racial differences in overall survival after adjuvant therapy have been observed, without differences in disease-free survival, suggesting that comorbid conditions play a role in survival outcome in different patient populations.[25]

Risk Factors

Because of the frequency of the disease, ability to identify high-risk groups, demonstrated slow growth of primary lesions, better survival of patients with early-stage lesions, and relative simplicity and accuracy of screening tests, screening for colon cancer should be a part of routine care for all adults starting at age 50 years, especially for those with first-degree relatives with colorectal cancer. Groups that have a high incidence of colorectal cancer include those with hereditary conditions, such as familial polyposis, HNPCC or Lynch syndrome variants I and II, and those with a personal history of ulcerative colitis or Crohn's colitis.[26,27] Together they account for 10% to 15% of colorectal cancers. Patients with HNPCC reportedly have better prognoses in stage-stratified survival analysis than patients with sporadic colorectal cancer, but the retrospective nature of the studies and possibility of selection factors make this observation difficult to interpret.[28] [Level of evidence: 3iiiA] More common conditions with an increased risk include a personal history of colorectal cancer or adenomas; first-degree family history of colorectal cancer or adenomas; and a personal history of ovarian, endometrial, or breast cancer.[29,30] These high-risk groups account for only 23% of all colorectal cancers. Limiting screening or early cancer detection to only these high-risk groups would miss the majority of colorectal cancers.[31] (Refer to the PDQ summaries on *Screening for Colorectal Cancer* and *Prevention of Colorectal Cancer* for more information.)

Follow-up

Following treatment of colon cancer, periodic evaluations may lead to the earlier identification and management of recurrent disease.[32-35] The impact of such monitoring on overall mortality of patients with recurrent colon cancer, however, is limited by the relatively small proportion of patients in whom localized, potentially curable metastases, are found. To date, no large-scale randomized trials have documented the efficacy of a standard, postoperative monitoring program.[36-40] CEA is a serum glycoprotein frequently used in the management of patients with colon cancer. A review of the use of this tumor marker suggests the following:[41]

- A CEA level is not a valuable screening test for colorectal cancer because of the large numbers of false-positive and false-negative reports.
- Postoperative CEA testing should be restricted to patients who would be candidates for resection of liver or lung metastases.
- Routine use of CEA levels alone for monitoring response to treatment should not be recommended.

The optimal regimen and frequency of follow-up examinations are not well defined, however, because the impact on patient survival is not clear and the quality of data is poor.[38-40] New surveillance methods, including CEA immunoscintigraphy[42] and positron emission tomography,[43] are under clinical evaluation.

Gastrointestinal stromal tumors can occur in the colon. (Refer to the PDQ summary on *Adult Soft Tissue Sarcoma Treatment* for more information.)

REFERENCES

1. American Cancer Society. *Cancer Facts and Figures 2005.* Atlanta, GA: American Cancer Society, 2005. Also available online. Last accessed November 1, 2005.
2. Steinberg SM, Barkin JS, Kaplan RS, et al. Prognostic indicators of colon tumors. The Gastrointestinal Tumor Study Group experience. *Cancer.* 1986;57(9):1866-1870.
3. Filella X, Molina R, Grau JJ, et al. Prognostic value of CA 19.9 levels in colorectal cancer. *Ann Surg.* 1992;216(1):55-59.
4. Colon and rectum. In: American Joint Committee on Cancer. *AJCC Cancer Staging Manual.* 6th ed. New York, NY: Springer, 2002, pp 113-124.
5. Compton CC, Greene FL. The staging of colorectal cancer: 2004 and beyond. *CA Cancer J Clin.* 2004;54(6):295-308.
6. Nelson H, Petrelli N, Carlin A, et al. Guidelines 2000 for colon and rectal cancer surgery. *J Natl Cancer Inst.* 2001; 93(8):583-596.
7. Swanson RS, Compton CC, Stewart AK, et al. The prognosis of T3N0 colon cancer is dependent on the number of lymph nodes examined. *Ann Surg Oncol.* 2003;10(1):65-71.
8. Le Voyer TE, Sigurdson ER, Hanlon AL, et al. Colon cancer survival is associated with increasing number of lymph nodes analyzed: a secondary survey of intergroup trial INT-0089. *J Clin Oncol.* 2003;21(15): 2912-2919.
9. Prandi M, Lionetto R, Bini A, et al. Prognostic evaluation of stage B colon cancer patients is improved by an adequate lymphadenectomy: results of a secondary analysis of a large scale adjuvant trial. *Ann Surg.* 2002;235(4):458-463.
10. Tepper JE, O'Connell MJ, Niedzwiecki D, et al. Impact of number of nodes retrieved on outcome in patients with rectal cancer. *J Clin Oncol.* 2001;19(1):157-163.
11. McLeod HL, Murray GI. Tumour markers of prognosis in colorectal cancer. *Br J Cancer.* 1999;79(2):191-203.
12. Jen J, Kim H, Piantadosi S, et al. Allelic loss of chromosome 18q and prognosis in colorectal cancer. *N Engl J Med.* 1994;331(4):213-221.
13. Lanza G, Matteuzzi M, Gafá R, et al. Chromosome 18q allelic loss and prognosis in stage II and III colon cancer. *Int J Cancer.* 1998;79(4):390-395.
14. Griffin MR, Bergstralh EJ, Coffey RJ, et al. Predictors of survival after curative resection of carcinoma of the colon and rectum. *Cancer.* 1987;60(9):2318-2324.
15. Johnston PG, Fisher ER, Rockette HE, et al. The role of thymidylate synthase expression in prognosis and outcome of adjuvant chemotherapy in patients with rectal cancer. *J Clin Oncol.* 1994;12(12):2640-2647.
16. Shibata D, Reale MA, Lavin P, et al. The DCC protein and prognosis in colorectal cancer. *N Engl J Med.* 1996;335 (23):1727-1732.
17. Bauer KD, Lincoln ST, Vera-Roman JM, et al. Prognostic implications of proliferative activity and DNA aneuploidy in colonic adenocarcinomas. *Lab Invest.* 1987;57(3):329-335.
18. Bauer KD, Bagwell CB, Giaretti W, et al. Consensus review of the clinical utility of DNA flow cytometry in colorectal cancer. *Cytometry* 1993;14(5):486-491.
19. Sun XF, Carstensen JM, Zhang H, et al. Prognostic significance of cytoplasmic p53 oncoprotein in colorectal adenocarcinoma. *Lancet.* 1992;340(8832):1369-1373.
20. Roth JA. p53 prognostication: paradigm or paradox? *Clin Cancer Res.* 1999;5(11):3345.
21. Gryfe R, Kim H, Hsieh ET, et al. Tumor microsatellite

instability and clinical outcome in young patients with colorectal cancer. *N Engl J Med.* 2000;342(2):69-77.

22. Iwashyna TJ, Lamont EB. Effectiveness of adjuvant fluorouracil in clinical practice: a population-based cohort study of elderly patients with stage III colon cancer. *J Clin Oncol.* 2002;20(19):3992-3998.

23. Chiara S, Nobile MT, Vincenti M, et al. Advanced colorectal cancer in the elderly: results of consecutive trials with 5-fluorouracil-based chemotherapy. *Cancer Chemother Pharmacol.* 1998;42(4):336-340.

24. Popescu RA, Norman A, Ross PJ, et al. Adjuvant or palliative chemotherapy for colorectal cancer in patients 70 years or older. *J Clin Oncol.* 1999;17(8):2412-2418.

25. Dignam JJ, Colangelo L, Tian W, et al. Outcomes among African-Americans and Caucasians in colon cancer adjuvant therapy trials: findings from the National Surgical Adjuvant Breast and Bowel Project. *J Natl Cancer Inst.* 1999;91(22):1933-1940.

26. Thorson AG, Knezetic JA, Lynch HT. A century of progress in hereditary nonpolyposis colorectal cancer (Lynch syndrome). *Dis Colon Rectum.* 1999;42(1):1-9.

27. Smith RA, von Eschenbach AC, Wender R, et al. American Cancer Society guidelines for the early detection of cancer: update of early detection guidelines for prostate, colorectal, and endometrial cancers. Also: update 2001—testing for early lung cancer detection. *CA Cancer J Clin.* 51 2001; Jan-Feb(1):38-75;quiz 77-80.

28. Watson P, Lin KM, Rodriguez-Bigas MA, et al. Colorectal carcinoma survival among hereditary nonpolyposis colorectal carcinoma family members. *Cancer.* 1998;83(2):259-266.

29. Ransohoff DF, Lang CA. Screening for colorectal cancer. *N Engl J Med.* 1991;325(1):37-41.

30. Fuchs CS, Giovannucci EL, Colditz GA, et al. A prospective study of family history and the risk of colorectal cancer. *N Engl J Med.* 1994;331(25):1669-1674.

31. Winawer SJ. Screening for colorectal cancer. Cancer: *Principles and Practice of Oncology Updates.* 1987;2(1):1-16.

32. Martin EW Jr, Minton JP, Carey LC. CEA-directed second-look surgery in the asymptomatic patient after primary resection of colorectal carcinoma. *Ann Surg.* 1985;202(3): 310-317.

33. Bruinvels DJ, Stiggelbout AM, Kievit J, et al. Follow-up of patients with colorectal cancer. A meta-analysis. *Ann Surg.* 1994;219(2):174-182.

34. Lautenbach E, Forde KA, Neugut AI. Benefits of colonoscopic surveillance after curative resection of colorectal cancer. *Ann Surg.* 1994;220 (2):206-211.

35. Khoury DA, Opelka FG, Beck DE, et al. Colon surveillance after colorectal cancer surgery. *Dis Colon Rectum.* 1996; 39(3):252-256.

36. Safi F, Link KH, Beger HG. Is follow-up of colorectal cancer patients worthwhile? *Dis Colon Rectum.* 1993;36(7):636-43;discussion 643-644.

37. Moertel CG, Fleming TR, Macdonald JS, et al. An evaluation of the carcinoembryonic antigen (CEA) test for monitoring patients with resected colon cancer. *JAMA.* 1993;270(8): 943-947.

38. Rosen M, Chan L, Beart RW Jr, et al. Follow-up of colorectal cancer: a meta-analysis. *Dis Colon Rectum.* 1998;41(9):1116-1126.

39. Desch CE, Benson AB 3rd, Smith TJ, et al. Recommended colorectal cancer surveillance guidelines by the American Society of Clinical Oncology. *J Clin Oncol.* 1999;17(4): 1312.

40. Benson AB 3rd, Desch CE, Flynn PJ, et al. 2000 update of American Society of Clinical Oncology colorectal cancer surveillance guidelines. *J Clin Oncol.* 2000;18(20):3586-3588.

41. Clinical practice guidelines for the use of tumor markers in breast and colorectal cancer. Adopted on May 17, 1996 by the American Society of Clinical Oncology. *J Clin Oncol.* 1996;14(10):2843-2877.

42. Lechner P, Lind P, Goldenberg DM. Can postoperative surveillance with serial CEA immunoscintigraphy detect resectable rectal cancer recurrence and potentially improve tumor-free survival? *J Am Coll Surg.* 2000;191 (5):511-518.

43. Lonneux M, Reffad AM, Detry R, et al. FDG-PET improves the staging and selection of patients with recurrent colorectal cancer. *Eur J Nucl Med Mol Imaging.* 2002;29 (7): 915-921.

CELLULAR CLASSIFICATION

Histologic types of colon cancer include the following:

- Adenocarcinoma (most colon cancers)
  - Mucinous (colloid) adenocarcinoma
  - Signet ring adenocarcinoma
- Scirrhous tumors
- Neuroendocrine[1]; tumors with neuroendocrine differentiation typically have a poorer prognosis than pure adenocarcinoma variants.

REFERENCES

1. Saclarides TJ, Szeluga D, Staren ED. Neuroendocrine cancers of the colon and rectum. Results of a ten-year experience. *Dis Colon Rectum.* 1994;37(7):635-642.

STAGE INFORMATION

Treatment decisions should be made with reference to the TNM classification,[1] rather than to the older Dukes' or the Modified Astler-Coller classification schema.

The American Joint Committee on Cancer (AJCC) and a National Cancer Institute-sponsored panel recommended that at least 12 lymph nodes be examined in patients with colon and rectal cancer to confirm the absence of nodal involvement by tumor.[1-3] This recommendation takes into consideration that the number of lymph nodes examined is a reflection of the aggressiveness of lymphovascular mesenteric dissection at the time of surgical resection and the pathologic identification of nodes in the specimen. Retrospective studies demonstrated that the number of lymph nodes examined in colon and rectal surgery may be associated with patient outcome.[4-7]

The AJCC has designated staging by TNM classification.[1]

TNM Definitions

Primary tumor (T)
- TX: Primary tumor cannot be assessed
- T0: No evidence of primary tumor
- Tis: Carcinoma in situ: intraepithelial or invasion of the lamina propria*
- T1: Tumor invades submucosa
- T2: Tumor invades muscularis propria
- T3: Tumor invades through the muscularis propria into the subserosa or into nonperitonealized pericolic or perirectal tissues
- T4: Tumor directly invades other organs or structures and/or perforates visceral peritoneum**.***

* [*Note: Tis includes cancer cells confined within the glandular basement membrane (intraepithelial) or lamina propria (intramucosal) with no extension through the muscularis mucosae into the submucosa.*]
** [*Note: Direct invasion in T4 includes invasion of other segments of the colorectum by way of the serosa, for example, invasion of the sigmoid colon by a carcinoma of the cecum.*]
*** [*Note: Tumor that is adherent macroscopically to other organs or structures is classified T4. If no tumor is present in the adhesion microscopically, however, the classification should be pT3. The V and L substaging should be used to identify the presence or absence of vascular or lymphatic invasion.*]

Regional lymph nodes (N)

- NX: Regional nodes cannot be assessed
- N0: No regional lymph node metastasis
- N1: Metastasis in 1 to 3 regional lymph nodes
- N2: Metastasis in 4 or more regional lymph nodes

[*Note: A tumor nodule in the pericolorectal adipose tissue of a primary carcinoma, without histologic evidence of residual lymph node in the nodule, is classified in the pN category as a regional lymph node metastasis if the nodule has the form and smooth contour of a lymph node. If the nodule has an irregular contour, it should be classified in the T category, and also coded as V1 (microscopic venous invasion) or as V2 (if it was grossly evident), because there is a strong likelihood that is represents venous invasion.*]

Distant metastasis (M)

- MX: Distant metastasis cannot be assessed
- M0: No distant metastasis
- M1: Distant metastasis

AJCC Stage Groupings

Stage 0
- Tis, N0, M0

Stage I
- T1, N0, M0
- T2, N0, M0

Stage IIA
- T3, N0, M0

Stage IIB
- T4, N0, M0

Stage IIIA
- T1, N1, M0
- T2, N1, M0

Stage IIIB
- T3, N1, M0
- T4, N1, M0

Stage IIIC
- Any T, N2, M0

Stage IV
- Any T, Any N, M1

REFERENCES

1. Colon and rectum. American Joint Committee on Cancer. *AJCC Cancer Staging Manual.* 6th ed. New York, NY: Springer, 2002, pp 113-124.
2. Compton CC, Greene FL. The staging of colorectal cancer: 2004 and beyond. *CA Cancer J Clin.* 2004;54(6):295-308.
3. Nelson H, Petrelli N, Carlin A, et al. Guidelines 2000 for colon and rectal cancer surgery. *J Natl Cancer Inst.* 2001; 93(8):583-596.
4. Swanson RS, Compton CC, Stewart AK, et al. The prognosis of T3N0 colon cancer is dependent on the number of lymph nodes examined. *Ann Surg Oncol.* 2003;10(1):65-71.
5. Le Voyer TE, Sigurdson ER, Hanlon AL, et al. Colon cancer survival is associated with increasing number of lymph nodes analyzed: a secondary survey of intergroup trial INT-0089. *J Clin Oncol.* 2003;21(15):2912-219.
6. Prandi M, Lionetto R, Bini A, et al. Prognostic evaluation of stage B colon cancer patients is improved by an adequate lymphadenectomy: results of a secondary analysis of a large scale adjuvant trial. *Ann Surg.* 2002;235(4):458-463.
7. Tepper JE, O'Connell MJ, Niedzwiecki D, et al. Impact of number of nodes retrieved on outcome in patients with rectal cancer. *J Clin Oncol.* 2001;19(1):157-163.

TREATMENT OPTION OVERVIEW

[Note: Some citations in the text of this section are followed by a level of evidence. The PDQ editorial boards use a formal ranking system to help the reader judge the strength of evidence linked to the reported results of a therapeutic strategy. (Refer to the PDQ summary on *Levels of Evidence* for more information.)]

Drug combinations described in this section:

- AIO regimen (folic acid, fluorouracil (5-FU), irinotecan):
  - Irinotecan (100 mg/m^2) as a two-hour infusion day 1; leucovorin (500 mg/m^2) as a two-hour infusion day 1; followed by 5-FU (2,000 mg/m^2) intravenous (IV) bolus via ambulatory pump over 24 hours weekly x 4 every 52 weeks.
- FOLFOX4 regimen (oxaliplatin, leucovorin, 5-FU):
  - Oxaliplatin (85 mg/m^2) as a two-hour infusion day 1; leucovorin (200 mg/m^2) as a two-hour infusion days 1 and 2; followed by a loading dose of 5-FU (400 mg/m^2)

IV bolus, then 5-FU (600 mg/m^2) via ambulatory pump over 22 hours, days 1 and 2 every two weeks.

- FOLFOX6 regimen (oxaliplatin, leucovorin, 5-FU):
  - Oxaliplatin (85-100 mg/m^2) as a two-hour infusion day 1; leucovorin (400 mg/m^2) as a two-hour infusion day 1; followed by a loading dose of 5-FU (400 mg/m^2) IV bolus on day 1, then 5-FU (2,400-3,000 mg/m^2) via ambulatory pump over 46 hours every two weeks.
- FOLFIRI regimen (folic acid, 5-FU, irinotecan):
  - Irinotecan (180 mg/m^2) as a two-hour infusion day 1; leucovorin (400 mg/m^2) as a two-hour infusion day 1; followed by a loading dose of 5-FU (400 mg/m^2) IV bolus on day 1, then 5-FU (2,400-3,000 mg/m^2) via ambulatory pump over 46 hours every two weeks.
- IFL (or Saltz) regimen (irinotecan, 5-FU, leucovorin):
  - Irinotecan (125 mg/m^2), 5-FU (500 mg/m^2) IV bolus and leucovorin (20 mg/m^2) IV bolus weekly for four out of six weeks.
- NCCTG regimen (5-FU, levamisole):
  - Bolus 5-FU (450 mg/m^2 per day) days 1 to 5, then weekly 28 days later plus levamisole (50 mg) orally three times a day for three days every two weeks.
- NCCTG regimen (5-FU, low-dose leucovorin):
  - Bolus 5-FU (450 mg/m^2) plus leucovorin (20 mg/m^2) daily for five days every 28 days.
- NSABP regimen (5-FU, high-dose leucovorin):
  - Bolus 5-FU (500 mg/m^2) plus

leucovorin (500 mg/m^2) weekly for six consecutive weeks every eight weeks.

Primary Surgical Therapy

Standard treatment for patients with colon cancer has been open surgical resection of the primary and regional lymph nodes for localized disease. The role of laparoscopic techniques[1-4] in the treatment of colon cancer has been examined in two studies. A multicenter prospective randomized noninferiority trial compared laparoscopic-assisted colectomy (LAC) to open colectomy in 872 patients.[5] At a median follow-up of 4.4 years, three-year recurrence rates (16% LAC vs 18% open; hazard ratio [HR] for recurrence, 0.86; 95% confidence interval [CI], 0.63-1.17; P=.32) and three-year overall survival rates (86% LAC vs. 85% open colectomy; HR for death in LAC, 0.91; 95% CI, 0.68-1.21; P=.51) were similar in both groups for all stages of disease evaluated.[6] [Level of evidence: 1iiA]. Tumor recurrence in surgical incisions was <1% for both groups. Decreased hospital stay (five days LAC vs. six days open colectomy, P < .001) and decreased use of analgesics were reported in the LAC group. A 21% conversion rate from LAC to open procedure was shown. This study excluded patients with locally advanced disease, transverse colon and rectal tumor locations, and perforated lesions. Each of the 66 surgeons participating in the trial had performed at least 20 LACs and were accredited for study participation after independent videotape review assured appropriate oncologic and surgical principles were maintained.[6] The quality-of-life component of this trial was published separately and report-ed minimal short-term quality-of-life benefits with LAC.[7] [Level of evidence: 1iiC] One small, single-institution randomized study of 219 patients showed that the LAC procedure was independently associated with reduced tumor recurrence on multivariate analysis.[8] [Level of evidence: 1iiB] The role of sentinel lymph node mapping is also under clinical evaluation.[9,10]

Surgery is also curative in 25% to 40% of patients who develop resectable metastases in the liver and lung. Improved surgical techniques and advances in preoperative imaging have allowed for better patient selection for resection.

Adjuvant Chemotherapy

Chemotherapy regimens based on fluorouracil, leucovorin, and levamisole

Many early trials of adjuvant chemotherapy failed to show a significant improvement in either overall or disease-free survival for patients receiving treatment compared to concurrently randomized control patients receiving no adjuvant therapy.[11-14] These trials employed 5-FU alone or 5-FU plus semustine (methyl-CCNU). The North Central Cancer Treatment Group (NCCTG) conducted a randomized trial comparing surgical resection alone with postoperative levamisole or 5-FU-levamisole.[15] [Level of evidence: 1iiA] A significant improvement in disease-free survival was observed for patients with stage III (Dukes' C) colon cancer who received 5-FU-levamisole, but overall survival benefits were of borderline statistical significance. An absolute survival benefit of approximately 12% (49% vs 37%) was seen in patients with stage III disease treated with 5-FU-levamisole.

In a large, confirmatory intergroup trial, 5-FU-levamisole prolonged disease-free and overall survival in patients with stage III colon cancer, compared to patients who received no treatment after surgery.[16] [Level of evidence: 1iiA] Levamisole alone did not confer these benefits. Subsequent studies tested the combination of 5-FU and leucovorin in the adjuvant treatment of patients with resected carcinoma of the colon. Results of multiple randomized trials that have enrolled over 4,000 patients comparing adjuvant chemotherapy with 5-FU-leucovorin to surgery or 5-FU-semustine-vincristine demonstrate a relative reduction in mortality of between 22% and 33% (three-year overall survival of 71% to 78% increased to 75% to 84%).[17-19]

Subsequently, four additional trials have explored whether shorter treatments and combinations of chemotherapy with leucovorin and levamisole or interferon impact survival. These studies have shown that treatment for six to eight months with 5-FU-leucovorin is equivalent to 12 months, and that the addition of interferon does increase toxic effects without improving efficacy.[20-22] At this time, patients with stage III (Dukes' C) colon cancer should be considered for adjuvant therapy with 5-FU-leucovorin for six to eight months.[21,23]

The NCCTG performed a trial comparing six months to 12 months of treatment using either 5-FU and levamisole or 5-FU, levamisole, and leucovorin for patients with stages II and III (Dukes' B and C or MAC B2, B3, and C1-3) colon cancer.[24] [Level of evidence: 1iiA] The trial showed that for equivalent survival benefit, the 5-FU plus levamisole regimen must be given for 12 months, while the three-drug regimen could be administered over

just six months. An intergroup trial with four treatment arms, including 5-FU-levamisole, 5-FU plus low-dose leucovorin (the NCCTG regimen), 5-FU plus high-dose leucovorin (the NSABP regimen), or 5-FU-leucovorin-levamisole, has been reported in preliminary fashion.[25] [Level of evidence: 1iiA] This study also demonstrated that seven to eight months of 5-FU-leucovorin is at least as effective as 12 months of 5-FU-levamisole. The NSABP C-04 study found equivalent results in overall survival for one year of 5-FU plus high-dose leucovorin when compared to one year of 5-FU-levamisole.[21] The addition of levamisole to 5-FU and leucovorin did not improve disease-free or overall survival. Mature data from NSABP C-05 suggest no survival benefit from the addition of interferon alfa-2a to 5-FU and high-dose leucovorin but did note a substantial increase in grade 3 or higher toxic effects.[20]

Based on the outcomes of all of these trials, a recommendation was made at the 1997 American Society of Clinical Oncology meeting that any one of three regimens could be considered for postoperative treatment of patients with stage III colon cancer, all of which have resulted in a survival advantage over no postoperative chemotherapy. These include the following:

- NCCTG regimen (5-FU, levamisole) for one year.
- NCCTG regimen (5-FU, low-dose leucovorin) for six months.
- NSABP regimen (5-FU, high-dose leucovorin) for seven to eight months (four cycles).

At this time, no data suggest any advantage to the three-drug combination of 5-FU and leucovorin and levamisole over any of the previously noted two-drug regimens. Also, insufficient data are available to prove whether high-dose, intermediate-dose, or low-dose leucovorin is most advantageous as a modulator of 5-FU. However, the data suggest increased toxic effects with a five-day schedule (Mayo Clinic) without evidence of an improved therapeutic benefit compared with the weekly regimen (Roswell Park). Pooled analysis of randomized trials indicate that elderly patients (>70 years) derived equal benefit from adjuvant treatment as younger individuals and should not be excluded from these treatments based solely on age.[26]

The potential value of adjuvant therapy for patients with stage II (Dukes' B or MAC B2 or B3) colon cancer also remains controversial. Investigators from the NSABP have indicated that the reduction in risk of recurrence by adjuvant therapy in patients with stage II disease is of similar magnitude to the benefit seen in patients with stage III disease treated with adjuvant therapy, though an overall survival advantage has not been established.[27] A randomized trial of postoperative 5-FU plus levamisole compared to surgery alone, however, showed no survival advantage to postoperative adjuvant chemotherapy.[28] A meta-analysis of 1,000 stage II patients whose experience was amalgamated from a series of trials indicates a 2% advantage in disease-free survival at five years when adjuvant therapy-treated patients treated with 5-FU-leucovorin are compared to untreated controls.[29] [Level of evidence: 1iiDi][30] Patients with stage II colon cancer remain candidates for clinical trials in which either surgery alone or 5-FU-leucovorin represent standard therapy.[31-33]

Chemotherapy regimens based on irinotecan and oxaliplatin

After the development and approval of irinotecan and oxaliplatin for the treatment of patients with advanced colorectal cancer (see *Stage IV and Recurrent Colon Cancer* section), these drugs are now being tested in patients with local or recurrent disease. Irinotecan is a topoisomerase-I inhibitor with a 10% to 20% partial response rate in patients with metastatic colon cancer.[34-37] Phase III trials have demonstrated improved response rates and prolonged overall survival with irinotecan combined with 5-FU-leucovorin when compared with 5-FU-leucovorin alone.[38,39]

The MOSAIC study compared the toxic effects and efficacy of FOLFOX4 with a 5-FU-leucovorin regimen administered for six months in 2,246 patients with resected stage II or stage III colon cancer. The preliminary results of the study with 37 months of follow-up demonstrated a significant improvement in disease-free survival at three years (77.8% vs. 72.9%, P=.01) in favor of FOLFOX4.[40] Patients treated with FOLFOX4 experienced more frequent toxic effects consisting mainly of neutropenia (41% >grade 3) and reversible peripheral sensorial neuropathy (12.4% >grade 3). These results are still preliminary, however, information is lacking with regard to overall survival suggesting that FOLFOX4 is a therapeutic option for patients with resected stage III colon cancer.[40]

Adjuvant Radiation Therapy

While combined modality therapy with chemotherapy and radiation therapy has a significant role in the management of patients with rectal cancer (below the peritoneal reflection), the role of adjuvant radiation therapy for patients with colon cancer (above the peritoneal reflection) is not well-defined. Patterns-of-care analyses and single-institution retrospective reviews suggest a role for radiation therapy in certain high-risk subsets of colon cancer patients (T4, tumor location in immobile sites, local perforation, obstruction, and residual disease postresection).[41-46] Such observations led to the development of a phase III randomized Intergroup study designed to test the benefit of adding radiation therapy to surgery and chemotherapy with 5-FU-levamisole for selected high-risk colon cancer patients (T4; or T3, N1-N2 ascending/descending colon).[47] This clinical trial closed early secondary to inadequate patient accrual, and analysis of 222 enrolled patients (the original goal was 700 patients) demonstrated no relapse or overall survival benefit for the group receiving radiation therapy, though the sample size and statistical power were inadequate to exclude benefit. Adjuvant radiation therapy therefore has no current standard role in the management of patients with colon cancer following curative resection, though it may have a role for patients with residual disease.

Recurrent or Advanced Disease

Treatment of patients with recurrent or advanced colon cancer depends on the location of the disease. For patients with locally recurrent and/or liver-only and/or lung-only metastatic disease, surgical resection, if feasible, is the only potentially curative treatment. Patients with unresectable disease are treated with systemic chemotherapy.

Chemotherapy trials in patients with locally advanced, unresectable, or metastatic disease, typically with 5-FU-based regimens, demonstrate partial responses and prolongation of the time-to-progression of disease,[48,49] as well as improved survival and quality of life for patients receiving chemotherapy, compared to best supportive care.[50-52] Several trials have analyzed the activity and toxic effects of various 5-FU-leucovorin regimens using different doses and administration schedules and showed essentially equivalent results with a median survival time in the 12-month range.[53] Subsequent studies incorporated irinotecan and oxaliplatin in the treatment of patients with advanced colorectal cancer. These new regimens have improved the response rate, time-to-tumor progression, and median survival of patients with advanced disease, with tolerable side effects. The median survival of these patients has improved from approximately 12 months in the mid 1990s to over 20 months in 2003.[38,39,54-56]

Irinotecan combined with 5-FU-leucovorin has demonstrated improved survival in patients with advanced or metastatic disease compared with 5-FU-leucovorin alone, albeit with increased, yet controllable, toxic effects.[34-37] Interim results from ongoing studies of oxaliplatin, alone or combined with 5-FU-leucovorin, may lead to further improvements in time-to-progression of disease and improved survival.[55,57-59] Continued participation in clinical trials is appropriate.

Currently several first-line and second-line chemotherapy regimens are available that can be used in patients with recurrent or advanced colorectal carcinoma.[36,38,39,50,54-56,60-65]

First-line chemotherapy treatment

With the lack of comparative head-to-head studies between many first-line and second-line regimens, the choice of one regimen versus another for first-line treatment depends on factors such as physician and patient preferences, comorbidities, and convenience, rather than efficacy parameters. In addition, the newer colorectal cancer chemotherapy schemas are serving as the platform on which combined novel targeted agents such as inhibitors of the epidermal growth factor receptor and vascular endothelial growth factor are based. Accepted first-line regimens are either irinotecan-based (IFL, FOLFIRI, AIO) or oxaliplatin-based (FOLFOX4, FOLFOX6).

Second-line chemotherapy treatment

Second-line regimens depend on which first-line regimens the patient already received. Patients who were treated with irinotecan-based regimens are commonly treated with a FOLFOX combination. Because of the lack of activity of single-agent oxaliplatin alone, use of this drug is recommended in combination with infusional 5-FU regardless of whether patients received infusional 5-FU as their first-line regimen.[65] Patients who had been treated with a FOLFOX-based regimen as part of their first-line regimen should receive irinotecan-based chemotherapy for second-line treatment. Treatment with irinotecan alone is reasonable in this situation because no data are available to support that the combination of irinotecan and 5-FU is superior to irinotecan alone in patients previously treated with 5-FU, and because irinotecan has single-agent activity in this setting.[36,38] The combination of irinotecan and infusional 5-FU, however, should be considered in patients who received bolus 5-FU as their first-line treatment considering the trend towards superior activity of infusional 5-FU as compared to bolus regimen.[54]

The designations in PDQ that treatments are "standard" or "under clinical evaluation" are not to be used as a basis for reimbursement determinations.

REFERENCES

1. Bokey EL, Moore JW, Chapuis PH, et al. Morbidity and mortality following laparoscopic-assisted right hemicolectomy for cancer. *Dis Colon Rectum*. 1996;39(10 Suppl):S24-28.
2. Franklin ME Jr, Rosenthal D, Abrego-Medina D, et al. Prospective comparison of open vs. laparoscopic colon surgery for carcinoma. Five-year results. *Dis Colon Rectum*. 1996;39(10 Suppl):S35-46.
3. Fleshman JW, Nelson H, Peters WR, et al. Early results of laparoscopic surgery for colorectal cancer. Retrospective analysis of 372 patients treated by Clinical Outcomes of Surgical Therapy (COST) Study Group. *Dis Colon Rectum*. 1996;39(10 Suppl):S53-58.
4. Schwenk W, Böhm B, Müller JM. Postoperative pain and fatigue after laparoscopic or conventional colorectal resections. A prospective randomized trial. *Surg Endosc*. 1998; 12(9): 1131-1136.
5. Nelson H, North Central Cancer Treatment Group. NCI HIGH PRIORITY CLINICAL TRIAL—Phase III Randomized Study of Laparoscopic-Assisted Colectomy Versus Open Colectomy for Colon Cancer, NCCTG-934653, Clinical trial, Closed.
6. Clinical Outcomes of Surgical Therapy Study Group. A comparison of laparoscopically assisted and open colectomy for colon cancer. *N Engl J Med*. 2004;350(20):2050-2059.
7. Weeks JC, Nelson H, Gelber S, et al. Short-term quality-of-life outcomes following laparoscopic-assisted colectomy vs open colectomy for colon cancer: a randomized trial. *JAMA*. 2002;287(3):321-328.
8. Lacy AM, García-Valdecasas JC, Delgado S, et al. Laparoscopy-assisted colectomy versus open colectomy for treatment of non-metastatic colon cancer: a randomised trial. *Lancet*. 2002;359(9325):2224-2229.
9. Esser S, Reilly WT, Riley LB, et al. The role of sentinel lymph node mapping in staging of colon and rectal cancer. *Dis Colon Rectum*. 2001;44(6):850-854; discussion 854-856.
10. Bilchik AJ, Nora DT, Sobin LH, et al. Effect of lymphatic mapping on the new tumor-node-metastasis classification for colorectal cancer. *J Clin Oncol*. 2003;21(4):668-672.
11. Panettiere FJ, Goodman PJ, Costanzi JJ, et al. Adjuvant therapy in large bowel adenocarcinoma: long-term results of a Southwest Oncology Group Study. *J Clin Oncol*. 1988; 6(6):947-954.
12. Adjuvant therapy of colon cancer—results of a prospectively randomized trial. Gastrointestinal Tumor Study Group. *N Engl J Med*.1984;310(12):737-743.
13. Higgins GA Jr, Amadeo JH, McElhinney J, et al. Efficacy of prolonged intermittent therapy with combined 5-fluorouracil and methyl-CCNU following resection for carcinoma of the large bowel. A Veterans Administration Surgical Oncology Group report. *Cancer*. 1984;53(1):1-8.
14. Buyse M, Zeleniuch-Jacquotte A, Chalmers TC. Adjuvant therapy of colorectal cancer. Why we still don't know. *JAMA*. 1988;259(24):3571-3578.
15. Laurie JA, Moertel CG, Fleming TR, et al. Surgical adjuvant therapy of large-bowel carcinoma: an evaluation of levamisole and the combination of levamisole and fluorouracil. The North Central Cancer Treatment Group and the Mayo Clinic. *J Clin Oncol*. 1989;7(10):1447-1456.

16. Moertel CG, Fleming TR, Macdonald JS, et al. Levamisole and fluorouracil for adjuvant therapy of resected colon carcinoma. *N Engl J Med.* 1990;322(6):352-358.

17. Wolmark N, Rockette H, Fisher B, et al. The benefit of leucovorin-modulated fluorouracil as postoperative adjuvant therapy for primary colon cancer: results from National Surgical Adjuvant Breast and Bowel Project protocol C-03. *J Clin Oncol.* 1993;11(10):1879-1887.

18. Efficacy of adjuvant fluorouracil and folinic acid in colon cancer. International Multicentre Pooled Analysis of Colon Cancer Trials (IMPACT) investigators. *Lancet.* 1995;345(8955):939-944.

19. O'Connell M, Mailliard J, Macdonald J, et al. An intergroup trial of intensive course 5FU and low dose leucovorin as surgical adjuvant therapy for high risk colon cancer. *Proceedings of the American Society of Clinical Oncology.* 1993;12:A-552,190.

20. Wolmark N, Bryant J, Smith R, et al. Adjuvant 5-fluorouracil and leucovorin with or without interferon alfa-2a in colon carcinoma: National Surgical Adjuvant Breast and Bowel Project protocol C-05. *J Natl Cancer Inst.* 1998; 90(23):1810-1816.

21. Wolmark N, Rockette H, Mamounas E, et al. Clinical trial to assess the relative efficacy of fluorouracil and leucovorin, fluorouracil and levamisole, and fluorouracil, leucovorin, and levamisole in patients with Dukes' B and C carcinoma of the colon: results from National Surgical Adjuvant Breast and Bowel Project C-04. *J Clin Oncol.* 1999;17(11):3553-3559.

22. Okuno SH, Woodhouse CL, Loprinzi CL, et al. Phase III placebo-controlled clinical trial evaluation of glutamine for decreasing mucositis in patients with 5FU (fluorouracil)-base chemotherapy. [Abstract] *Proceedings of the American Society of Clinical Oncology.* 17: A-256, 1998.

23. NIH consensus conference. Adjuvant therapy for patients with colon and rectal cancer. *JAMA.* 1990;264(11):1444-1450.

24. O'Connell MJ, Laurie JA, Kahn M, et al. Prospectively randomized trial of postoperative adjuvant chemotherapy in patients with high-risk colon cancer. *J Clin Oncol.* 1998;16(1):295-300.

25. Haller DG, Catalano PJ, Macdonald JS, et al. Fluorouracil (FU), leucovorin (LV) and levamisole (LEV) adjuvant therapy for colon cancer: five-year final report of INT-0089. [Abstract] *Proceedings of the American Society of Clinical Oncology.* 17:A-982, 256a, 1998.

26. Sargent DJ, Goldberg RM, Jacobson SD, et al. A pooled analysis of adjuvant chemotherapy for resected colon cancer in elderly patients. *N Engl J Med.* 2001;345(15):1091-1097.

27. Mamounas E, Wieand S, Wolmark N, et al. Comparative efficacy of adjuvant chemotherapy in patients with Dukes' B versus Dukes' C colon cancer: results from four National Surgical Adjuvant Breast and Bowel Project adjuvant studies (C-01, C-02, C-03, and C-04) *J Clin Oncol.* 1999; 17(5):1349-13455.

28. Moertel CG, Fleming TR, Macdonald JS, et al. Intergroup study of fluorouracil plus levamisole as adjuvant therapy for stage II/Dukes' B2 colon cancer. *J Clin Oncol.* 1995;13 (12): 2936-2943.

29. Efficacy of adjuvant fluorouracil and folinic acid in B2 colon cancer. International Multicentre Pooled Analysis of B2 Colon Cancer Trials (IMPACT B2) Investigators. *J Clin Oncol.* 1999;17(5):1356-1363.

30. Harrington DP. The tea leaves of small trials. *J Clin Oncol.* 1999;17(5):1336-1338.

31. Colaccio TA, Cancer and Leukemia Group B. Phase III Randomized Study of Adjuvant Edrecolomab Versus No Adjuvant Therapy After Resection in Patients With Stage II Adenocarcinoma of the Colon, CLB-9581, Clinical trial, Closed.

32. Pazdur R, National Surgical Adjuvant Breast and Bowel Project. Phase III Randomized Study of Oral Uracil/Tegafur (UFT) With Leucovorin vs Fluorouracil with Leucovorin Following Resection for Stage II/III Adenocarcinoma of the Colon (Summary Last Modified 05/1999), NSABP-C-06, Clinical trial, Closed.

33. Poplin EA, Southwest Oncology Group. Phase III Randomized Study of Bolus Fluorouracil and Leucovorin Calcium With Levamisole vs Continuous Infusion Fluorouracil with Levamisole as Adjuvant Therapy in Patients with High Risk Colon Cancer (Summary Last Modified 04/2000), SWOG-9415, Clinical trial, Closed.

34. Rothenberg ML, Eckardt JR, Kuhn JG, et al. Phase II of irinotecan in patients with progressive or rapidly recurrent colorectal cancer. *J Clin Oncol* 1996;14(4):1128-1135.

35. Conti JA, Kemeny NE, Saltz LB, et al. Irinotecan is an active agent in untreated patients with metastatic colorectal cancer. *J Clin Oncol.* 1996;14(3):709-715.

36. Rougier P, Van Cutsem E, Bajetta E, et al. Randomised trial of irinotecan versus fluorouracil by continuous infusion after fluorouracil failure in patients with metastatic colorectal cancer. *Lancet.* 1998;352(9138): 1407-1412.

37. Cunningham D, Pyrhönen S, James RD, et al. Randomised trial of irinotecan plus supportive care versus supportive care alone after fluorouracil failure for patients with metastatic colorectal cancer. *Lancet.* 1998;352(9138): 1413-1418.

38. Saltz LB, Cox JV, Blanke C, et al. Irinotecan plus fluorouracil and leucovorin for metastatic colorectal cancer. Irinotecan Study Group. *N Engl J Med.* 2000;343(13): 905-914.

39. Douillard JY, Cunningham D, Roth AD, et al. Irinotecan combined with fluorouracil compared with fluorouracil alone as first-line treatment for metastatic colorectal cancer: a multicentre randomised trial. *Lancet.* 2000;355 (9209):1041-1047.

40. De Gramont A, Banzi M, Navarro M, et al. Oxaliplatin/ 5-FU/LV in adjuvant colon cancer: results of the international randomized MOSAIC trial. [Abstract] Proceedings of the *American Society of Clinical Oncology.* 2003;22:A-1015.

41. Willett C, Tepper JE, Cohen A, et al. Local failure following curative resection of colonic adenocarcinoma. *Int J Radiat Oncol Biol Phys.* 1984;10(5):645-651.

42. Willett C, Tepper JE, Cohen A, et al. Obstructive and perforative colonic carcinoma: patterns of failure. *J Clin Oncol.* 1985;3(3):379-384.

43. Gunderson LL, Sosin H, Levitt S. Extrapelvic colonareas of failure in a reoperation series: implications for adjuvant therapy. *Int J Radiat Oncol Biol Phys.* 1985;11 (4):731-741.

44. Willett CG, Fung CY, Kaufman DS, et al. Postoperative radiation therapy for high-risk colon carcinoma. *J Clin Oncol.* 1993;11(6):1112-1117.

45. Willett CG, Goldberg S, Shellito PC, et al. Does postoperative irradiation play a role in the adjuvant therapy of stage T4 colon cancer? *Cancer J Sci Am.* 1999 Jul-Aug;5 (4): 242-247.

46. Schild SE, Gunderson LL, Haddock MG, et al. The treatment of locally advanced colon cancer. *Int J Radiat Oncol Biol Phys.* 1997;37(1):51-58.

47. Martenson J, Willett C, Sargent D, et al. Phase III study of adjuvant chemotherapy and radiation therapy compared with chemotherapy alone in the surgical adjuvant treatment of colon cancer: results of intergroup protocol 0130. *J Clin Oncol.* 2004;22:3277-3283.

48. Petrelli N, Herrera L, Rustum Y, et al. A prospective randomized trial of 5-fluorouracil versus 5-fluorouracil and high-dose leucovorin versus 5-fluorouracil and methotrexate in previously untreated patients with advanced colorectal carcinoma. *J Clin Oncol.* 1987;5(10):1559-1565.

49. Petrelli N, Douglass HO Jr, Herrera L, et al. The modulation of fluorouracil with leucovorin in metastatic colorectal carcinoma: a prospective randomized phase III trial. Gastrointestinal Tumor Study Group. *J Clin Oncol.* 1989; 7(10):1419-1426.

50. Scheithauer W, Rosen H, Kornek GV, et al. Randomised comparison of combination chemotherapy plus supportive care with supportive care alone in patients with metastatic colorectal cancer. *BMJ.* 1993;306(6880):752-755.

51. Expectancy or primary chemotherapy in patients with advanced asymptomatic colorectal cancer: a randomized trial. Nordic Gastrointestinal Tumor Adjuvant Therapy Group. *J Clin Oncol.* 1992;10(6):904-911.

52. Buyse M, Thirion P, Carlson RW, et al. Relation between tumour response to first-line chemotherapy and survival in advanced colorectal cancer: a meta-analysis. Meta-Analysis Group in Cancer. *Lancet.* 2000;356(9227):373-378.

53. Leichman CG, Fleming TR, Muggia FM, et al. Phase II study of fluorouracil and its modulation in advanced

colorectal cancer: a Southwest Oncology Group study. *J Clin Oncol.* 1995;13(6):1303-1311.

54. de Gramont A, Bosset JF, Milan C, et al. Randomized trial comparing monthly low-dose leucovorin and fluorouracil bolus with bimonthly high-dose leucovorin and fluorouracil bolus plus continuous infusion for advanced colorectal cancer: a French intergroup study. *J Clin Oncol.* 1997;15(2):808-815.

55. Giacchetti S, Perpoint B, Zidani R, et al. Phase III multicenter randomized trial of oxaliplatin added to chronomodulated fluorouracil-leucovorin as first-line treatment of metastatic colorectal cancer. *J Clin Oncol.* 2000;18(1): 136-147.

56. Goldberg RM, Sargent DJ, Morton RF, et al. A randomized controlled trial of fluorouracil plus leucovorin, irinotecan, and oxaliplatin combinations in patients with previously untreated metastatic colorectal cancer. *J Clin Oncol.* 2004;22(1):23-30.

57. de Gramont A, Vignoud J, Tournigand C, et al. Oxaliplatin with high-dose leucovorin and 5-fluorouracil 48-hour continuous infusion in pretreated metastatic colorectal cancer. *Eur J Cancer.* 1997;33(2):214-219.

58. Bleiberg H, de Gramont A. Oxaliplatin plus 5-fluorouracil: clinical experience in patients with advanced colorectal cancer. *Semin Oncol.* 1998;25(2 Suppl 5):32-39.

59. Cvitkovic E, Bekradda M. Oxaliplatin: a new therapeutic option in colorectal cancer. *Semin Oncol.* 1999;26(6):647-662.

60. Rougier P, Laplanche A, Huguier M, et al. Hepatic arterial infusion of floxuridine in patients with liver metastases from colorectal carcinoma: long-term results of a prospective randomized trial. *J Clin Oncol.* 1992;10 (7):1112-1118.

61. de Gramont A, Figer A, Seymour M, et al. Leucovorin and fluorouracil with or without oxaliplatin as first-line treatment in advanced colorectal cancer. *J Clin Oncol.* 2000;18 (16):2938-2947.

62. Cunningham D, Humblet Y, Siena S, et al. Cetuximab (C225) alone or in combination with irinotecan (CPT-11) in patients with epidermal growth factor receptor (EGFR)-positive, irinotecan-refractory metastatic colorectal cancer (MCRC). [Abstract] *Proceedings of the American Society of Clinical Oncology.* 22:A-1012, 252, 2003.

63. Hurwitz H, Fehrenbacher L, Cartwright T, et al. Bevacizumab (a monoclonal antibody to vascular endothelial growth factor) prolongs survival in first-line colorectal cancer (CRC): results of a phase III trial of bevacizumab in combination with bolus IFL (irinotecan, 5-fluorouracil, leucovorin) as first-line therapy in subjects with metastatic CRC. [Abstract] *Proceedings of the American Society of Clinical Oncology.* 22:A-3646, 2003.

64. Rothenberg ML, Oza AM, Burger B, et al. Final results of a phase III trial of 5-FU/leucovorin versus oxaliplatin versus the combination in patients with metastatic colorectal cancer following irinotecan, 5-FU, and leucovorin. [Abstract] *Proceedings of the American Society of Clinical Oncology.* 22:A-1011, 2003.

65. Rothenberg ML, Oza AM, Bigelow RH, et al. Superiority of oxaliplatin and fluorouracil-leucovorin compared with either therapy alone in patients with progressive colorectal cancer after irinotecan and fluorouracil-leucovorin: interim results of a phase III trial. *J Clin Oncol.* 2003;21 (11): 2059-2069.

STAGE 0 COLON CANCER

Stage 0 colon cancer is the most superficial of all the lesions and is limited to the mucosa without invasion of the lamina propria. Because of its superficial nature, the surgical procedure may be limited.

Treatment options:

- Local excision or simple polypectomy with clear margins.
- Colon resection for larger lesions not amenable to local excision.

STAGE I COLON CANCER

Stage I (Old Staging: Dukes' A or Modified Astler-Coller A and B1)

Because of its localized nature, stage I has a high cure rate.

Treatment options:

- Wide surgical resection and anastomosis. The role of laparoscopic techniques[1-4] in the treatment of colon cancer is under evaluation in a multicenter prospective randomized trial comparing laparoscopic-assisted colectomy (LAC) with open colectomy.[5] The quality-of-life component of this trial has been published and reported minimal short-term quality-of-life benefits with LAC.[6] [Level of evidence: 1iiC]

REFERENCES

1. Bokey EL, Moore JW, Chapuis PH, et al. Morbidity and mortality following laparoscopic-assisted right hemicolectomy for cancer. *Dis Colon Rectum.* 1996;39(10 Suppl):S24-28.

2. Franklin ME Jr, Rosenthal D, Abrego-Medina D, et al. Prospective comparison of open vs. laparoscopic colon surgery for carcinoma. Five-year results. *Dis Colon Rectum.* 1996;39(10 Suppl):S35-46.

3. Fleshman JW, Nelson H, Peters WR, et al. Early results of laparoscopic surgery for colorectal cancer. Retrospective analysis of 372 patients treated by Clinical Outcomes of Surgical Therapy (COST) Study Group. *Dis Colon Rectum.* 1996;39(10 Suppl):S53-58.

4. Schwenk W, Böhm B, Müller JM. Postoperative pain and fatigue following laparoscopic or conventional colorectal resections. A prospective randomized trial. *Surg Endosc.* 1998; 12(9): 1131-1136.

5. Nelson H, North Central Cancer Treatment Group. NCI HIGH PRIORITY CLINICAL TRIAL—Phase III Randomized Study of Laparoscopic-Assisted Colectomy Versus Open Colectomy for Colon Cancer, NCCTG-934653, Clinical trial, Closed.

6. Weeks JC, Nelson H, Gelber S, et al. Short-term quality-of-life outcomes following laparoscopic-assisted colectomy vs open colectomy for colon cancer: a randomized trial. *JAMA.* 2002;287 (3): 321-328.

STAGE II COLON CANCER

Stage II (Old Staging: Dukes' B or Modified Astler-Coller B2 and B3)

Treatment options:

1. Wide surgical resection and anastomosis. The role of laparoscopic techniques[1-4] in the treatment of colon cancer is under evaluation in a multicenter prospective randomized trial comparing laparoscopic-assisted colectomy (LAC) to open colectomy.[5] The quality-of-life component of this trial has been published and reported minimal short-term quality-of-life benefits with LAC.[4] [Level of evidence: 1iiC]

2. Following surgery, patients should be considered for entry into carefully controlled clinical trials evaluating the use of systemic or regional chemotherapy, or biologic therapy.[6,7] Information about ongoing clinical trials is available from the NCI website. Adjuvant therapy is not indicated for most patients unless they are entered into a clinical trial.

Adjuvant therapy

The potential value of adjuvant therapy for patients with stage II (Dukes' B or MAC B2 or B3) colon cancer also remains controversial. Although subgroups of patients with stage II colon cancer may be at higher-than-average risk for recurrence (including those with anatomic features such as tumor adherence to adjacent structures, perforation, complete obstruction, or with biologic characteristics such as aneuploidy, high S-phase analysis, or deletion of 18q),[8-10] evidence is inconsistent that adjuvant 5-fluorouracil (5-FU)-based chemotherapy is associated with an overall improved survival compared to surgery alone.[11] Investigators from the National Surgical Adjuvant Breast and Bowel Project have indicated that the reduction in risk of recurrence by adjuvant therapy in patients with stage II disease is of similar magnitude to the benefit seen in patients with stage III disease treated with adjuvant therapy, though an overall survival advantage has not been established.[12] A randomized trial of postoperative fluorouracil plus levamisole compared to surgery alone showed no survival advantage to postoperative adjuvant chemotherapy.[11] A meta-analysis of 1,000 stage II patients, whose experience was amalgamated from a series of trials, indicates a 2% advantage in disease-free survival at five years when adjuvant therapy-treated patients treated with 5-FU-leucovorin are compared to untreated controls.[13] [Level of evidence: 1iiDi][14] Patients with stage II colon cancer remain candidates for clinical trials in which either surgery alone or 5-FU-leucovorin represent standard therapy.[15-17]

Improved outcomes with postoperative radiation therapy have been suggested in single-institution retrospective reviews for certain high-risk subsets of colon cancer patients (T3 or T4, tumor location in immobile sites, local perforation, obstruction, and residual disease postresection).[18-23] A phase III randomized Intergroup trial designed to test the benefit of adding radiation therapy to surgery and chemotherapy with 5-FU-levamisole for selected high-risk colon cancer patients (T4; or T3, N1-N2 ascending/descending colon) was closed early secondary to inadequate patient accrual,[24] and preliminary analysis of 222 enrolled patients (the original goal was 700 patients) demonstrated no relapse or overall survival benefit for the group receiving radiation therapy.

REFERENCES

1. Bokey EL, Moore JW, Chapuis PH, et al. Morbidity and mortality following laparoscopic-assisted right hemicolectomy for cancer. *Dis Colon Rectum.* 1996;39(10 Suppl): S24-28.
2. Franklin ME Jr, Rosenthal D, Abrego-Medina D, et al. Prospective comparison of open vs. laparoscopic colon surgery for carcinoma. Five-year results. *Dis Colon Rectum.* 1996;39(10 Suppl):S35-46.
3. Fleshman JW, Nelson H, Peters WR, et al. Early results of laparoscopic surgery for colorectal cancer. Retrospective analysis of 372 patients treated by Clinical Outcomes of Surgical Therapy (COST) Study Group. *Dis Colon Rectum.* 1996;39(10 Suppl):S53-58.
4. Weeks JC, Nelson H, Gelber S, et al. Short-term quality-of-life outcomes following laparoscopic-assisted colectomy vs open colectomy for colon cancer: a randomized trial. *JAMA.* 2002;287(3):321-328.
5. Nelson H, North Central Cancer Treatment Group. NCI HIGH PRIORITY CLINICAL TRIAL—Phase III Randomized Study of Laparoscopic-Assisted Colectomy Versus Open Colectomy for Colon Cancer, NCCTG-934653, Clinical trial, Closed.
6. Focan CNJ, Groupe Regional d'Etudes du Cancer Colorectal—Belgium. Phase III Randomized Study of Adjuvant Chronomodulated Versus Standard Schedule Fluorouracil and Leucovorin Calcium With or Without Carboplatin in Patients With Completely Resected Stage IIB or III Colon Cancer, GRECCR-03, Clinical trial, Active.
7. Williams N, National Cancer Research Institute. Phase III Randomized Study of Adjuvant Chemotherapy With L-leucovorin and Fluorouracil Versus Observation in Patients With Resected Colorectal Cancer, NCRI-QUASAR1, Clinical trial, Active.
8. Lanza G, Matteuzzi M, Gafá R, et al. Chromosome 18q allelic loss and prognosis in stage II and III colon cancer. *Int J Cancer.* 1998;79(4):390-395.
9. Jen J, Kim H, Piantadosi S, et al. Allelic loss of chromosome 18q and prognosis in colorectal cancer. *N Engl J Med.* 331. 1994;331:213-221.
10. Merkel S, Wein A, Günther K, et al. High-risk groups of patients with Stage II colon carcinoma. *Cancer.* 2001;92 (6):1435-1443.
11. Moertel CG, Fleming TR, Macdonald JS, et al. Intergroup study of fluorouracil plus levamisole as adjuvant therapy for stage II/Dukes' B2 colon cancer. *J Clin Oncol.* 1995;13 (12):2936-2943.
12. Mamounas E, Wieand S, Wolmark N, et al. Comparative efficacy of adjuvant chemotherapy in patients with Dukes' B versus Dukes' C colon cancer: results from four National Surgical Adjuvant Breast and Bowel Project adjuvant studies (C-01, C-02, C-03, and C-04) *J Clin Oncol.* 1999; 17(5):1349-1355.
13. Efficacy of adjuvant fluorouracil and folinic acid in B2 colon cancer. International Multicentre Pooled Analysis of B2 Colon Cancer Trials (IMPACT B2) Investigators. *J Clin Oncol.* 1999;17(5):1356-1363.
14. Harrington DP. The tea leaves of small trials. *J Clin Oncol.* 1999;17(5):1336-1338.
15. Colacchio TA, Cancer and Leukemia Group B. Phase III Randomized Study of Adjuvant Edrecolomab Versus No Adjuvant Therapy After Resection in Patients With Stage II Adenocarcinoma of the Colon, CLB-9581, Clinical trial, Closed.
16. Pazdur R, National Surgical Adjuvant Breast and Bowel Project: Phase III Randomized Study of Oral Uracil/ Tegafur (UFT) With Leucovorin vs Fluorouracil with Leucovorin Following Resection for Stage II/III Adenocarcinoma of the Colon (Summary Last Modified

05/1999), NSABP-C-06, Clinical trial, Closed.
17. Poplin EA, Southwest Oncology Group: Phase III Randomized Study of Bolus Fluorouracil and Leucovorin Calcium with Levamisole vs Continuous Infusion Fluorouracil with Levamisole as Adjuvant Therapy in Patients with High Risk Colon Cancer (Summary Last Modified 04/2000), SWOG-9415, Clinical trial, Closed.
18. Willett C, Tepper JE, Cohen A, et al. Local failure following curative resection of colonic adenocarcinoma. *Int J Radiat Oncol Biol Phys.* 1984;10(5):645-651.
19. Willett C, Tepper JE, Cohen A, et al. Obstructive and perforative colonic carcinoma: patterns of failure. *J Clin Oncol.* 1985;3(3):379-384.
20. Gunderson LL, Sosin H, Levitt S. Extrapelvic colon—areas of failure in a reoperation series: implications for adjuvant therapy. *Int J Radiat Oncol Biol Phys.* 1985;11 (4):731-741.
21. Willett CG, Fung CY, Kaufman DS, et al. Postoperative radiation therapy for high-risk colon carcinoma. *J Clin Oncol.* 1993;11(6):1112-1117.
22. Willett CG, Goldberg S, Shellito PC, et al. Does postoperative irradiation play a role in the adjuvant therapy of stage T4 colon cancer? *Cancer J Sci Am.* 1999;5(4):242-247.
23. Schild SE, Gunderson LL, Haddock MG, et al. The treatment of locally advanced colon cancer. *Int J Radiat Oncol Biol Phys.* 1997;37(1):51-58.
24. Martenson J, Willett C, Sargent D, et al. Phase III study of adjuvant chemotherapy and radiation therapy compared with chemotherapy alone in the surgical adjuvant treatment of colon cancer: results of intergroup protocol 0130. *J Clin Oncol.* 2004;22:3277-3283.

STAGE III COLON CANCER

Note: Some citations in the text of this section are followed by a level of evidence. The PDQ editorial boards use a formal ranking system to help the reader judge the strength of evidence linked to the reported results of a therapeutic strategy. (Refer to the PDQ summary on *Levels of Evidence* for more information.)

Stage III (Old Staging: Dukes' C or Modified Astler-Coller C1-C3)

Stage III colon cancer denotes lymph node involvement. Studies have indicated that the number of lymph nodes involved affects prognosis; patients with one to three involved nodes have a significantly better survival than those with four or more involved nodes.

Treatment options:

1. Wide surgical resection and anastomosis.

The role of laparoscopic techniques [14] in the treatment of colon cancer is under evaluation in a multicenter prospective randomized trial comparing laparoscopic-assisted colectomy (LAC) with open colectomy.[5] The quality-of-life component of this trial has been published and reported minimal short-term quality-of-life benefits with LAC.[6] [Level of evidence: 1iiC]

For patients who are not candidates for clinical trials, postoperative chemotherapy with fluorouracil (5-FU)-leucovorin for six months. Based on preliminary results from the MOSAIC trial presented at the American Society of Clinical Oncology meeting in 2003, adjuvant FOLFOX4 (oxaliplatin, leucovorin, 5-FU) demonstrated prolonged three-year survival but did not demonstrate an overall survival advantage.[7]

2. Eligible patients should be considered for entry into carefully controlled clinical trials comparing various postoperative chemotherapy regimens that are now also including oxaliplatin-based and irinotecan-based chemotherapy with new targeted agents, postoperative radiation therapy, or biological therapy, alone or in combination.[8,9] Information about ongoing clinical trials is available from the NCI website.[12]

Adjuvant therapy

Improved outcomes with postoperative radiation therapy have been suggested in single-institution retrospective reviews for certain high-risk subsets of colon cancer patients (T3 or T4, tumor location in immobile sites, local perforation, obstruction,

and residual disease postresection).[10-15] A phase III randomized Intergroup trial designed to test the benefit of adding radiation therapy to surgery and 5-FU-levamisole chemotherapy for selected high-risk colon cancer patients (T4; or T3, N1-N2 ascending/descending colon)[16] was closed early secondary to inadequate patient accrual, and preliminary analysis of 222 patients demonstrated no relapse or overall survival benefit for the group receiving radiation therapy. (Refer to the discussion of adjuvant therapy in the *Treatment Option Overview* section of this summary.)

In the late 1980s, a passive immunotherapy approach to adjuvant treatment of stage III colorectal cancer demonstrated encouraging results in a single randomized trial.[17] This trial compared postoperative administration of a murine monoclonal antibody to 17-1A antigen (MOAB 17-1A), a cell surface glycoprotein of uncertain function expressed on both normal and malignant epithelial cells, to surgery alone. Treated patients appeared to have a survival benefit comparable to that seen in adjuvant chemotherapy trials, with a relative reduction in mortality of 32% (95% confidence interval [CI], 8-51).[17] [Level of evidence: 1iiA] The small size of this trial, however, was associated with a wide CI for the observed benefit and the result remains to be confirmed. Other adjuvant immunotherapeutic approaches, including autologous tumor vaccines,[18] are also under clinical evaluation.

REFERENCES

1. Bokey EL, Moore JW, Chapuis PH, et al. Morbidity and mortality following laparoscopic-assisted right hemicolectomy for cancer. *Dis Colon Rectum.* 1996;39(10 Suppl): S24-28.
2. Franklin ME Jr, Rosenthal D, Abrego-Medina D, et al.

Prospective comparison of open vs. laparoscopic colon surgery for carcinoma. Five-year results. *Dis Colon Rectum.* 1996;39(10 Suppl):S35-46.

3. Fleshman JW, Nelson H, Peters WR, et al. Early results of laparoscopic surgery for colorectal cancer. Retrospective analysis of 372 patients treated by Clinical Outcomes of Surgical Therapy (COST) Study Group. *Dis Colon Rectum.* 1996;39(10 Suppl):S53-58.

4. Schwenk W, Böhm B, Müller JM. Postoperative pain and fatigue after laparoscopic or conventional colorectal resections. A prospective randomized trial. *Surg Endosc.* 1998; 12(9):1131-1136.

5. Nelson H, North Central Cancer Treatment Group: NCI HIGH PRIORITY CLINICAL TRIAL—Phase III Randomized Study of Laparoscopic-Assisted Colectomy Versus Open Colectomy for Colon Cancer, NCCTG-934653, Clinical trial, Closed.

6. Weeks JC, Nelson H, Gelber S, et al. Short-term quality-of-life outcomes following laparoscopic-assisted colectomy vs open colectomy for colon cancer: a randomized trial. *JAMA.* 2002;287(3):321-328.

7. De Gramont A, Banzi M, Navarro M, et al. Oxaliplatin/5-FU/LV in adjuvant colon cancer: results of the international randomized MOSAIC trial. [Abstract] *Proceedings of the American Society of Clinical Oncology.* 2003;22: A-1015.

8. Pazdur R, GlaxoSmithKline: Phase III Randomized Study of Adjuvant MOAB 17-1A plus 5-FU-Based Chemotherapy vs. 5-FU-Based Chemotherapy Alone for Surgically Resected Stage III Adenocarcinoma of the Colon (Summary Last Modified 08/1999), GW-157-001, Clinical trial, Closed.

9. Rougier P, Nordlinger B. Large scale trial for adjuvant treatment in high risk resected colorectal cancers. Rationale to test the combination of loco-regional and systemic chemotherapy and to compare l-leucovorin + 5-FU to levamisole + 5-FU. *Ann Oncol.* 1993;4(Suppl 2):21-28.

10. Willett C, Tepper JE, Cohen A, et al. Local failure following curative resection of colonic adenocarcinoma. *Int J Radiat Oncol Biol Phys.* 1984;10(5):645-651.

11. Willett C, Tepper JE, Cohen A, et al. Obstructive and perforative colonic carcinoma: patterns of failure. *J Clin Oncol.* 1985;3(3):379-384.

12. Gunderson LL, Sosin H, Levitt S. Extrapelvic colon—areas of failure in a reoperation series: implications for adjuvant therapy. *Int J Radiat Oncol Biol Phys.* 1985; 11(4):731-741.

13. Willett CG, Fung CY, Kaufman DS, et al. Postoperative radiation therapy for high-risk colon carcinoma. *J Clin Oncol.* 1993;11(6):1112-1117.

14. Willett CG, Goldberg S, Shellito PC, et al. Does postoperative irradiation play a role in the adjuvant therapy of stage T4 colon cancer? *Cancer J Sci Am.* 1999;5(4):242-247.

15. Schild SE, Gunderson LL, Haddock MG, et al. The treatment of locally advanced colon cancer. *Int J Radiat Oncol Biol Phys.* 1997;37(1):51-58.

16. Martenson J, Willett C, Sargent D, et al. Phase III study of adjuvant chemotherapy and radiation therapy compared with chemotherapy alone in the surgical adjuvant treatment of colon cancer: results of intergroup protocol 0130. *J Clin Oncol.* 2004;22:3277-3283.

17. Riethmüller G, Holz E, Schlimok G, et al. Monoclonal antibody therapy for resected Dukes' C colorectal cancer: seven-year outcome of a multicenter randomized trial. *J Clin Oncol.* 1998;16(5):1788-1794.

18. Benson AB, Eastern Cooperative Oncology Group: Phase III Comparison of Adjuvant 5-FU/LEV vs. 5-FU/LEV plus Autologous Tumor Cell Vaccination in Patients with Potentially Curatively Resected Stage C1-3 Adenocarcinoma of the Colon (Summary Last Modified 11/94), E-1290, Clinical trial, Closed.

STAGE IV AND RECURRENT COLON CANCER

Note: Some citations in the text of this section are followed by a level of evidence. The PDQ editorial boards use a formal ranking system to help the reader judge the strength of evidence linked to the reported results of a therapeutic strategy. (Refer to the PDQ summary on *Levels of Evidence* for more information.)

Stage IV (Old Staging: Modified Astler-Coller D) and Recurrent Colon Cancer

Stage IV colon cancer denotes distant metastatic disease. Treatment of recurrent colon cancer depends on the sites of recurrent disease demonstrable by physical examination and/or radiographic studies. In addition to standard radiographic procedures, radioimmunoscintography may add clinical information which may affect management.[1] Such approaches, however, have not led to improvements in long-term outcome measures such as survival.

Treatment options:

1. Surgical resection of locally recurrent cancer.

2. Surgical resection/anastomosis or bypass of obstructing or bleeding primary lesions in selected metastatic cases.

3. Resection of liver metastases in selected metastatic patients (five-year cure rate for resection of solitary or combination metastases exceeds 20%) or ablation in selected patients.[2-11]

4. Resection of isolated pulmonary or ovarian metastases in selected patients.[12]

5. Palliative radiation therapy.

6. Palliative chemotherapy.

7. Clinical trials evaluating new drugs and biological therapy.

8. Clinical trials comparing various

chemotherapy regimens or biological therapy, alone or in combination.

Locally Recurrent Colon Cancer

Locally recurrent colon cancer, such as a suture line recurrence, may be resectable.

Liver Metastasis

Approximately 50% of colon cancer patients will be diagnosed with hepatic metastases, either at the time of initial presentation or as a result of disease recurrence. Although only a small proportion of patients with hepatic metastases are candidates for surgical resection, advances in tumor ablation techniques and in both regional and systemic chemotherapy administration provide for a number of treatment options.

For patients with hepatic metastasis considered to be resectable (based on limited number of lesions, intrahepatic locations of lesions, lack of major vascular involvement, absent or limited extrahepatic disease, and sufficient functional hepatic reserve), a negative margin resection has resulted in five-year survival rates of 25% to 40% in mostly nonrandomized studies.[5,7,13-16] Improved surgical techniques and advances in preoperative imaging have allowed for better patient selection for resection.

For patients with hepatic metastases deemed unresectable, radiofrequency ablation has emerged as a safe technique (2% major morbidity, and <1% mortality rate) that may provide for long-term tumor control.[17-22] Radiofrequency ablation and cryosurgical ablation[24-26] remain options for patients with tumors that can not be resected.

Other local ablative techniques that have been used to manage liver metastases include embolization and interstitial radiation therapy.[27,28] Patients with limited pulmonary metastases, and patients with both pulmonary and hepatic metastases, may also be considered for surgical resection, with five-year survival possible in highly-selected patients.[12,29,30]

The role of adjuvant chemotherapy after potentially curative resection of liver metastases is uncertain. A trial of hepatic arterial floxuridine plus systemic fluorouracil (5-FU) plus leucovorin was shown to result in improved two-year disease-free and overall survival (86% vs. 72%, P=.03), but did not show a significant statistical difference in median survival, compared with systemic 5-FU therapy alone.[31] [Level of evidence: 1iiA] A second trial preoperatively randomized 109 patients who had one to three potentially resectable colorectal hepatic metastases to either no further therapy or postoperative hepatic arterial floxuridine plus systemic 5-FU.[32] Of those randomized, 27% were deemed ineligible at the time of surgery, leaving only 75 patients evaluable for recurrence and survival. While liver recurrence was decreased, median or four-year survival was not significantly different. Further studies are required to evaluate this treatment approach and to determine if more effective systemic combination chemotherapy alone may provide similar results compared with hepatic intra-arterial therapy plus systemic treatment.

Hepatic intra-arterial chemotherapy with floxuridine for liver metastases has produced higher overall response rates but no consistent improvement in survival when compared with systemic chemotherapy.[2,33-37] Controversy regarding the efficacy of regional chemotherapy has led to initiation of a large multicenter phase III trial (CLB-9481) of hepatic arterial infusion versus systemic chemotherapy. The use of the combination of intra-arterial chemotherapy with hepatic irradiation, especially employing focal radiation of metastatic lesions, is under evaluation.[38] Several studies show increased local toxic effects with hepatic infusional therapy, including liver function abnormalities and fatal biliary sclerosis.

Other drug combinations described in this section:

- AIO regimen (folic acid, 5-FU, irinotecan):

  Irinotecan (100 mg/m^2) as a 2-hour infusion day 1; leucovorin (500 mg/m^2) as a 2-hour infusion day 1; followed by 5-FU (2,000 mg/m^2) intravenous (IV) bolus via ambulatory pump over 24 hours weekly x 4 every 52 weeks.

- Douillard regimen (folic acid, 5-FU, irinotecan):

  Irinotecan (180 mg/m^2) as a 2-hour infusion day 1; leucovorin (200 mg/m^2) as a 2-hour infusion days 1 and 2; followed by a loading dose of 5-FU (400 mg/m^2) IV bolus, then 5-FU (600 mg/m^2) via ambulatory pump over 22 hours days 1 and 2 every two weeks.

- FOLFOX4 regimen (oxaliplatin, leucovorin, 5-FU):

  Oxaliplatin (85 mg/m^2) as a 2-hour infusion day 1; leucovorin (200 mg/m^2) as a 2-hour infusion days 1 and 2; followed by a loading dose of 5-FU (400 mg/m^2) IV bolus, then 5-FU (600 mg/m^2) via ambulatory pump over 22 hours days 1 and 2 every two weeks.

- FOLFOX6 regimen (oxaliplatin, leucovorin, 5-FU):

  Oxaliplatin (85-100 mg/m^2) as a 2-hour infusion day 1; leucovorin (400 mg/m^2) as a 2-hour infusion day 1; followed by a loading dose of 5-FU (400 mg/m^2) IV bolus on day 1, then 5-FU (2,400-3,000 mg/m^2) via ambulatory pump over 46 hours every two weeks.

- FOLFIRI regimen (folic acid, 5-FU, irinotecan):

  Irinotecan (180 mg/m^2) as a 2-hour infusion day 1; leucovorin (400 mg/m^2) as a 2-hour infusion day 1; followed by a loading dose of 5-FU (400 mg/m^2) IV bolus on day 1, then 5-FU (2,400-3,000 mg/m^2) via ambulatory pump over 46 hours every two weeks.

- IFL (or Saltz) regimen (irinotecan, 5-FU, leucovorin):

  Irinotecan (125 mg/m^2), 5-FU (500 mg/m^2) IV bolus, and leucovorin (20 mg/m^2) IV bolus weekly for four out of six weeks.

First-line chemotherapy treatment

In stage IV and recurrent colon cancer, chemotherapy has been used for palliation. Combinations of 5-FU and leucovorin with irinotecan (FOLFIRI, AIO, IFL) or oxaliplatin (FOLFOX4, FOLFOX6) are considered to be standard.

A randomized study of first-line treatment for advanced colorectal cancers compared IFL to 5-FU (425 mg/m^2 daily times five days) administered with leucovorin (20 mg/m^2 daily times five days consecutively every four weeks).[39] The IFL regimen demonstrated significantly longer progression-free survival (7.9 vs. 4.3 months, P=.004), a higher response rate (39% vs. 21%,

P<.001), and prolonged overall survival (median 14.8 months vs. 12.6 months, *P*=.04).

Another trial compared irinotecan, using the Douillard or AIO regimen, with infusional 5-FU and leucovorin using the same schedule. The patients receiving the irinotecan-based IFL treatment demonstrated significantly longer time to progression (median 6.7 months vs. 4.4 months, *P*<.001), a higher response rate, and a higher overall survival (median 17.4 vs. 14.1 months, *P*=.031). On the basis of these randomized trials, these three regimens are licensed for use in the United States as first-line therapy.

The toxic effects of the IFL regimen became a matter of some concern in 2001 when two randomized National Cancer Institute-sponsored trials, one in advanced-stage disease and one in the adjuvant setting for stage III colon cancer, each demonstrated a higher 60-day death rate in the IFL arms.[40] Subsequent analyses suggested that such toxic effects may be characteristic of regimens based on bolus 5-FU, whether or not they incorporate irinotecan. Nonetheless, the issue of toxic effects with bolus IFL has necessitated careful consideration of patient eligibility for this approach, balancing the trade-offs inherent in this type of combination chemotherapy, and close patient follow-up and management of early signs of side effects.

First-line chemotherapy studies also tested the combinations of oxaliplatin with 5-FU and leucovorin in patients with advanced colorectal cancer. One study compared the FOL-FOX4 regimen to the same regimen of infusional 5-FU and leucovorin without oxaliplatin in patients with advanced colorectal cancer. Patients treated with FOLFOX4 had a signifi-

cantly longer progression-free survival (nine months vs. 6.2 months) and response rate (50.7% vs 22.3%), but no improvement in overall survival.[40] Similar results were observed in a second randomized trial using a chronomodulated schedule.[42] Based on these results, the FOLFOX4 regimen was approved for first-line treatment of patients with advanced colorectal cancer in Europe and other countries.

The next generation of studies compared irinotecan-based and oxaliplatin-based chemotherapy in patients with newly diagnosed advanced colorectal cancer. The V308 study conducted by the GERCOR group compared FOLFOX6 with FOLFIRI in patients with advanced colorectal cancer.[43] In this study, patients were crossed-over from one regimen to the other at the time of progression. These two first-line treatments for metastatic and advanced colorectal cancer have demonstrated similar response rates and acceptable toxic effects profiles with no differences in median time-to-first progression (eight months vs. 8.5 months) or overall survival (20.6 months vs. 21.5 months) for FOLFOX6 followed by FOLFIRI regimen versus FOLFIRI followed by FOL-FOX regimen, respectively.

The U.S. Cooperative Groups completed a randomized intergroup clinical trial sponsored by NCI for the initial treatment of advanced colorectal cancer.[44] This trial was originally launched to compare the IFL regimen, the FOLFOX4 regimen, and several other regimens to the previous standard Mayo five-day bolus 5-FU/leucovorin regimen. When the randomized data became available demonstrating superiority of IFL over the Mayo regimen[39] and IFL was approved, the intergroup study (N9741) was modified to a three-arm trial with the Mayo regimen dropped (along with several other arms) and IFL became the standard arm. The FOLFOX4 regimen and a combination of oxaliplatin and irinotecan were compared in this study.[45]

A planned interim analysis of N9741 was performed in April 2002 and pre-specified stopping boundaries were crossed in the comparison between IFL and FOLFOX (but not in comparisons involving the oxaliplatin-irinotecan arm). A total of 795 patients were randomized among the different study arms. With a median follow-up of 20.4 months, all outcome measures for patients receiving FOLFOX4 were significantly better than for those receiving the standard IFL regimen, including a significantly better time-to-tumor progression for FOLFOX4 compared to IFL (8.7 months vs. 6.9 months; $P=.0014$), higher response rates (45% vs. 31%; $P=.002$), and improved overall survival (19.5 months vs. 15 months; $P=.0001$). Patients treated with irinotecan and oxaliplatin (IROX) had a significantly lower median time-to-progression (6.5 months) and response rate (35%) compared to FOLFOX4 ($P=.001$ and $P=.03$, respectively); median survival, however, did not differ significantly between the two regimens (19.5 months vs. 17.4 months, $P=.09$).[46]

The results of this study establish the FOLFOX4 regimen as a first-line treatment option in advanced colorectal cancer that is at least as effective, and perhaps more so, than others available. The N9741 study, however, cannot be considered definitive because of asymmetry in availability of potentially effective second-line therapy for patients on this trial. Whereas most patients who did not respond or stopped responding to FOLFOX4 would have access to irinotecan alone or in combination (and about 50% did receive it), oxaliplatin was not commercially available in the United States at that time, so only a minority of patients coming off the IFL arm because of progression received this agent. This means that the difference in overall survival observed in N9741 may have been somewhat magnified by differential access to effective second-line treatment. The progression-free survival, response rates, and toxic-effects outcomes also favored the FOLFOX4 regimen, however, and these would not have been affected by this issue of second-line treatment.

Based on these data, recommended first-line regimens for patients with advanced colorectal cancer include FOLFOX4, FOLFOX6, FOLFIRI, Douillard, AIO, and Avastin.

Second-line chemotherapy treatment

Treatment of patients who progress after first-line chemotherapy is guided by which treatment was used for first-line treatment. Patients who were treated with a FOLFOX-based regimen should be treated with an irinotecan-based regimen and patients who already received an irinotecan-based regimen should be treated with a FOLFOX-based regimen.

The data from the GERCOR V308 study showed a 15% response rate and 4.5 months median progression-free survival in patients who progress to FOLFIRI chemotherapy when treated with FOLFOX, and a 4% response rate and 2.5 months median progression-free survival for the reverse sequence.[43] Treatment with FOLFOX was found superior in response rate (9.6%) to oxaliplatin (1.1%) and 5-FU-leucovorin (0.7%) alone in the EFC4584 phase III study.[47] Mature data from this study, however, failed to show a statistically significant improvement in median survival (9.8, 8.1, and 8.7 months, respectively, $P=.07$). Toxic effects, particularly neutropenia and neuropathy were higher in the FOLFOX arm.[48] Whether these results applied to patients who have received first-line irinotecan-based chemotherapy, which has been a common situation, is not known.

For patients who are clinically unlikely to tolerate aggressive combination chemotherapy, or who have unacceptable pre-existing comorbid disease, an infusional single-agent 5-FU-based regimen without either oxaliplatin or irinotecan remains a reasonable treatment option.[49] A phase III trial (GERCOR C96.1) demonstrated that infusional 5-FU-leucovorin administered on the same schedule as that used in the Douillard regimen was less toxic and more active in terms of response rate and progression-free survival than low-dose bolus daily times five days 5-FU-leucovorin in patients with advanced or metastatic colorectal cancer.[50]

New Therapies and Combinations

At the American Society of Clinical Oncology 2003 meeting, the results of two randomized trials incorporating novel therapies in patients with colorectal cancer were presented. The results of a randomized trial were presented that compared IFL-placebo with IFL-bevacizumab, a monoclonal antibody, against the vascular endothelial growth factor receptor in 925 patients with advanced colorectal cancer. Bevacizumab was administered at a dose of 5 mg/kg every other week. The median progression-free survival of patients treated with IFL plus bevacizumab was 10.6, versus 6.2 months ($P=.00001$) for patients treated with IFL and placebo, and the median overall survival was 20.3 versus 15.6 months ($P=.00003$), respectively. Overall response rates were also superior for the bevacizumab-containing regimen (44.9 vs. 34.7%, $P=.029$). Patients treated with bevacizumab and IFL had a higher overall incidence of grade 3 to 4 toxic effects (85% vs. 74%, $P<.01$).[51]

The second study compared cetuximab, a monoclonal antibody, against epidermal growth factor receptor, alone or in combination with irinotecan in 329 patients with irinotecan-refractory colorectal cancer. Patients treated with the combination regimen had a significantly higher response rate of 22.9% compared to 10.8% for patients treated with cetuximab alone ($P=.0074$) and a longer time to treatment failure (4.1 months vs. 1.5 months, $P<.0001$), but no significant improvement was observed in median survival between arms.[52]

REFERENCES

1. Serafini AN, Klein JL, Wolff BG, et al. Radio-immunoscintigraphy of recurrent, metastatic, or occult colorectal cancer with technetium 99m-labeled totally human monoclonal antibody 88BV59: results of pivotal, phase III multicenter studies. *J Clin Oncol.* 1998;16(5):1777-1787.
2. Wagman LD, Kemeny MM, Leong L, et al. A prospective, randomized evaluation of the treatment of colorectal cancer metastatic to the liver. *J Clin Oncol.* 1990;8(11):1885-1893.
3. Scheele J, Stangl R, Altendorf-Hofmann A. Hepatic metastases from colorectal carcinoma: impact of surgical resection on the natural history. *Br J Surg.* 1990;77(11):1241-1246.
4. Scheele J, Stangl R, Altendorf-Hofmann A, et al. Indicators of prognosis after hepatic resection for colorectal secondaries. *Surgery.* 1991;110(1):13-29.
5. Adson MA, van Heerden JA, Adson MH, et al. Resection of hepatic metastases from colorectal cancer. *Arch Surg.* 1984;119(6):647-651.
6. Coppa GF, Eng K, Ranson JH, et al. Hepatic resection for metastatic colon and rectal cancer. An evaluation of preoperative and postoperative factors. *Ann Surg.* 1985;202(2):203-208.
7. Gayowski TJ, Iwatsuki S, Madariaga JR, et al. Experience in hepatic resection for metastatic colorectal cancer: analysis of clinical and pathologic risk factors. *Surgery.* 1994;116(4):703-710; discussion 710-711.
8. Fernández-Trigo V, Shamsa F, Sugarbaker PH. Repeat liver resections from colorectal metastasis. Repeat Hepatic Metastases Registry. *Surgery.* 1995;117(3):296-304.
9. Jaeck D, Bachellier P, Guiguet M, et al. Long-term sur-

vival following resection of colorectal hepatic metastases. Association Française de Chirurgie. *Br J Surg.* 1997;84 (7):977-980.

10. Taylor M, Forster J, Langer B, et al. A study of prognostic factors for hepatic resection for colorectal metastases. *Am J Surg.* 1997;173(6):467-471.

11. Elias D, Cavalcanti A, Sabourin JC, et al. Resection of liver metastases from colorectal cancer: the real impact of the surgical margin. *Eur J Surg Oncol.* 1998;24(3):174-179.

12. Girard P, Ducreux M, Baldeyrou P, et al. Surgery for lung metastases from colorectal cancer: analysis of prognostic factors. *J Clin Oncol.* 1996;14(7):2047-2053.

13. Hughes KS, Simon R, Songhorabodi S, et al. Resection of the liver for colorectal carcinoma metastases: a multi-institutional study of patterns of recurrence. *Surgery.* 1986;100(2):278-284.

14. Schlag P, Hohenberger P, Herfarth C. Resection of liver metastases in colorectal cancer—competitive analysis of treatment results in synchronous versus metachronous metastases. *Eur J Surg Oncol.* 1990;16(4):360-365.

15. Rosen CB, Nagorney DM, Taswell HF, et al. Perioperative blood transfusion and determinants of survival after liver resection for metastatic colorectal carcinoma. *Ann Surg.* 1992;216(4):493-504; discussion 504-505.

16. Fong Y, Fortner J, Sun RL, et al. Clinical score for predicting recurrence after hepatic resection for metastatic colorectal cancer: analysis of 1001 consecutive cases. *Ann Surg.* 1999; 230(3):309-318; discussion 318-321.

17. Rossi S, Buscarini E, Garbagnati F, et al. Percutaneous treatment of small hepatic tumors by an expandable RF needle electrode. *AJR Am J Roentgenol.* 1998;170(4):1015-1022.

18. Solbiati L, Livraghi T, Goldberg SN, et al. Percutaneous radio-frequency ablation of hepatic metastases from colorectal cancer: long-term results in 117 patients. *Radiology.* 2001;221(1):159-166.

19. Lencioni R, Goletti O, Armillotta N, et al. Radio-frequency thermal ablation of liver metastases with a cooled-tip electrode needle: results of a pilot clinical trial. *Eur Radiol.* 1998;8(7):1205-1211.

20. Curley SA, Izzo F, Delrio P, et al. Radiofrequency ablation of unresectable primary and metastatic hepatic malignancies: results in 123 patients. *Ann Surg.* 1999;230(1):1-8.

21. Oshowo A, Gillams A, Harrison E, et al. Comparison of resection and radiofrequency ablation for treatment of solitary colorectal liver metastases. *Br J Surg.* 2003;90(10):1240-1243.

22. Livraghi T, Solbiati L, Meloni F, et al. Percutaneous radiofrequency ablation of liver metastases in potential candidates for resection: the "test-of-time approach". *Cancer.* 2003;97 (12):3027-3035.

23. Pawlik TM, Izzo F, Cohen DS, et al. Combined resection and radiofrequency ablation for advanced hepatic malignancies: results in 172 patients. *Ann Surg Oncol.* 2003;10:1059-1069.

24. Jarnagin WR, Fong Y, Ky A, et al. Liver resection for metastatic colorectal cancer: assessing the risk of occult irresectable disease. *J Am Coll Surg.* 1999;188(1): 33-42.

25. Ravikumar TS, Kaleya R, Kishinevsky A. Surgical ablative therapy of liver tumors. *Cancer: Principles and Practice of Oncology Updates.* 2000;14(3):1-12.

26. Seifert JK, Morris DL. Prognostic factors after cryotherapy for hepatic metastases from colorectal cancer. *Ann Surg.* 1998; 228(2):201-208.

27. Thomas DS, Nauta RJ, Rodgers JE, et al. Intraoperative high-dose rate interstitial irradiation of hepatic metastases from colorectal carcinoma. Results of a phase I-II trial. *Cancer.* 1993;71(6):1977-1981.

28. Ravikumar TS. Interstitial therapies for liver tumors. *Surg Oncol Clin N Am.* 1996;5(2):365-377.

29. McAfee MK, Allen MS, Trastek VF, et al. Colorectal lung metastases: results of surgical excision. *Ann Thorac Surg.* 1992;53(5):780-785; discussion 785-786.

30. Headrick JR, Miller DL, Nagorney DM, et al. Surgical treatment of hepatic and pulmonary metastases from colon cancer. *Ann Thorac Surg.* 2001;71(3):975-979; discussion 979-980.

31. Kemeny N, Huang Y, Cohen AM, et al. Hepatic arterial infusion of chemotherapy after resection of hepatic metastases from colorectal cancer. *N Engl J Med.* 1999;341(27):2039-2048.

32. Kemeny MM, Adak S, Gray B, et al. Combined-modality treatment for resectable metastatic colorectal carcinoma to the liver: surgical resection of hepatic metastases in combination with continuous infusion of chemotherapy—an intergroup study. *J Clin Oncol.* 2002;20(6):1499-1505.

33. Kemeny N, Daly J, Reichman B, et al. Intrahepatic or systemic infusion of fluorodeoxyuridine in patients with liver metastases from colorectal carcinoma. A randomized trial. *Ann Intern Med.* 1987;107(4):459-465.

34. Chang AE, Schneider PD, Sugarbaker PH, et al. A prospective randomized trial of regional versus systemic continuous 5-fluorodeoxyuridine chemotherapy in the treatment of colorectal liver metastases. *Ann Surg.* 1987;206(6):685-693.

35. Rougier P, Laplanche A, Huguier M, et al. Hepatic arterial infusion of floxuridine in patients with liver metastases from colorectal carcinoma: long-term results of a prospective randomized trial. *J Clin Oncol.* 1992;10(7):1112-1118.

36. Kemeny N, Cohen A, Seiter K, et al. Randomized trial of hepatic arterial floxuridine, mitomycin, and carmustine versus floxuridine alone in previously treated patients with liver metastases from colorectal cancer. *J Clin Oncol.* 1993;11(2):330-335.

37. Reappraisal of hepatic arterial infusion in the treatment of nonresectable liver metastases from colorectal cancer. Meta-Analysis Group in Cancer. *J Natl Cancer Inst.* 1996;88 (5):252-258.

38. McGinn CJ, Lawrence TS. Clinical Results of the Combination of Radiation and Fluoropyrimidines in the Treatment of Intrahepatic Cancer. *Semin Radiat Oncol.* 1997;7(4):313-323.

39. Saltz LB, Cox JV, Blanke C, et al. Irinotecan plus fluorouracil and leucovorin for metastatic colorectal cancer. Irinotecan Study Group. *N Engl J Med.* 2000;343(13):905-914.

40. Rothenberg ML, Meropol NJ, Poplin EA, et al. Mortality associated with irinotecan plus bolus fluorouracil/leucovorin: summary findings of an independent panel. *J Clin Oncol.* 2001; 19(18):3801-3807.

41. de Gramont A, Bosset JF, Milan C, et al. Randomized trial comparing monthly low-dose leucovorin and fluorouracil bolus with bimonthly high-dose leucovorin and fluorouracil bolus plus continuous infusion for advanced colorectal cancer: a French intergroup study. *J Clin Oncol.* 1997;15(2):808-815.

42. Giacchetti S, Perpoint B, Zidani R, et al. Phase III multicenter randomized trial of oxaliplatin added to chronomodulated fluorouracil-leucovorin as first-line treatment of metastatic colorectal cancer. *J Clin Oncol.* 2000;18(1):136-147.

43. Tournigand C, André T, Achille E, et al. FOLFIRI followed by FOLFOX6 or the reverse sequence in advanced colorectal cancer: a randomized GERCOR study. *J Clin Oncol.* 2004;22 (2):229-237.

44. Pitot HC, North Central Cancer Treatment Group: Phase III Randomized Study of Combinations of Oxaliplatin, Fluorouracil, Leucovorin Calcium, and Irinotecan as Initial Therapy in Patients With Advanced Adenocarcinoma of the Colon and Rectum, NCCTG-N9741, Clinical trial, Completed.

45. Wasserman E, Kalla S, Misset JL, et al. Oxaliplatin (L-OHP) and irinotecan (CPT11) phase I/II studies: results in 5 FU refractory (FR) colorectal cancer (CRC) patients (pts). [Abstract] *Proceedings of the American Society of Clinical Oncology.* 1999;18:A-913.

46. Goldberg RM, Sargent DJ, Morton RF, et al. A randomized controlled trial of fluorouracil plus leucovorin, irinotecan, and oxaliplatin combinations in patients with previously untreated metastatic colorectal cancer. *J Clin Oncol.* 2004;22(1):23-30.

47. Rothenberg ML, Oza AM, Bigelow RH, et al. Superiority of oxaliplatin and fluorouracil-leucovorin compared with either therapy alone in patients with progressive colorectal cancer after irinotecan and fluorouracil-leucovorin: interim results of a phase III trial. *J Clin Oncol.* 2003;21(11):2059-2069.

48. Rothenberg ML, Oza AM, Burger B, et al. Final results of a phase III trial of 5-FU/leucovorin versus oxaliplatin versus the combination in patients with metastatic colorectal cancer following irinotecan, 5-FU, and leucovorin. [Abstract] *Proceedings of the American Society of Clinical Oncology.* 2003;22:A-1011.

49. de Gramont A, Bosset JF, Milan C, et al. Randomized trial comparing monthly low-dose leucovorin and fluorouracil bolus with bimonthly high-dose leucovorin and fluorouracil bolus plus continuous infusion for advanced colorectal cancer: a French intergroup study. *J Clin Oncol.* 1997;15: 808-815.

50. Andre T, Colin T, Louvet C, et al. Phase III trial (GERCOR C96.1) comparing bimonthly LV5FU2 to monthly 5FU-leucoverin high dose (LV hd) in patients with Dukes B2 and C colon cancer. [Abstract] *Proceedings of the American Society of Clinical Oncology.* 2002;21: A-529.

51. Hurwitz H, Fehrenbacher L, Cartwright T, et al. Bevacizumab (a monoclonal antibody to vascular endothelial growth factor) prolongs survival in first-line colorectal

cancer (CRC): results of a phase III trial of bevacizumab in combination with bolus IFL (irinotecan, 5-fluorouracil, leucovorin) as first-line therapy in subjects with metastatic CRC. [Abstract] *Proceedings of the American Society of Clinical Oncology.* 2003;22:A-3646.

52. Cunningham D, Humblet Y, Siena S, et al. Cetuximab (C225) alone or in combination with irinotecan (CPT-11) in patients with epidermal growth factor receptor (EGFR)-positive, irinotecan-refractory metastatic colorectal cancer (MCRC). [Abstract] *Proceedings of the American Society of Clinical Oncology.* 2003;22:A-1012, 252.

RECTAL CANCER (PDQ®): TREATMENT HEALTH PROFESSIONAL VERSION

GENERAL INFORMATION

[Note: Separate PDQ summaries on *Screening for Colorectal Cancer*, *Prevention of Colorectal Cancer*, and *Genetics of Colorectal Cancer* are also available. Information about colon cancer in children is available in the PDQ summary on *Unusual Cancers of Childhood: Treatment*.

Note: Estimated new cases and deaths from rectal cancer in the United States in 2005:[1]

- New cases: 40,340
- Deaths (colon and rectal cancers combined): 56,290

Note: Some citations in the text of this section are followed by a level of evidence. The PDQ editorial boards use a formal ranking system to help the reader judge the strength of evidence linked to the reported results of a therapeutic strategy. (Refer to the PDQ summary on *Levels of Evidence* for more information.)] **(Table 1.)**

Cancer of the rectum is a highly treatable and often curable disease when localized. Surgery is the primary treatment and results in cure in approximately 45% of all patients. The prognosis of rectal cancer is clearly related to the degree of penetration of the tumor through the bowel wall and the presence or absence of nodal involvement. These two characteristics

Table 1. PDQ Levels of Evidence

Level of evidence 1iiA
Randomized, controlled, nonblinded clinical trial with total mortality as an endpoint

Level of evidence 1iiB
Randomized, controlled, nonblinded clinical trial with cause-specific mortality as an endpoint.

Level of evidence 1iiC
Randomized, controlled, nonblinded clinical trial with carefully assessed quality of life as an endpoint.

Level of evidence 1iiDiii
Randomized, controlled, nonblinded clinical trial with tumor response rate as an endpoint.

Level of evidence 3iiiA
Nonconsecutive case series with total mortality as an endpoint.

Level of evidence 3iiiDi
Nonconsecutive case series with total disease-free survival as an endpoint.

form the basis for all staging systems developed for this disease. Preoperative staging procedures include digital rectal examination, computed tomographic scan or magnetic resonance imaging scan of the abdomen and pelvis, endoscopic evaluation with biopsy, and endoscopic ultrasound (EUS).[2] EUS is an accurate method of evaluating tumor stage (up to 95% accuracy) and the status of the perirectal nodes (up to 74% accuracy). Accurate staging can influence therapy by helping to determine which patients may be candidates for local excision rather than more extensive surgery and which patients may be candidates for preoperative chemotherapy and radiation therapy to maximize the likelihood of resection with clear margins.

The American Joint Committee on Cancer and a National Cancer Institute-sponsored panel recommended that at least 12 lymph nodes be examined in patients with colon and rectal cancer to confirm the absence of nodal involvement by tumor.[3-5] This recommendation takes into consideration that the number of lymph nodes examined is a reflection of both the aggressiveness of lymphovascular mesenteric dissection at the time of surgical resection and the pathologic identification of nodes in the specimen. Retrospective studies demonstrated that the number of lymph nodes examined in colon and rectal surgery may be associated with patient outcome.[6-9] Many other prognostic markers have been evaluated retrospectively in the prognosis of patients with rectal cancer, though most, including allelic loss of chromosome 18q or thymidylate synthase expression, have not been prospectively validated.[10-12] Microsatellite instability, also associated with hereditary

nonpolyposis rectal cancer, has been shown to be associated with improved survival independent of tumor stage in a population-based series of 607 patients less than 50 years of age with colorectal cancer.[13] Racial differences in overall survival after adjuvant therapy have been observed, without differences in disease-free survival, suggesting that comorbid conditions play a role in survival outcome in different patient populations.[14] A major limitation of surgery is the inability to obtain wide radial margins because of the presence of the bony pelvis. In those patients with disease penetration through the bowel wall and/or spread into lymph nodes at the time of diagnosis, local recurrence following surgery is a major problem and often ultimately results in death.[15] The radial margin of resection of rectal primaries may also predict for local recurrence.[16]

Because of the frequency of the disease, the demonstrated slow growth of primary lesions, the better survival of patients with early-stage lesions, and the relative simplicity and accuracy of screening tests, screening for rectal cancer should be a part of routine care for all adults over the age of 50 years, especially those with first-degree relatives with colorectal cancer.[17] There are groups that have a high incidence of colorectal cancer. These groups include those with hereditary conditions, such as familial polyposis, hereditary nonpolyposis colon cancer (HNPCC) or Lynch Syndrome Variants I and II, and those with a personal history of ulcerative colitis or Crohn's colitis.[18,19] (Refer to the PDQ summary on *Genetics of Colorectal Cancer* for more information.) Together they account for 10% to 15% of colorectal cancers. Patients with

HNPCC reportedly have better prognoses in stage-stratified survival analysis than patients with sporadic colorectal cancer, but the retrospective nature of the studies and the possibility of selection factors make this observation difficult to interpret.[20] [Level of evidence: 3iiiA] More common conditions with an increased risk include: a personal history of colorectal cancer or adenomas, first degree family history of colorectal cancer or adenomas, and a personal history of ovarian, endometrial, or breast cancer.[21,22] These high-risk groups account for only 23% of all colorectal cancers. Limiting screening or early cancer detection to only these high-risk groups would miss the majority of colorectal cancers.[23] (Refer to the PDQ summaries on *Screening for Colorectal Cancer* and *Prevention of Colorectal Cancer* for more information.)

Following treatment of rectal cancer, periodic evaluations may lead to the earlier identification and management of recurrent disease.[24-27] However, the impact of such monitoring on overall mortality of patients with recurrent rectal cancer is limited by the relatively small proportion of patients in whom localized, potentially curable metastases are found. To date, there have been no large-scale randomized trials documenting the efficacy of a standard, postoperative monitoring program.[28-32] Carcinoembryonic antigen (CEA) is a serum glycoprotein frequently used in the management of patients with rectal cancer. A review of the use of this tumor marker suggests: that CEA is not useful as a screening test; that postoperative CEA testing be restricted to patients who would be candidates for resection of liver or lung metastases; and that routine use of CEA alone for monitoring response to treatment not be recommended.[33] However, the optimal regimen and frequency of follow-up examinations are not well defined, since the impact on patient survival is not clear and the quality of data is poor.[30-32] New surveillance methods including CEA immunoscintigraphy and positron tomography are under clinical evaluation.[34]

Although a large number of studies have evaluated various clinical, pathological, and molecular parameters with prognosis, as yet, none have had a major impact on prognosis or therapy.[35] Clinical stage remains the most important prognostic indicator.

Gastrointestinal stromal tumors can occur in the rectum. (Refer to the PDQ summary on *Adult Soft Tissue Sarcoma Treatment* for more information.)

Adjuvant Therapy

Patients with stage II or stage III rectal cancer are at high risk for local and systemic relapse. Adjuvant therapy should address both problems. Most trials of preoperative or postoperative radiation therapy alone have shown a decrease in the local recurrence rate but no definite effect on survival[24,36-39]; although a Swedish trial has shown a survival advantage from preoperative radiation therapy compared to surgery alone.[40] [Level of evidence: 1iiA] Two trials have confirmed that fluorouracil (5-FU) plus radiation therapy is effective and may be considered standard treatment.[36-38] In these trials, combined modality adjuvant treatment with radiation therapy and chemotherapy following surgery also resulted in local failure rates lower than with either radiation therapy or chemotherapy alone. An analysis of patients treated with postoperative chemotherapy and radiation therapy suggests that these patients may have more chronic bowel dysfunction compared to those who undergo surgical resection alone.[41] Improved radiation planning and techniques can be used to minimize treatment-related complications. These techniques include the use of multiple pelvic fields, prone positioning, customized bowel immobilization molds (belly boards), bladder distention, visualization of the small bowel with oral contrast, and the incorporation of three-dimensional or comparative treatment planning.[42,43] Ongoing clinical trials comparing preoperative and postoperative adjuvant chemoradiotherapy should further clarify the impact of either approach on bowel function and other important quality-of-life issues (eg, sphincter preservation) in addition to the more conventional endpoints of disease-free and overall survival.

Advanced Disease

Radiation therapy in rectal cancer is palliative in most situations but may have greater impact when used perioperatively. Palliation may be achieved in approximately 10% to 20% of patients with 5-FU. Several studies suggest an advantage when leucovorin is added to 5-FU in terms of response rate and palliation of symptoms but not always in terms of survival.[44-50] Irinotecan (CPT-11) has been approved by the U.S. Food and Drug Administration for the treatment of patients whose tumors are refractory to 5-FU.[51-54] Participation in clinical trials is appropriate. A number of other drugs are undergoing evaluation for the treatment of colon cancer.[55] Oxaliplatin, alone or combined with 5-FU and leucovorin, has also shown activity in 5-FU refractory patients.[56-59]

REFERENCES

1. American Cancer Society. *Cancer Facts and Figures 2005.* Atlanta, GA: American Cancer Society, 2005. Also available online. Last accessed November 1, 2005.
2. Snady H, Merrick MA. Improving the treatment of colorectal cancer: the role of EUS. *Cancer Invest.* 1998;16(8):572-581.
3. Colon and rectum. In: American Joint Committee on Cancer. *AJCC Cancer Staging Manual.* 6th ed. New York, NY: Springer, 2002, pp 113-124.
4. Compton CC, Greene FL. The staging of colorectal cancer: 2004 and beyond. *CA Cancer J Clin.* 2004;54(6):295-308.
5. Nelson H, Petrelli N, Carlin A, et al. Guidelines 2000 for colon and rectal cancer surgery. *J Natl Cancer Inst.* 2001;93(8):583-596.
6. Swanson RS, Compton CC, Stewart AK, et al. The prognosis of T3N0 colon cancer is dependent on the number of lymph nodes examined. *Ann Surg Oncol.* 2003;10(1):65-71.
7. Le Voyer TE, Sigurdson ER, Hanlon AL, et al. Colon cancer survival is associated with increasing number of lymph nodes analyzed: a secondary survey of intergroup trial INT-0089. *J Clin Oncol.* 2003;21(15):2912-2919.
8. Prandi M, Lionetto R, Bini A, et al. Prognostic evaluation of stage B colon cancer patients is improved by an adequate lymphadenectomy: results of a secondary analysis of a large scale adjuvant trial. *Ann Surg.* 2002;235(4):458-463.
9. Tepper JE, O'Connell MJ, Niedzwiecki D, et al. Impact of number of nodes retrieved on outcome in patients with rectal cancer. *J Clin Oncol.* 2001;19(1):157-163.
10. McLeod HL, Murray GI. Tumour markers of prognosis in colorectal cancer. *Br J Cancer.* 1999;79(2):191-203.
11. Jen J, Kim H, Piantadosi S, et al. Allelic loss of chromosome 18q and prognosis in colorectal cancer. *N Engl J Med.* 1994;331(4):213-221.
12. Lanza G, Matteuzzi M, Gafà R, et al. Chromosome 18q allelic loss and prognosis in stage II and III colon cancer. *Int J Cancer.* 1998;79(4):390-395.
13. Gryfe R, Kim H, Hsieh ET, et al. Tumor microsatellite instability and clinical outcome in young patients with colorectal cancer. *N Engl J Med.* 2000;342(2):69-77.
14. Dignam JJ, Colangelo L, Tian W, et al. Outcomes among African-Americans and Caucasians in colon cancer adjuvant therapy trials: findings from the National Surgical Adjuvant Breast and Bowel Project. *J Natl Cancer Inst.* 1999;91(22):1933-1940.
15. Heald RJ, Ryall RD. Recurrence and survival after total mesorectal excision for rectal cancer. *Lancet.* 1986;1(8496):1479-1482.
16. de Haas-Kock DF, Baeten CG, Jager JJ, et al. Prognostic significance of radial margins of clearance in rectal cancer. *Br J Surg.* 1996;83(6):781-785.
17. Cannon-Albright LA, Skolnick MH, Bishop DT, et al. Common inheritance of susceptibility to colonic adenomatous polyps and associated colorectal cancers. *N Engl J Med.* 1988;319(9):533-537.
18. Thorson AG, Knezetic JA, Lynch HT. A century of progress in hereditary nonpolyposis colorectal cancer (Lynch syndrome). *Dis Colon Rectum.* 1999;42(1):1-9.
19. Smith RA, von Eschenbach AC, Wender R, et al. American Cancer Society guidelines for the early detection of cancer: update of early detection guidelines for prostate, colorectal, and endometrial cancers. Also: update 2001--testing for early lung cancer detection. *CA Cancer J Clin.* 2001;51(1):38-75; quiz 77-80.
20. Watson P, Lin KM, Rodriguez-Bigas MA, et al. Colorectal carcinoma survival among hereditary nonpolyposis colorectal carcinoma family members. *Cancer.* 1998;83(2):259-266.
21. Ransohoff DF, Lang CA. Screening for colorectal cancer. *N Engl J Med.* 1991;325(1):37-41.
22. Fuchs CS, Giovannucci EL, Colditz GA, et al. A prospective study of family history and the risk of colorectal cancer. *N Engl J Med.* 1994;331(25):1669-1674.
23. Winawer SJ. Screening for colorectal cancer. *Cancer: Principles and Practice of Oncology Updates.* 1987;2(1):1-16.
24. Martin EW Jr, Minton JP, Carey LC. CEA-directed second-look surgery in the asymptomatic patient after primary

resection of colorectal carcinoma. *Ann Surg.* 1985;202 (3):310-317.

25. Bruinvels DJ, Stiggelbout AM, Kievit J, et al. Follow-up of patients with colorectal cancer. A meta-analysis. *Ann Surg.* 1994;219(2):174-182.

26. Lautenbach E, Forde KA, Neugut AI. Benefits of colonoscopic surveillance after curative resection of colorectal cancer. *Ann Surg.* 1994;220(2):206-211.

27. Khoury DA, Opelka FG, Beck DE, et al. Colon surveillance after colorectal cancer surgery. *Dis Colon Rectum.* 1996; 39(3):252-256.

28. Safi F, Link KH, Beger HG. Is follow-up of colorectal cancer patients worthwhile? *Dis Colon Rectum.* 1993;36(7):636-643; discussion 643-644.

29. Moertel CG, Fleming TR, Macdonald JS, et al. An evaluation of the carcinoembryonic antigen (CEA) test for monitoring patients with resected colon cancer. *JAMA.* 1993;270(8):943-947.

30. Rosen M, Chan L, Beart RW Jr, et al. Follow-up of colorectal cancer: a meta-analysis. *Dis Colon Rectum.* 1998; 41(9):1116-1126.

31. Desch CE, Benson AB 3rd, Smith TJ, et al. Recommended colorectal cancer surveillance guidelines by the American Society of Clinical Oncology. *J Clin Oncol.* 1999;17(4): 1312.

32. Benson AB 3rd, Desch CE, Flynn PJ, et al. 2000 update of American Society of Clinical Oncology colorectal cancer surveillance guidelines. *J Clin Oncol.* 2000;18(20):3586-3588.

33. Clinical practice guidelines for the use of tumor markers in breast and colorectal cancer. Adopted on May 17, 1996 by the American Society of Clinical Oncology. *J Clin Oncol.* 1996;14(10):2843-2877.

34. Lechner P, Lind P, Goldenberg DM. Can postoperative surveillance with serial CEA immunoscintigraphy detect resectable rectal cancer recurrence and potentially improve tumor-free survival? *J Am Coll Surg.* 2000;191 (5):511-518.

35. Roth JA. p53 prognostication: paradigm or paradox? *Clin Cancer Res.* 1999;5(11):3345.

36. O'Connell M, Wieand H, Krook J, et al. Lack of value for methyl-CCNU (MeCCNU) as a component of effective rectal cancer surgical adjuvant therapy: interim analysis of intergroup protocol 86-47-51. [Abstract] *Proceedings of the American Society of Clinical Oncology.* 1991; 10:A-403, 134.

37. Radiation therapy and fluorouracil with or without semustine for the treatment of patients with surgical adjuvant adenocarcinoma of the rectum. Gastrointestinal Tumor Study Group. *J Clin Oncol.* 1992;10(4):549-557.

38. Moertel CG Chemotherapy for colorectal cancer. *N Engl J Med.* 1994;330(16):1136-1142.

39. Kachnic LA, Willett CG. Radiation therapy in the management of rectal cancer. *Curr Opin Oncol.* 2001;13(4): 300-306.

40. Improved survival with preoperative radiotherapy in resectable rectal cancer. Swedish Rectal Cancer Trial. *N Engl J Med.* 1997;336(14):980-987.

41. Kollmorgen CF, Meagher AP, Wolff BG, et al. The long-term effect of adjuvant postoperative chemoradiotherapy for rectal carcinoma on bowel function. *Ann Surg.* 1994; 220(5):676-682.

42. Koelbl O, Richter S, Flentje M. Influence of patient positioning on dose-volume histogram and normal tissue complication probability for small bowel and bladder in patients receiving pelvic irradiation: a prospective study using a 3D planning system and a radiobiological model. *Int J Radiat Oncol Biol Phys.* 1999;45(5):1193-1198.

43. Gunderson LL, Russell AH, Llewellyn HJ, et al. Treatment planning for colorectal cancer: radiation and surgical techniques and value of small-bowel films. *Int J Radiat Oncol Biol Phys.* 1985;11(7):1379-1393.

44. Petrelli N, Douglass HO Jr, Herrera L, et al. The modulation of fluorouracil with leucovorin in metastatic colorectal carcinoma: a prospective randomized phase III trial. Gastrointestinal Tumor Study Group. *J Clin Oncol.* 1989;7(10):1419-1426.

45. Erlichman C, Fine S, Wong A, et al. A randomized trial of fluorouracil and folinic acid in patients with metastatic colorectal carcinoma. *J Clin Oncol.* 1988;6(3):469-475.

46. Doroshow JH, Multhauf P, Leong L, et al. Prospective randomized comparison of fluorouracil versus fluorouracil and high-dose continuous infusion leucovorin calcium for the treatment of advanced measurable colorectal cancer in patients previously unexposed to chemotherapy. *J Clin Oncol.* 1990;8(3):491-501.

47. Poon MA, O'Connell MJ, Wieand HS, et al. Biochemical modulation of fluorouracil with leucovorin: confirmatory evidence of improved therapeutic efficacy in advanced colorectal cancer. *J Clin Oncol.* 1991;9(11):1967-1972.

48. Valone FH, Friedman MA, Wittlinger PS, et al. Treatment of patients with advanced colorectal carcinomas with fluorouracil alone, high-dose leucovorin plus fluorouracil, or sequential methotrexate, fluorouracil, and leucovorin: a randomized trial of the Northern California Oncology Group. *J Clin Oncol.* 1989;7(10):1427-1436.

49. Borner MM, Castiglione M, Bacchi M, et al. The impact of adding low-dose leucovorin to monthly 5-fluorouracil in advanced colorectal carcinoma: results of a phase III trial. Swiss Group for Clinical Cancer Research (SAKK). *Ann Oncol.* 1998;9(5):535-541.

50. Modulation of fluorouracil by leucovorin in patients with advanced colorectal cancer: evidence in terms of response rate. Advanced Colorectal Cancer Meta-Analysis Project. *J Clin Oncol.* 1992;10(6):896-903.

51. Rothenberg ML, Eckardt JR, Kuhn JG, et al. Phase II trial of irinotecan in patients with progressive or recurrent colorectal cancer. *J Clin Oncol.* 1996;14(4): 1128-1135.

52. Conti JA, Kemeny NE, Saltz LB, et al. Irinotecan is an active agent in untreated patients with metastatic colorectal cancer. *J Clin Oncol.* 1996;14(3):709-715.

53. Rougier P, Van Cutsem E, Bajetta E, et al. Randomised trial of irinotecan versus fluorouracil by continuous infusion after fluorouracil failure in patients with metastatic colorectal cancer. *Lancet.* 1998;352(9138):1407-1412.

54. Cunningham D, Pyrhönen S, James RD, et al. Randomised trial of irinotecan plus supportive care versus supportive care alone after fluorouracil failure for patients with metastatic colorectal cancer. *Lancet.* 1998; 352(9138):1413-1418.

55. Von Hoff DD. Promising new agents for treatment of patients with colorectal cancer. *Semin Oncol.* 1998;25 (5 Suppl 11):47-52.

56. de Gramont A, Vignoud J, Tournigand C, et al. Oxaliplatin with high-dose leucovorin and 5-fluorouracil 48-hour continuous infusion in pretreated metastatic colorectal cancer. *Eur J Cancer.* 1997;33(2):214-219.

57. Bleiberg H, de Gramont A. Oxaliplatin plus 5-fluorouracil: clinical experience in patients with advanced colorectal cancer. *Semin Oncol.* 1998;25(2 Suppl 5):32-39.

58. Cvitkovic E, Bekradda M. Oxaliplatin: a new therapeutic option in colorectal cancer. *Semin Oncol.* 1999;26(6): 647-662.

59. Giacchetti S, Perpoint B, Zidani R, et al. Phase III multicenter randomized trial of oxaliplatin added to chronomodulated fluorouracil-leucovorin as first-line treatment of metastatic colorectal cancer. *J Clin Oncol.* 2000;18(1):136-147.

CELLULAR CLASSIFICATION

Histologic types of rectal cancer include:

- Adenocarcinoma (most rectal cases).
  - Mucinous (colloid) adenocarcinoma.
  - Signet ring adenocarcinoma.
- Scirrhous tumors.
- Neuroendocrine:[1] Tumors with neuroendocrine differentiation typically have a poorer prognosis

than pure adenocarcinoma variants.

- Carcinoid tumors. (Refer to the PDQ summary on *Gastrointestinal Carcinoid Tumor Treatment* for more information.)

REFERENCES

1. Saclarides TJ, Szeluga D, Staren ED. Neuroendocrine cancers of the colon and rectum. Results of a ten-year experience. *Dis Colon Rectum.* 1994;37(7):635-642.

STAGE INFORMATION

Treatment decisions should be made with reference to the TNM classification, rather than the older Dukes' or the Modified Astler-Coller (MAC) classification schema.

The American Joint Committee on Cancer and a National Cancer Institute-sponsored panel recommended that at least 12 lymph nodes be examined in patients with colon and rectal cancer to confirm the absence of nodal involvement by tumor.[1-3] This recommendation takes into consideration that the number of lymph nodes examined is a reflection of both the aggressiveness of lymphovascular mesenteric dissection at the time of surgical resection and the pathologic identification of nodes in the specimen. Retrospective studies demonstrated that the number of lymph nodes examined in colon and rectal surgery may be associated with patient outcome.[4-7]

The AJCC has designated staging by TNM classification.

TNM Definitions

Primary tumor (T)

- TX: Primary tumor cannot be assessed
- T0: No evidence of primary tumor
- Tis: Carcinoma in situ: intraepithelial or invasion of the lamina propria*
- T1: Tumor invades submucosa
- T2: Tumor invades muscularis propria
- T3: Tumor invades through the muscularis propria into the subserosa, or into nonperitonealized pericolic or perirectal tissues
- T4: Tumor directly invades other organs or structures, and/or perforates the visceral peritoneum**.***

* [*Note: Tis includes cancer cells confined within the glandular basement membrane (intraepithelial) or lamina propria (intramucosal) with no extension through the muscularis mucosae into the submucosa.*]

** [*Note: Direct invasion in T4 includes invasion of other segments of the colorectum by way of the serosa; for example, invasion of the sigmoid colon by a carcinoma of the cecum.*]

*** [*Note: Tumor that is adherent to other organs or structures, macroscopically, is classified T4. However, if no tumor is present in the adhesion, microscopically, the classification should be pT3. The V and L substaging should be used to identify the presence or absence of vascular or lymphatic invasion.*]

Regional lymph nodes (N)

- NX: Regional lymph nodes cannot be assessed
- N0: No regional lymph node metastasis
- N1: Metastasis in 1 to 3 regional lymph nodes
- N2: Metastasis in 4 or more regional lymph nodes

Note: A tumor nodule in the pericolorectal adipose tissue of a primary carcinoma without histologic evidence of residual lymph node in the nodule is classified in the pN category as a regional lymph node metastasis if the nodule has the form and smooth contour of a lymph node. If the nodule has an irregular contour, it should be classified in the T category and also coded as V1 (microscopic venous invasion) or as V2 (if it was grossly evident), because there is a strong likelihood that it represents venous invasion.]

Distant metastasis (M)

- MX: Distant metastasis cannot be assessed
- M0: No distant metastasis
- M1: Distant metastasis

AJCC stage groupings

Stage 0
- Tis, N0, M0

Stage I
- T1, N0, M0
- T2, N0, M0

Stage IIA
- T3, N0, M0

Stage IIB
- T4, N0, M0

Stage IIIA
- T1, N1, M0
- T2, N1, M0

Stage IIIB
- T3, N1, M0
- T4, N1, M0

Stage IIIC
- Any T, N2, M0

Stage IV
- Any T, any N, M1

REFERENCES

1. Colon and rectum. In: American Joint Committee on Cancer. *AJCC Cancer Staging Manual.* 6th ed. New York, NY: Springer, 2002, pp 113-124.
2. Compton CC, Greene FL. The staging of colorectal cancer: 2004 and beyond. *CA Cancer J Clin.* 2004 Nov-Dec;54 (6):295-308.
3. Nelson H, Petrelli N, Carlin A, et al. Guidelines 2000 for colon and rectal cancer surgery. *J Natl Cancer Inst.* 2001; 93(8):583-596.
4. Swanson RS, Compton CC, Stewart AK, et al. The prognosis of T3N0 colon cancer is dependent on the number of lymph nodes examined. *Ann Surg Oncol.* 2003;Feb; 10(1):65-71.
5. Le Voyer TE, Sigurdson ER, Hanlon AL, et al. Colon cancer survival is associated with increasing number of lymph nodes analyzed: a secondary survey of intergroup trial INT-0089. *J Clin Oncol.* 2003;21(15):2912-2919.
6. Prandi M, Lionetto R, Bini A, et al. Prognostic evaluation of stage B colon cancer patients is improved by an adequate lymphadenectomy: results of a secondary analysis of a large scale adjuvant trial. *Ann Surg.* 2002;235(4):458-463.
7. Tepper JE, O'Connell MJ, Niedzwiecki D, et al. Impact of number of nodes retrieved on outcome in patients with rectal cancer. *J Clin Oncol.* 2001;19(1):157-163.

TREATMENT OPTION OVERVIEW

[Note: Some citations in the text of this section are followed by a level of evidence. The PDQ editorial boards use a formal ranking system to help the reader judge the strength of evidence linked to the reported results of a therapeutic strategy. (Refer to the PDQ summary on *Levels of Evidence* for more information.)]

Treatment of rectal cancer is surgical resection of the primary tumor and regional lymph nodes for localized disease. The technique of rectal excision may impact the rate of local recurrence. Local failure rates in the range of 4% to 8% following rectal resection with appropriate mesorectal excision (total mesorectal excision for low/middle rectal tumors and mesorectal excision at least 5 centimeters below the tumor for high rectal tumors) have been reported.[1-5] The low incidence of local relapse following meticulous mesorectal excision has led some investigators to question the routine use of adjuvant radiation therapy. Total mesorectal excision combined with low stapled colorectal or coloanal anastomosis obviates the need, in many patients, for abdominoperineal resection and associated permanent stoma. The risk of anastomotic dehiscence with these sphincter-preserving procedures, however, is considerable (>15%), frequently requiring temporary proximal diversion. The role of sentinel lymph node mapping in regional nodal staging for rectal cancer is under clinical evaluation.[6] Because of an increased tendency for first failure in locoregional sites only, the impact of perioperative irradiation is greater in rectal cancer than in colon cancer.[7] Both preoperative and postoperative radiation therapy alone decrease local failure.[8-11] Substantial improvement in overall survival has not been demonstrated with pre- or postoperative radiation therapy alone, except in a single European trial.[10] [Level of evidence: 1iiA]

Recent progress in adjuvant postoperative treatment regimens relates to the integration of systemic therapy to radiation, as well as redefining the techniques for both modalities. The efficacy of postoperative radiation and 5-FU-based chemotherapy for stage II and III rectal cancer was established by a series of prospective, randomized clinical trials (the Gastrointestinal Tumor Study Group (GITSG) Protocol 7175, the Mayo/North Central Cancer Treatment Group (NCCTG) Protocol 79-47-51, and the National Surgical Adjuvant Breast and Bowel Project (NSABP) R-01).[12-14] [Level of evidence: 1iiA] These studies demonstrated an increase in both disease-free interval and overall survival when radiation therapy is combined with chemotherapy following surgical resection. Following the publication of these trials, the National Cancer Institute (NCI) concluded at a Consensus Development Conference in 1990 that postoperative combined modality treatment is recommended for patients with stage II and stage III rectal carcinoma.[15]

Subsequent studies have attempted to increase the survival benefit by improving radiation sensitization and by identifying the optimal chemotherapeutic agents and delivery systems. The chemotherapy associated with the first successful combined modality treatments was fluorouracil (5-FU) and semustine. Semustine is not commercially available, and previous studies have linked this drug to increased risks of renal toxic effects and leukemia.

A follow-up randomized trial from GITSG demonstrated that semustine does not produce an additive survival benefit to radiotherapy and 5-FU.[16] [Level of evidence: 1iiA] The Intergroup 86-47-51 trial has demonstrated a 10% improved overall survival with the use of continuous-infusion 5-FU (225 mg/m^2/day) throughout the course of radiation therapy when compared with bolus 5-FU (500 mg/m^2 times three injections in the first and fifth weeks of radiation).[17] [Level of evidence: 1iiA] The final results of Intergroup trial 0114 show no survival or local control benefit to the addition of leucovorin, levamisole, or both, to 5-FU administered postoperatively for stage II and stage III rectal cancers at a median follow-up of 7.4 years.[18] [Level of evidence: 1iiA] Intergroup 0144 is a three-arm randomized trial designed to determine whether continuous-infusion 5-FU throughout the entire standard adjuvant six-cycle chemotherapy course is more effective than continuous 5-FU only during pelvic radiation.[19] [Level of evidence: 1iiA] This trial is now closed and results are pending.

While the above data demonstrate a benefit of postoperative radiation and 5-FU chemotherapy for stage II and stage III rectal cancer, a follow-up study to the R-01 study, the NSABP R-02, addressed whether the addition of radiation therapy to chemotherapy would enhance the survival advantage reported in R-01.[20] [Level of evidence: 1iiA] The addition of radiation while significantly reducing local recurrence at 5 years (8% for chemotherapy and radiation vs 13% for chemotherapy alone, P=.02), demonstrated no significant benefit in survival. The interpretation of the interaction of radiotherapy with prognostic factors, however, was challenging. Radiation appeared to improve survival in patients younger than 60 years, as well as in patients who received abdominoperineal resection. This trial has initiated discussion in the oncologic community as to the proper role of postoperative radiation therapy. Omission of radiotherapy seems premature, since locoregional recurrence remains a clinically relevant problem. Using current surgical techniques, including total mesorectal excision (TME), it may be possible to identify subsets of patients whose chance of pelvic failure is low enough to omit postoperative radiation. A Dutch trial (CKVO 95-04) randomizing patients with resectable rectal cancers (stages I-IV) to a short course of radiation (500 cGy x 5) followed by TME compared to TME alone demonstrated no difference in overall survival at two years (82% for both arms).[21] [Level of evidence: 1iiA] Local recurrence rates were significantly reduced in the radiation therapy plus TME arm (2.4%) as compared to the TME only arm (8.2%, P<.001). At present, acceptable postoperative therapy for patients with stage II or stage III

rectal cancer not enrolled in clinical trials includes continuous-infusion 5-FU during 45 Gy to 55 Gy pelvic radiation, followed by four cycles of maintenance chemotherapy with bolus 5-FU with or without modulation with leucovorin.

An analysis of patients treated with postoperative chemotherapy and radiation therapy suggests that these patients may have more chronic bowel dysfunction compared to those who undergo surgical resection alone.[22] Improved radiation planning and techniques can be used to minimize treatment-related complications. These techniques include the use of multiple pelvic fields, prone positioning, customized bowel immobilization molds (belly boards), bladder distention, visualization of the small bowel through oral contrast, and the incorporation of three-dimensional or comparative treatment planning.[23,24]

Although combined chemoradiotherapy is standard in the United States, European centers typically use preoperative radiation therapy alone. Several studies suggest that in selected patients with low rectal tumors, high-dose preoperative radiation therapy may permit resection of the primary tumor with a high rate of preservation of sphincter function.[25-29] Such treatment results in survival rates similar to those observed with more radical surgery without increasing the risk of pelvic or perineal recurrences. In a randomized trial evaluating the optimal timing of surgery following radiation therapy, a longer interval of surgery (six to eight weeks) following radiation therapy of 39 Gy in 13 fractions produced significantly better tumor response rates (53% vs 72%, P=.007) and pathologic downstaging (10% vs 26%, P=.005) when compared to the shorter interval of surgery (two weeks) following radiation therapy.[30] [Level of evidence: 1iiDiii] A trend toward more sphincter-preserving surgery was noted for the longer-interval arm (76%) compared to the shorter-interval arm (68%, P=.27). An ongoing trial is addressing whether chemotherapy adds to the benefits of preoperative radiation.[31]

Because of the suggestion of enhanced sphincter preservation with preoperative radiation with or without chemotherapy for clinically resectable T3 rectal cancers, ongoing randomized trials comparing preoperative and postoperative adjuvant combined modality therapy should further clarify the impact of either approach on bowel function, as well as on the endpoints of local control and overall survival. An interval analysis of the first 116 patients enrolled on the NSABP R-03 randomized trial of pre- versus postoperative chemoradiation revealed a similar incidence of postoperative complications in both arms.[32] This trial closed in 1999 and preliminary results are expected. A similar trial from Germany (COA/ARO/AIO 94) is ongoing. Preliminary results in 417 patients indicate lower rates of acute toxicity and higher rates of sphincter-preserving surgery and complete resection with negative margins in patients receiving preoperative chemoradiation versus postoperative chemoradiation.[33]

The designations in PDQ that treatments are "standard" or "under clinical evaluation" are not to be used as a basis for reimbursement determinations.

REFERENCES

1. MacFarlane JK, Ryall RD, Heald RJ. Mesorectal excision for rectal cancer. *Lancet.* 1993;341(8843):457-460.
2. Enker WE, Thaler HT, Cranor ML, et al. Total mesorectal excision in the operative treatment of carcinoma of the rectum. *J Am Coll Surg.* 1995;181(4):335-346.
3. Zaheer S, Pemberton JH, Farouk R, et al. Surgical treatment of adenocarcinoma of the rectum. *Ann Surg.* 1998; 227(6):800-811.
4. Heald RJ, Smedh RK, Kald A, et al. Abdominoperineal excision of the rectum—an endangered operation. Norman Nigro Lectureship. *Dis Colon Rectum.* 1997;40(7):747-751.
5. Lopez-Kostner F, Lavery IC, Hool GR, et al. Total mesorectal excision is not necessary for cancers of the upper rectum. *Surgery.* 1998;124(4):612-617; discussion 617-618.
6. Esser S, Reilly WT, Riley LB, et al. The role of sentinel lymph node mapping in staging of colon and rectal cancer. *Dis Colon Rectum.* 2001;44(6):850-854; discussion 854-856.
7. Gunderson LL, Sosin H. Areas of failure found at reoperation (second or symptomatic look) following "curative surgery" for adenocarcinoma of the rectum. Clinicopathologic correlation and implications for adjuvant therapy. *Cancer.* 1974;34(4):1278-1292.
8. Randomised trial of surgery alone versus radiotherapy followed by surgery for potentially operable locally advanced rectal cancer. Medical Research Council Rectal Cancer Working Party. *Lancet.* 1996;348(9042):1605-1610.
9. Randomised trial of surgery alone versus surgery followed by radiotherapy for mobile cancer of the rectum. Medical Research Council Rectal Cancer Working Party. *Lancet.* 1996;348(9042):1610-1614.
10. Martling A, Holm T, Johansson H, et al. The Stockholm II trial on preoperative radiotherapy in rectal carcinoma: long-term follow-up of a population-based study. *Cancer.* 2001;92(4):896-902.
11. Dahlberg M, Glimelius B, Påhlman L. Improved survival and reduction in local failure rates after preoperative radiotherapy: evidence for the generalizability of the results of Swedish Rectal Cancer Trial. *Ann Surg.* 1999; 229(4):493-497.
12. Thomas PR, Lindblad AS. Adjuvant postoperative radiotherapy and chemotherapy in rectal carcinoma: a review of the Gastrointestinal Tumor Study Group experience. *Radiother Oncol.* 1988;13(4):245-252.
13. Krook JE, Moertel CG, Gunderson LL, et al. Effective surgical adjuvant therapy for high-risk rectal carcinoma. *N Engl J Med.* 1991;324(11):709-715.
14. Fisher B, Wolmark N, Rockette H, et al. Postoperative adjuvant chemotherapy or radiation therapy for rectal cancer: results from NSABP protocol R-01. *J Natl Cancer Inst.* 1988;80(1):21-29.
15. NIH consensus conference. Adjuvant therapy for patients with colon and rectal cancer. *JAMA.* 1990;264(11):1444-1450.
16. Radiation therapy and fluorouracil with or without semustine for the treatment of patients with surgical adjuvant adenocarcinoma of the rectum. Gastrointestinal Tumor Study Group. *J Clin Oncol* 1992;10(4):549-557.
17. O'Connell MJ, Martenson JA, Wieand HS, et al. Improving adjuvant therapy for rectal cancer by combining protracted-infusion fluorouracil with radiation therapy after curative surgery. *N Engl J Med.* 1994;331(8):502-507.
18. Tepper JE, O'Connell M, Niedzwiecki D, et al. Adjuvant therapy in rectal cancer: analysis of stage, sex, and local control—final report of intergroup 0114. *J Clin Oncol.* 2002;20(7):1744-1750.
19. Smalley SR, Southwest Oncology Group. Phase III Randomized Study of Three Different Regimens Containing Fluorouracil in Patients with Stage II or III Rectal Cancer, SWOG-9304, Clinical trial, Closed.
20. Wolmark N, Wieand HS, Hyams DM, et al. Randomized trial of postoperative adjuvant chemotherapy with or without radiotherapy for carcinoma of the rectum: National Surgical Adjuvant Breast and Bowel Project Protocol R-02. *J Natl Cancer Inst.* 2000;92(5):388-396.
21. Kapiteijn E, Marijnen CA, Nagtegaal ID, et al. Preoperative radiotherapy combined with total mesorectal

excision for resectable rectal cancer. *N Engl J Med.* 2001;345(9):638-646.

22. Kollmorgen CF, Meagher AP, Wolff BG, et al. The long-term effect of adjuvant postoperative chemoradiotherapy for rectal carcinoma on bowel function. *Ann Surg.* 1994; 220(5):676-682.

23. Koelbl O, Richter S, Flentje M. Influence of patient positioning on dose-volume histogram and normal tissue complication probability for small bowel and bladder in patients receiving pelvic irradiation: a prospective study using a 3D planning system and a radiobiological model. *Int J Radiat Oncol Biol Phys.* 1999;45(5):1193-1198.

24. Gunderson LL, Russell AH, Llewellyn HJ, et al. Treatment planning for colorectal cancer: radiation and surgical techniques and value of small-bowel films. *Int J Radiat Oncol Biol Phys.* 1985;11(7):1379-1393.

25. Mohiuddin M, Marks G. High dose preoperative irradiation for cancer of the rectum, 1976-1988. *Int J Radiat Oncol Biol Phys.* 1991;20(1):37-43.

26. Ng AK, Recht A, Busse PM. Sphincter preservation therapy for distal rectal carcinoma: a review. *Cancer.* 1997;79 (4):671-683.

27. Mohiuddin M, Marks G, Bannon J. High-dose preoperative radiation and full thickness local excision: a new option for selected T3 distal rectal cancers. *Int J Radiat Oncol Biol Phys.* 1994;30(4):845-849.

28. Willett CG. Organ preservation in anal and rectal cancers. *Curr Opin Oncol.* 1996;8(4):329-333.

29. Harms BA, Starling JR. Current status of sphincter preservation in rectal cancer. *Oncology* (Huntingt). 1990;4(8):53-60; discussion 65.

30. Francois Y, Nemoz CJ, Baulieux J, et al. Influence of the interval between preoperative radiation therapy and surgery on downstaging and on the rate of sphincter-sparing surgery for rectal cancer: the Lyon R90-01 randomized trial. *J Clin Oncol.* 1999;17(8):2396.

31. Bosset J, European Organization for Research and Treatment of Cancer: Phase III Randomized Study of Preoperative Radiotherapy With or Without Fluorouracil (5-FU) Combined With Leucovorin Calcium (CF) and/or Postoperative 5-FU/CF in Patients With Resectable Adenocarcinoma of the Rectum, EORTC-22921, Clinical trial, Closed.

32. Hyams DM, Mamounas EP, Petrelli N, et al. A clinical trial to evaluate the worth of preoperative multimodality therapy in patients with operable carcinoma of the rectum: a progress report of National Surgical Breast and Bowel Project Protocol R-03. *Dis Colon Rectum.* 1997; 40(2):131-139.

33. Sauer R, Fietkau R, Martus P, et al. Adjuvant and neoadjuvant radiochemotherapy for advanced rectal cancer—first results of the German multicenter phase III trial. *Int J Radiat Oncol Biol Phys.* 2000;48(suppl 119): #17.

STAGE 0 RECTAL CANCER

Stage 0 rectal cancer is the most superficial of all the lesions and is limited to the mucosa without invasion of the lamina propria. Because of its superficial nature, surgical and other procedures may be limited.

Standard treatment options:

1. Local excision or simple polypectomy.[1]
2. Full thickness rectal resection by the transanal or transcoccygeal route for large lesions not amenable to local excision.
3. Endocavitary irradiation.[2-4]
4. Local radiation therapy.[2]

REFERENCES

1. Bailey HR, Huval WV, Max E, et al. Local excision of carcinoma of the rectum for cure. *Surgery.* 1992;111(5):555-561.
2. Kodner IJ, Gilley MT, Shemesh EI, et al. Radiation therapy as definitive treatment for selected invasive rectal cancer. *Surgery.* 1993;114(4):850-6; discussion 856-857.
3. Mendenhall WM, Rout WR, Vauthey JN, et al. Conservative treatment of rectal adenocarcinoma with endocavitary irradiation or wide local excision and postoperative irradiation. *J Clin Oncol.* 1997;15(10):3241-3248.
4. Aumock A, Birnbaum EH, Fleshman JW, et al. Treatment of rectal adenocarcinoma with endocavitary and external beam radiotherapy: results for 199 patients with localized tumors. *Int J Radiat Oncol Biol Phys.* 2001;51(2):363-370.

STAGE I RECTAL CANCER

Stage I (Old Stage: Dukes' A or Modified Astler-Coller A and B1)

Because of its localized nature, stage I has a high cure rate.

Standard treatment options:

1. Wide surgical resection and anastomosis when an adequate low anterior resection (LAR) can be performed with sufficient distal rectum to allow a conventional anastomosis or coloanal anastomosis.
2. Wide surgical resection with abdominoperineal resection (APR) for lesions too distal to permit low anterior resection (LAR).
3. Local transanal or other resection[1,2] with or without perioperative external beam radiation plus fluorouracil (5-FU). No randomized trials are available to compare local excision with or without postoperative chemoradiation treatments to wide surgical resection (LAR and APR). One prospective multicenter phase II

study and several larger retrospective series suggest that well-staged patients with small (<4 centimeters) tumors with good histologic prognostic features (well- to moderately differentiated adenocarcinomas), mobile, and no lymphatic, venous, or perineural invasion, treated with full-thickness local excision that results in negative margins may have outcomes equivalent to APR or LAR with the selective post-operative use chemoradiation therapy.[3-5] Endoscopic ultrasound studies have been helpful in defining these patients. Patients with tumors that are pathologically T1 may not need postoperative therapy. Patients with tumors that are T2 or greater have lymph node involvement of 20% or more and require additional therapy, such as radiation and chemotherapy, or more standard surgical resection.[6] Patients with poor histologic features should consider LAR or APR and postoperative treatment as dictated by full surgical staging. The selection of patients for local excision may also be improved by newer imaging techniques, such as endorectal magnetic resonance imaging and endorectal ultrasound.

4. Endocavitary, with or without external beam, radiation in selected patients with tumors less than 3 centimeters in size, with well-differentiated tumors, and without deep ulceration, tumor fixation, or palpable lymph nodes.[7-10] Special equipment and experience are required to achieve results equivalent to surgery.

REFERENCES

1. Bailey HR, Huval WV, Max E, et al. Local excision of carcinoma of the rectum for cure. *Surgery*. 1992;111(5): 555-561.

2. Benson R, Wong CS, Cummings BJ, et al. Local excision and postoperative radiotherapy for distal rectal cancer. *Int J Radiat Oncol Biol Phys*. 2001;50(5):1309-1316.
3. Willett CG, Compton CC, Shellito PC, et al. Selection factors for local excision or abdominoperineal resection of early stage rectal cancer. *Cancer*. 1994;73(11):2716-2720.
4. Russell AH, Harris J, Rosenberg PJ, et al. Anal sphincter conservation for patients with adenocarcinoma of the distal rectum: long-term results of radiation therapy oncology group protocol 89-02. *Int J Radiat Oncol Biol Phys*. 2000;46(2):313-322.
5. Steele GD Jr, Herndon JE, Bleday R, et al. Sphincter-sparing treatment for distal rectal adenocarcinoma. *Ann Surg Oncol*. 1999 Jul-Aug;6(5):433-441.
6. Sitzler PJ, Seow-Choen F, Ho YH, et al. Lymph node involvement and tumor depth in rectal cancers: an analysis of 805 patients. *Dis Colon Rectum*. 1997;40(12): 1472-1476.
7. Sischy B, Graney MJ, Hinson EJ. Endocavitary irradiation for adenocarcinoma of the rectum. *CA Cancer J Clin*. 1984;34(6):333-339.
8. Kodner IJ, Gilley MT, Shemesh EI, et al. Radiation therapy as definitive treatment for selected invasive rectal cancer. *Surgery*. 1993;114(4):850-856; discussion 856-857.
9. Maingon P, Guerif S, Darsouni R, et al. Conservative management of rectal adenocarcinoma by radiotherapy. *Int J Radiat Oncol Biol Phys*. 1998;40(5):1077-1085.
10. Aumock A, Birnbaum EH, Fleshman JW, et al. Treatment of rectal adenocarcinoma with endocavitary and external beam radiotherapy: results for 199 patients with localized tumors. *Int J Radiat Oncol Biol Phys*. 2001;51(2): 363-370.

STAGE II RECTAL CANCER

[Note: Some citations in the text of this section are followed by a level of evidence. The PDQ editorial boards use a formal ranking system to help the reader judge the strength of evidence linked to the reported results of a therapeutic strategy. (Refer to the PDQ summary on *Levels of Evidence* for more information.)]

Stage II (Old Staging: Dukes' B or Modified Astler-Coller B2 and B3)

The uterus, vagina, parametria, ovaries, or prostate are sometimes involved. Studies employing preoperative or postoperative radiation therapy alone have demonstrated decreased locoregional failure rates.[1-3] Significant improvement in overall survival has not been demonstrated with radiation therapy alone except in a single trial of preoperative radiation therapy.[3] [Level of evidence: 1iiA]

A randomized trial by the Gastrointestinal Tumor Study Group demonstrated an increase in both disease-free interval and overall survival when radiation therapy is combined with chemotherapy following surgical resection in patients whose rectal cancer has penetrated through the bowel wall into the perirectal fat (stage II) or has metastasized to regional lymph nodes (stage III).[4] A disease-free survival advantage has been observed in patients with stage II and stage III rectal cancer treated with chemotherapy and radiation therapy compared to those treated with radiation therapy alone.[5] An Intergroup trial has demonstrated a 10% improved survival with the use of continuous-infusion fluorouracil (5-FU) throughout the course of radiation therapy when compared with bolus 5-FU. This method of 5-FU administration should be considered standard.[6] The final results of Intergroup trial 0114 showed no survival benefit with the addition of leucovorin, levamisole, or both, to 5-FU administered postoperatively at a median follow-up of 7.4 years.[7] Clinical trials further addressing 5-FU modulation are underway, including the use of oral 5-FU prodrugs.[8] The radiation should be delivered to high-dose levels (45 Gy to 55 Gy) either preoperatively or postoperatively, with meticulous attention to technique. An analysis of patients treated with postoperative chemotherapy and radiation therapy suggests that these patients may have more chronic bowel dysfunction compared to those who undergo surgical resection alone.[9] Improved radiation planning and techniques can be used to minimize treatment-related complications. These techniques include the use of multiple pelvic fields, prone positioning, customized bowel immobilization molds (belly

boards), bladder distention, visualization of the small bowel through oral contrast, and the incorporation of three-dimensional or comparative treatment planning.[10,11] Late effects of radiation have also been observed in patients receiving preoperative radiation alone with high doses per fraction. Results from the Swedish Rectal Cancer trial suggest an increase in long-term bowel dysfunction in patients treated with short-course, high-dose preoperative radiation therapy when compared to patients treated with surgery alone.[12] Ongoing clinical trials comparing preoperative and postoperative adjuvant chemoradiotherapy should further clarify the impact of either approach on bowel function and other important quality-of-life issues (eg, sphincter preservation) in addition to the more conventional endpoints of disease-free and overall survival.

Standard treatment options:

1. Wide surgical resection and low anterior resection with colorectal or coloanal reanastomosis when feasible, followed by chemotherapy and postoperative radiation therapy, preferably through participation in a clinical trial.[4,5,13-16]

2. Wide surgical resection with abdominoperineal resection with adjuvant chemotherapy and postoperative radiation therapy, preferably through participation in a clinical trial.[13,17-19]

3. Partial or total pelvic exenteration in the uncommon situation where bladder, uterus, vagina, or prostate are invaded, with adjuvant chemotherapy and postoperative radiation therapy, preferably through participation in a clinical trial.

4. Preoperative radiation therapy with

or without chemotherapy followed by surgery with an attempt to preserve sphincter function with subsequent adjuvant chemotherapy, preferably through participation in a clinical trial.[9,20-23]

5. Intraoperative electron beam radiation therapy (IORT) to the sites of residual microscopic or gross residual disease following surgical extirpation can be considered at institutions where the appropriate equipment is available. When combined with external-beam radiation therapy and chemotherapy in highly selected patients, IORT with or without 5-FU has resulted in improved local control in single institution experiences.[24] [Level of evidence: 3iiiDi].[25]

REFERENCES

1. Randomised trial of surgery alone versus radiotherapy followed by surgery for potentially operable locally advanced rectal cancer. Medical Research Council Rectal Cancer Working Party. *Lancet.* 1996;348(9042):1605-1610.
2. Randomised trial of surgery alone versus surgery followed by radiotherapy for mobile cancer of the rectum. Medical Research Council Rectal Cancer Working Party. *Lancet.* 1996;348(9042):1610-1614.
3. Improved survival with preoperative radiotherapy in resectable rectal cancer. Swedish Rectal Cancer Trial. *N Engl J Med.* 1997;336(14):980-987.
4. Thomas PR, Lindblad AS. Adjuvant postoperative radiotherapy and chemotherapy in rectal carcinoma: a review of the Gastrointestinal Tumor Study Group experience. *Radiother Oncol.* 1988;13(4):245-252.
5. Krook JE, Moertel CG, Gunderson LL, et al. Effective surgical adjuvant therapy for high-risk rectal carcinoma. *N Engl J Med.* 1991;324(11):709-715.
6. O'Connell MJ, Martenson JA, Wieand HS, et al. Improving adjuvant therapy for rectal cancer by combining protracted-infusion fluorouracil and radiation therapy after curative surgery. *N Engl J Med.* 1994;331(8):502-507.
7. Tepper JE, O'Connell M, Niedzwiecki D, et al. Adjuvant therapy in rectal cancer: analysis of stage, sex, and local control—final report of intergroup 0114. *J Clin Oncol.* 2002;20(7):1744-1750.
8. Min JS, Kim NK, Park JK, et al. A prospective randomized trial comparing intravenous 5-fluorouracil and oral doxifluridine as postoperative adjuvant treatment for advanced rectal cancer. *Ann Surg Oncol.* 2000;7(9):674-679.
9. Kollmorgen CF, Meagher AP, Wolff BG, et al. The long-term effect of adjuvant postoperative chemoradiotherapy for rectal carcinoma on bowel function. *Ann Surg.* 1994;220(5):676-682.
10. Koelbl O, Richter S, Flentje M. Influence of patient positioning on dose-volume histogram and normal tissue complication probability for small bowel and bladder in patients receiving pelvic irradiation: a prospective study using a 3D planning system and a radiobiological model. *Int J Radiat Oncol Biol Phys.* 1999;45(5):1193-1198.
11. Gunderson LL, Russell AH, Llewellyn HJ, et al. Treatment planning for colorectal cancer: radiation and surgical techniques and value of small-bowel films. *Int J Radiat Oncol Biol Phys.* 1985;11(7):1379-1393
12. Dahlberg M, Glimelius B, Graf W, et al. Preoperative irradiation affects functional results after surgery for rectal cancer: results from a randomized study. *Dis Colon Rectum.* 1998;41(5):543-549; discussion 549-551.
13. NIH consensus conference. Adjuvant therapy for patients with colon and rectal cancer. *JAMA.* 1990;264(11):1444-1450.
14. Moertel CG. Chemotherapy for colorectal cancer. *N Engl J Med.* 1994;330(16):1136-1142.
15. Smalley SR. Southwest Oncology Group: Phase III Randomized Study of Three Different Regimens Containing Fluorouracil in Patients With Stage II or III Rectal Cancer, SWOG-9304, Clinical trial, Closed.
16. Minsky BD, Coia L, Haller DG, et al. Radiation therapy for rectosigmoid and rectal cancer: results of the 1992-1994 Patterns of Care process survey. *J Clin Oncol.* 1998;16(7):2542-2547.
17. Tepper JE, O'Connell MJ, Petroni GR, et al. Adjuvant postoperative fluorouracil-modulated chemotherapy combined with pelvic radiation therapy for rectal cancer: initial results of intergroup 0114. *J Clin Oncol.* 1997;15(5):2030-2039.
18. Wolmark N, Fisher B. An analysis of survival and treatment failure following abdominoperineal and sphincter-saving resection in Dukes' B and C rectal carcinoma. A report of the NSABP clinical trials. National Surgical Adjuvant Breast and Bowel Project. *Ann Surg.* 1986;204(4):480-489.
19. Rougier P, Nordlinger B. Large scale trial for adjuvant treatment in high risk resected colorectal cancers. Rationale to test the combination of loco-regional and systemic chemotherapy and to compare l-leucovorin + 5-FU to levamisole + 5-FU. *Ann Oncol.* 1993;4(Suppl 2):21-28.
20. Mohiuddin M, Regine WF, Marks GJ, et al. High-dose preoperative radiation and the challenge of sphincter-preservation surgery for cancer of the distal 2 cm of the rectum. *Int J Radiat Oncol Biol Phys.* 1998;40(3):569-574.
21. Mohiuddin M, Marks G, Bannon J. High-dose preoperative radiation and full thickness local excision: a new option for selected T3 distal rectal cancers. *Int J Radiat Oncol Biol Phys.* 1994;30(4):845-849.
22. Minsky BD. Radiation Therapy Oncology Group. Phase III Intergroup Randomized Study of Preoperative vs Postoperative Combined 5-FU/CF and Radiotherapy for Resectable Rectal Adenocarcinoma (Summary Last Modified 01/98), RTOG-9401, Clinical trial, Completed.
23. Valentini V, Coco C, Cellini N, et al. Preoperative chemoradiation for extraperitoneal T3 rectal cancer: acute toxicity, tumor response, and sphincter preservation. *Int J Radiat Oncol Biol Phys.* 1998;40(5):1067-1075.
24. Gunderson LL, Nelson H, Martenson JA, et al. Locally advanced primary colorectal cancer: intraoperative electron and external beam irradiation +/- 5-FU. *Int J Radiat Oncol Biol Phys.* 1997;37(3):601-614.
25. Nakfoor BM, Willett CG, Shellito PC, et al. The impact of 5-fluorouracil and intraoperative electron beam radiation therapy on the outcome of patients with locally advanced primary rectal and rectosigmoid cancer. *Ann Surg.* 1998;228(2):194-200.

STAGE III RECTAL CANCER

[Note: Some citations in the text of this section are followed by a level of evidence. The PDQ editorial boards use a formal ranking system to help the reader judge the strength of evidence linked to the reported results of a therapeutic strategy. (Refer to the PDQ summary on *Levels of Evidence* for more information.)]

Stage III (Old Staging: Dukes' C or Modified Astler-Coller C1-C3)

Stage III rectal cancer denotes disease with lymph node involvement. The number of positive lymph nodes affects prognosis: patients with one to three involved nodes have superior survival to those with four or more involved nodes. Studies employing preoperative or postoperative radiation therapy alone have demonstrated decreased locoregional failure rates.[1-3] Significant improvement in overall survival has not been demonstrated with pre- or postoperative radiation therapy alone except in a single trial.[3] [Level of evidence: 1iiA]

A randomized trial by the Gastrointestinal Tumor Study Group demonstrated an increase in both disease-free interval and overall survival when radiation therapy is combined with chemotherapy following surgical resection in patients whose rectal cancer has penetrated through the bowel wall into the perirectal fat (stage II) or has metastasized to regional lymph nodes (stage III).[4] A similar survival advantage has been observed in patients with stage III rectal cancer treated with chemotherapy and radiation therapy compared to those treated with radiation alone.[5,6] These trials were reviewed at the National Institutes of Health Consensus Development Conference, and an advantage for combined-modality therapy with radiation and chemotherapy was confirmed.[6] The chemotherapy associated with these initial studies of successful combined-modality therapy was fluorouracil (5-FU) plus semustine. Subsequent trials confirmed that semustine can be omitted from the combined-modality therapy, and 5-FU alone with radiation therapy should be considered standard treatment.[7,8] An Intergroup trial has demonstrated 10% improved survival with the use of continuous-infusion 5-FU throughout the course of radiation therapy when compared with bolus 5-FU. This, or another modulation of 5-FU with leucovorin, should be considered standard.[9] Clinical trials addressing the use of oral 5-FU prodrugs are ongoing.[10] The radiation should be delivered to high-dose levels (45-55 Gy) either preoperatively or postoperatively, with meticulous attention to technique. An analysis of patients treated with postoperative chemotherapy and radiation therapy suggests that these patients may have more chronic bowel dysfunction compared to those who undergo surgical resection alone.[11] Late effects of radiation have also been observed in patients receiving preoperative radiation alone. Results from the Swedish Rectal Cancer trial suggest an increase in long-term bowel dysfunction in patients treated with short-course, high-dose preoperative radiation therapy when compared to patients treated with surgery alone.[12] Improved radiation planning and techniques can be used to minimize treatment-related complications. These techniques include the use of multiple pelvic fields, prone positioning, customized bowel immobilization molds (belly boards), bladder distention, visualization of the small bowel through oral contrast, and the incorporation of three-dimensional or comparative treatment planning.[13,14] A quality-of-life analysis, however, suggests that the increased early and late toxic effects associated with combined modality therapy are balanced by the decreased morbidity for delayed recurrence and increased survival.[15] [Level of evidence: 1iiA,1iiB,1iiC] Ongoing clinical trials comparing preoperative and postoperative adjuvant chemoradiotherapy should further clarify the impact of either approach on bowel function and other important quality-of-life issues (eg, sphincter preservation) in addition to the more conventional endpoints of disease-free and overall survival.[16]

Standard treatment options:

1. Wide surgical resection and low anterior resection with colorectal or coloanal reanastomosis when feasible, followed by chemotherapy and postoperative radiation therapy, preferably through participation in a clinical trial.[4-6,17,18]

2. Wide surgical resection with abdominoperineal resection with adjuvant chemotherapy and postoperative radiation therapy, preferably through participation in a clinical trial.[6,19-21]

3. Partial or total pelvic exenteration in the uncommon situation where bladder, uterus, vagina, or prostate are invaded, with adjuvant chemotherapy and postoperative radiation therapy, preferably through participation in a clinical trial.

4. Preoperative radiation therapy with or without chemotherapy followed by surgery with an attempt to preserve sphincter function with subsequent adjuvant chemotherapy, preferably through participation in a clinical trial.[22-24]

5. Intraoperative electron beam radiation therapy (IORT) to the sites of residual microscopic or gross residual disease following surgical extirpation can be considered at institutions where the appropriate equipment is available. When combined with external-beam radiation therapy and chemotherapy in highly selected patients, IORT has resulted in improved local control in

a single institution experience.[25] [Level of evidence: 3iiiDi].

6. Palliative chemoradiation.

REFERENCES

1. Randomised trial of surgery alone versus radiotherapy followed by surgery for potentially operable locally advanced rectal cancer. Medical Research Council Rectal Cancer Working Party. *Lancet.* 1996;348(9042):1605-1610.
2. Randomised trial of surgery alone versus surgery followed by radiotherapy for mobile cancer of the rectum. Medical Research Council Rectal Cancer Working Party. *Lancet.* 1996;348(9042):1610-1614.
3. Improved survival with preoperative radiotherapy in resectable rectal cancer. Swedish Rectal Cancer Trial. *N Engl J Med.* 1997;336(14):980-987.
4. Thomas PR, Lindblad AS. Adjuvant postoperative radiotherapy and chemotherapy in rectal carcinoma: a review of the Gastrointestinal Tumor Study Group experience. *Radiother Oncol.* 1988;13(4):245-252.
5. Krook JE, Moertel CG, Gunderson LL, et al. Effective surgical adjuvant therapy for high-risk rectal carcinoma. *N Engl J Med.* 1991;324(11):709-715.
6. NIH consensus conference. Adjuvant therapy for patients with colon and rectal cancer. *JAMA.* 1990;264(11):1444-1450.
7. O'Connell M, Wieand H, Krook J, et al. Lack of value for methyl-CCNU (MeCCNU) as a component of effective rectal cancer surgical adjuvant therapy: interim analysis of intergroup protocol 86-47-51. [Abstract] Proceedings of the *American Society of Clinical Oncology.* 1991;10:A-403, 134.
8. Radiation therapy and fluorouracil with or without semustine for the treatment of patients with surgical adjuvant adenocarcinoma of the rectum. Gastrointestinal Tumor Study Group. *J Clin Oncol.* 1992;10(4):549-557.
9. O'Connell MJ, Martenson JA, Wieand HS, et al. Improving adjuvant therapy for rectal cancer by combining protracted-infusion fluorouracil with radiation therapy after curative surgery. *N Engl J Med.* 1994;331(8):502-507.
10. Min JS, Kim NK, Park JK, et al. A prospective randomized trial comparing intravenous 5-fluorouracil and oral doxifluridine as postoperative adjuvant treatment for advanced rectal cancer. *Ann Surg Oncol.* 2000;7(9):674-679.
11. Kollmorgen CF, Meagher AP, Wolff BG, et al. The long-term effect of adjuvant postoperative chemoradiotherapy for rectal carcinoma on bowel function. *Ann Surg.* 1994; 220(5):676-682.
12. Dahlberg M, Glimelius B, Graf W, et al. Preoperative irradiation affects functional results after surgery for rectal cancer: results from a randomized study. *Dis Colon Rectum.* 1998;41(5):543-549; discussion 549-551.
13. Koelbl O, Richter S, Flentje M. Influence of patient positioning on dose-volume histogram and normal tissue complication probability for small bowel and bladder in patients receiving pelvic irradiation: a prospective study using a 3D planning system and a radiobiological model. *Int J Radiat Oncol Biol Phys.* 1999;45(5):1193-1104.
14. Gunderson LL, Russell AH, Llewellyn HJ, et al. Treatment planning for colorectal cancer: radiation and surgical techniques and value of small-bowel films. *Int J Radiat Oncol Biol Phys.* 1985;11(7):1379-1393.
15. Gelber RD, Goldhirsch A, Cole BF, et al. A quality-adjusted time without symptoms or toxicity (Q-TWiST) analysis of adjuvant radiation therapy and chemotherapy for resectable rectal cancer. *J Natl Cancer Inst.* 1996;88(15):1039-1045.
16. Wolmark N, National Surgical Adjuvant Breast and Bowel Project: Phase III Randomized Study of Preoperative vs Postoperative 5-FU/CF/Radiotherapy in Patients with Operable Adenocarcinoma of the Rectum (Summary Last Modified 09/1999), NSABP-R-03, Clinical trial, Closed.

17. Moertel CG. Chemotherapy for colorectal cancer. *N Engl J Med.* 1994;330(16):1136-1142.
18. Smalley SR. Southwest Oncology Group: Phase III Randomized Study of Three Different Regimens Containing Fluorouracil in Patients With Stage II or III Rectal Cancer, SWOG-9304, Clinical trial, Closed.
19. Tepper JE, O'Connell MJ, Petroni GR, et al. Adjuvant postoperative fluorouracil-modulated chemotherapy combined with pelvic radiation therapy for rectal cancer: initial results of intergroup 0114. *J Clin Oncol.* 1997;15(5): 2030-2039.
20. Wolmark N, Fisher B. An analysis of survival and treatment failure following abdominoperineal and sphincter-saving resection in Dukes' B and C rectal carcinoma. A report of the NSABP clinical trials. National Surgical Adjuvant Breast and Bowel Project. *Ann Surg.* 1986;204 (4):480-489.
21. Rougier P, Nordlinger B. Large scale trial for adjuvant treatment in high risk resected colorectal cancers. Rationale to test the combination of loco-regional and systemic chemotherapy and to compare l-leucovorin + 5-FU to levamisole + 5-FU. *Ann Oncol.* 1993;4(Suppl 2):21-28.
22. Mohiuddin M, Regine WF, Marks GJ, et al. High-dose preoperative radiation and the challenge of sphincter-preservation surgery for cancer of the distal 2 cm of the rectum. *Int J Radiat Oncol Biol Phys.* 1998;40(3):569-574.
23. Minsky BD, Radiation Therapy Oncology Group: Phase III Intergroup Randomized Study of Preoperative vs Postoperative Combined 5-FU/CF and Radiotherapy for Resectable Rectal Adenocarcinoma (Summary Last Modified 01/98), RTOG-9401, Clinical trial, Completed.
24. Valentini V, Coco C, Cellini N, et al. Preoperative chemoradiation for extraperitoneal T3 rectal cancer: acute toxicity, tumor response, and sphincter preservation. *Int J Radiat Oncol Biol Phys.* 1998;40(5):1067-1075.
25. Gunderson LL, Nelson H, Martenson JA, et al. Locally advanced primary colorectal cancer: intraoperative electron and external beam irradiation +/- 5-FU. *Int J Radiat Oncol Biol Phys.* 1997;37(3):601-614.

STAGE IV RECTAL CANCER

Note: Some citations in the text of this section are followed by a level of evidence. The PDQ editorial boards use a formal ranking system to help the reader judge the strength of evidence linked to the reported results of a therapeutic strategy. (Refer to the PDQ summary on *Levels of Evidence* for more information.)]

Stage IV (Old Staging: Modified Astler-Coller D)

Stage IV rectal cancer denotes distant metastatic disease. Local regional approaches to treating liver metastases include hepatic resection and/or intraarterial administration of chemotherapy with implantable infusion ports or pumps. For patients with limited (three or less) hepatic metastases, resection may be considered with five-year survival rates of 20% to 40%.[1-7] Other local ablative techniques that have been used to manage liver metastases include cryosurgery, embolization, and interstitial radiation therapy.[8,9] For those patients with hepatic metastases deemed unresectable (due to such factors as location, distribution, and excess number), cryosurgical ablation has been associated with long term tumor control.[10] Prognostic variables that predict a favorable outcome for cryotherapy are similar to those for hepatic resection, and include low preoperative carcinoembryonic antigen level, absence of extrahepatic disease, negative margins, and lymph node negative primary.[11] [Level of evidence: 3iiiA] Patients with limited pulmonary metastases, and patients with both pulmonary and hepatic metastases, may also be considered for surgical resection, with five-year survival possible in highly selected patients.[7,12,13] The role of additional systemic therapy after potentially curative resection of liver metastases is uncertain. A trial of hepatic arterial floxuridine plus systemic fluorouracil (5-FU) plus leucovorin was shown to result in improved two-year disease-free and overall survival (86% versus 72%, P=.03), but did not show a significant statistical difference in medial survival, compared to systemic 5-FU therapy alone.[14] [Level of evidence: 1iiA] Further follow-up is required to confirm these findings and to determine whether more effective combination chemotherapy alone may provide similar results compared to hepatic intra-arterial therapy plus systemic treatment.

Hepatic intraarterial chemotherapy with floxuridine for liver metastases has produced higher overall response rates but no improvement in survival when compared to systemic chemotherapy.[15-20] Controversy regarding the efficacy of regional chemotherapy has led to initiation of a large multicenter phase III trial (CALGB-9481) of hepatic arterial infusion versus systemic chemotherapy. Several studies show increased local toxic effects with hepatic infusional therapy, including liver function abnormalities and fatal biliary sclerosis.

In stage IV and recurrent rectal cancer, chemotherapy has been used for palliation with 5-FU-based treatment and is considered to be standard therapy.[21-23] 5-FU has been shown to be more cytotoxic, with increased response rates, but with variable effects on survival when modulated by leucovorin[24-30] or methotrexate.[31,32] Randomized clinical trials show that interferon alfa appears to add toxic effects but no clinical benefit to 5-FU therapy.[33,34] Continuous-infusion 5-FU regimens have also resulted in increased response rates in some studies, with a modest benefit in median survival.[35] The benefits of continuous-infusion 5-FU compared to bolus regimens have been summarized in a meta-analysis.[36] Oral regimens using prodrugs of 5-FU or inhibitors of dihydropyrimidine dehydrogenase (DPD) pharmacologically simulate continuous infusion and are under clinical evaluation.[37] The choice of a 5-FU-based chemotherapy regimen for an individual patient should be based on known response rates and toxic effects profile of the chosen regimen, as well as cost and quality-of-life issues.[38,39] In a meta-analysis of 1,219 patients in randomized trials where patients were assigned to receive 5-FU with or without leucovorin via either continuous infusion or bolus, neutropenia was noted in 4% of patients who received continuous infusion versus 31% of patients who received bolus and hand-foot syndrome was found in 34% of patients who received continuous infusion versus 13% of patients who received bolus. All other toxic effects were noted with similar frequency and severity, regardless of continuous infusion or bolus administration.[40]

DPD is the rate-limiting enzyme in the degradation pathway for 5-FU. While genetic polymorphism commonly results in considerable individual variability in levels of this enzyme, between 0.5% and 3% of the population are severely DPD deficient. Severe mucositis, neutropenia, diarrhea, and cerebellar dysfunction can result in toxic deaths among patients who are DPD deficient. Standard testing for DPD deficiency is not widely available, but one study found that patients with a pretreatment ratio of dihydrouracil to uracil of 1.8 or less were at risk of increased 5-FU toxic effects.[41-43]

Irinotecan (CPT-11) is a topoisomerase-I inhibitor with a 10% to 20% partial response rate in patients with metastatic rectal cancer, in patients who have received no prior chemotherapy, and in patients progressing on 5-FU therapy.[44,45] It is now considered standard therapy for patients with stage IV disease who do not respond to or progress on 5-FU.[46]

CPT-11 has been compared to either retreatment with 5-FU or best supportive care in a pair of randomized European trials of patients with colorectal cancer refractory to 5-FU.[47,48] [Level of evidence: 1iiA,1iiC]

Two phase III prospective randomized, controlled trials were designed to evaluate the combination of 5-FU, leucovorin, and CPT-11 to 5-FU and leucovorin alone. The first of these trials compared the bolus 5-FU, leucovorin, and CPT-11 to bolus 5-FU and leucovorin alone and to CPT-11; the primary endpoint was progression-free survival.[49] The trial demonstrated significant benefit in terms of confirmed response rates, time-to-tumor progression, and overall survival.[49] [Level of evidence: 1iiA] The combination treatment showed confirmed responses in 39% of patients, compared with 21% in patients treated with 5-FU and leucovorin alone and 18% in patients treated with CPT-11. This benefit was highly significant in favor of the combination. In addition, time-to-tumor progression was significantly prolonged with the combination (7.0 vs. 4.3 months, P=.004). Median survival was also improved with the combination; median survival was 14.8 months for patients on the combination arm and 12.6 months for patients on the 5-FU and leucovorin arm (P=.042).

The second pivotal trial of combination chemotherapy with CPT-11 compared two different regimens of infusional 5-FU and folinic acid (either the AIO [Arbeitsgemeinschaft Internische Onkologie] or the deGramont regimen).[50] Either weekly or biweekly CPT-11 was administered according to the schedule of the infusional 5-FU. This trial also demonstrated improvements in response rate, time-to-tumor progression, and median survival. For the most important endpoint, median survival, the combination arm was associated with a median survival of 17.4 months, compared with 14.1 months for the 5-FU and folinic acid arm (P=.032).[50] [Level of evidence: 1iiA] A combined analysis of the sur-

vival advantages seen in these two trials was presented at the 2000 American Society of Clinical Oncology meeting.[51] The combined survival for the combination of CPT-11, 5-FU, and leucovorin was 15.9 months, compared to 13.3 months for the non-CPT-11 regimen (P=.003). This represents a survival hazard ratio of 0.79.

Another drug, raltitrexed (Tomudex), is a specific thymidylate synthase inhibitor that has demonstrated activity similar to that of bolus 5-FU and leucovorin.[52] [Level of evidence: 1iiA][53] A number of other drugs are undergoing evaluation for the treatment of rectal cancer.[54]

Oxaliplatin, alone or combined with 5-FU and leucovorin, has shown promising activity in previously treated and untreated patients with metastatic colorectal cancer and in patients with 5-FU refractory disease.[55-57] One multicenter trial reported a response rate of 21%, a median progression-free survival of five months, and a median survival of 11 months.[58] Overall survival from the start of first-line chemotherapy was 19 months. In this trial, oxaliplatin was given first, followed by 48-hour infusion of 5-FU, with short leucovorin infusion.

The data and safety monitoring committees of the cooperative groups conducting studies comparing the value of 5-FU/leucovorin/CPT-11 to 5-FU/leucovorin in the adjuvant setting, and comparing the value to 5-FU/leucovorin/oxaliplatin or oxaliplatin/CPT-11 in the advanced disease setting, have suspended accrual to these trials because of an unexpectedly high death rate on the 5-FU/leucovorin/CPT-11 arms.[59] This three-drug regimen appears to be more toxic than initially reported. The majority of deaths in both studies were observed in the first 60 days, usually during the first chemotherapy cycle. This may imply increased sensitivity in a minority of patients, possibly based on genetic differences in key steps in the metabolic activation/deactivation of irinotecan, 5-FU, or both agents. Additional analyses may provide guidance in dose adjustment for the initial cycle and/or in patient selection. For the present, the use of this regimen should be accompanied by careful attention to early signs of diarrhea, dehydration, neutropenia, or other toxic effects, especially during the first chemotherapy cycle.

Standard treatment options:

1. Surgical resection/anastomosis or bypass of obstructing lesions in selected cases or resection for palliation.[60]

2. Surgical resection of isolated metastases (liver, lung, ovaries).[1,3,15,61-64]

3. Chemoradiation for local palliation.[65,66]

4. Chemotherapy alone for distant disease after resection of local disease.

5. Clinical trials evaluating new drugs and biologic therapy.

REFERENCES

1. Scheele J, Stangl R, Altendorf-Hofmann A. Hepatic metastases from colorectal carcinoma: impact of surgical resection on the natural history. *Br J Surg.* 1990;77(11):1241-1246.
2. Steele G Jr, Bleday R, Mayer RJ, et al. A prospective evaluation of hepatic resection for colorectal carcinoma metastases to the liver: Gastrointestinal Tumor Study Group Protocol 6584. *J Clin Oncol.* 1991;9(7):1105-1112.
3. Scheele J, Stangl R, Altendorf-Hofmann A, et al. Indicators of prognosis after hepatic resection for colorectal secondaries. *Surgery.* 1991;110(1):13-29.
4. Pedersen IK, Burcharth F, Roikjaer O, et al. Resection of liver metastases from colorectal cancer. Indications and results. *Dis Colon Rectum* 1994;37(11):1078-1082.
5. Harmon KE, Ryan JA Jr, Biehl TR, et al. Benefits and safety of hepatic resection for colorectal metastases. *Am J Surg.* 1999;177(5):402-404.
6. Fong Y, Cohen AM, Fortner JG, et al. Liver resection for colorectal metastases. *J Clin Oncol.* 1997;15(3):938-946.
7. Headrick JR, Miller DL, Nagorney DM, et al.: Surgical treatment of hepatic and pulmonary metastases from colon cancer. *Ann Thorac Surg.* 2001;71(3):975-979; discussion 979-980.
8. Thomas DS, Nauta RJ, Rodgers JE, et al. Intraoperative high-dose rate interstitial irradiation of hepatic metastases from colorectal carcinoma. Results of a phase I-II trial. *Cancer.* 1993;71(6):1977-1981.
9. Ravikumar TS. Interstitial therapies for liver tumors. *Surg Oncol Clin N Am.* 1996;5(2):365-377.
10. Ravikumar TS, Kaleya R, Kishinevsky A. Surgical ablative therapy of liver tumors. *Cancer: Principles and Practice of Oncology Updates.* 2000;14(3):1-12.
11. Seifert JK, Morris DL. Prognostic factors after cryotherapy for hepatic metastases from colorectal cancer. *Ann Surg.* 1998;228(2):201-208.
12. McAfee MK, Allen MS, Trastek VF, et al. Colorectal lung metastases: results of surgical excision. *Ann Thorac Surg.* 1992;53(5):780-785; discussion 785-786.
13. Girard P, Ducreux M, Baldeyrou P, et al. Surgery for lung metastases from colorectal cancer: analysis of prognostic factors. *J Clin Oncol.* 1996;14(7):2047-2053.
14. Kemeny N, Huang Y, Cohen AM, et al. Hepatic arterial infusion of chemotherapy after resection of hepatic metastases from colorectal cancer. *N Engl J Med.* 1999;341 (27):2039-2048.
15. Wagman LD, Kemeny MM, Leong L, et al. A prospective, randomized evaluation of the treatment of colorectal cancer metastatic to the liver. *J Clin Oncol.* 1990;8(11):1885-1893.
16. Kemeny N, Daly J, Reichman B, et al. Intrahepatic or systemic infusion of fluorodeoxyuridine in patients with liver metastases from colorectal carcinoma. A randomized trial. *Ann Intern Med.* 1987;107(4):459-465.
17. Chang AE, Schneider PD, Sugarbaker PH, et al. A prospective randomized trial of regional versus systemic continuous 5-fluorodeoxyuridine chemotherapy in the treatment of colorectal liver metastases. *Ann Surg.* 1987; 206(6):685-693.
18. Rougier P, Laplanche A, Huguier M, et al. Hepatic arterial infusion of floxuridine in patients with liver metastases from colorectal carcinoma: long-term results of a prospective randomized trial. *J Clin Oncol.* 1992;10(7):1112-1118.
19. Reappraisal of hepatic arterial infusion in the treatment of nonresectable liver metastases from colorectal cancer. Meta-Analysis Group in Cancer. *J Natl Cancer Inst.* 1996; 88(5):252-258.
20. Kemeny N, Cohen A, Seiter K, et al. Randomized trial of hepatic arterial floxuridine, mitomycin, and carmustine versus floxuridine alone in previously treated patients with liver metastases from colorectal cancer. *J Clin Oncol.* 1993;11(2):330-335.
21. Moertel CG. Chemotherapy for colorectal cancer. *N Engl J Med.* 1994;330 (16): 1136-1142.
22. Schmoll HJ, Büchele T, Grothey A, et al. Where do we stand with 5-fluorouracil? *Semin Oncol.* 1999;26(6):589-605.
23. Grothey A, Schmoll HJ. New chemotherapy approaches in colorectal cancer. *Curr Opin Oncol.* 2001;13(4):275-286.
24. Poon MA, O'Connell MJ, Wieand HS, et al. Biochemical modulation of fluorouracil with leucovorin: confirmatory evidence of improved therapeutic efficacy in advanced colorectal cancer. *J Clin Oncol.* 1991;9(11):1967-1972.
25. Valone FH, Friedman MA, Wittlinger PS, et al. Treatment of patients with advanced colorectal carcinomas with fluorouracil alone, high-dose leucovorin plus fluorouracil, or sequential methotrexate, fluorouracil, and leucovorin: a randomized trial of the Northern California Oncology Group. *J Clin Oncol.* 1989;7(10):1427-1436.
26. Petrelli N, Douglass HO Jr, Herrera L, et al. The modulation of fluorouracil with leucovorin in metastatic colorectal carcinoma: a prospective randomized phase III trial. Gastrointestinal Tumor Study Group. *J Clin Oncol.* 1989; 7(10):1419-1426.
27. Erlichman C, Fine S, Wong A, et al. A randomized trial of fluorouracil and folinic acid in patients with metastatic colorectal carcinoma. *J Clin Oncol.* 1988;6(3):469-475.
28. Doroshow JH, Multhauf P, Leong L, et al. Prospective randomized comparison of fluorouracil versus fluorouracil and high-dose continuous infusion leucovorin calcium for

the treatment of advanced measurable colorectal cancer in patients previously unexposed to chemotherapy. *J Clin Oncol.* 1990;8(3):491-501.

29. Buroker TR, O'Connell MJ, Wieand HS, et al. Randomized comparison of two schedules of fluorouracil and leucovorin in the treatment of advanced colorectal cancer. *J Clin Oncol.* 1994;12(1):14-20.

30. Jäger E, Heike M, Bernhard H, et al. Weekly high-dose leucovorin versus low-dose leucovorin combined with fluorouracil in advanced colorectal cancer: results of a randomized multicenter trial. Study Group for Palliative Treatment of Metastatic Colorectal Cancer Study Protocol 1. *J Clin Oncol.* 1996;14(8):2274-2279.

31. Meta-analysis of randomized trials testing the biochemical modulation of fluorouracil by methotrexate in metastatic colorectal cancer. Advanced Colorectal Cancer Meta-Analysis Project. *J Clin Oncol.* 1994;12(5):960-969.

32. Blijham G, Wagener T, Wils J, et al. Modulation of high-dose infusional fluorouracil by low-dose methotrexate in patients with advanced or metastatic colorectal cancer: final results of a randomized European Organization for Research and Treatment of Cancer Study. *J Clin Oncol.* 1996;14(8):2266-2273.

33. Kosmidis PA, Tsavaris N, Skarlos D, et al. Fluorouracil and leucovorin with or without interferon alfa-2b in advanced colorectal cancer: analysis of a prospective randomized phase III trial. Hellenic Cooperative Oncology Group. *J Clin Oncol.* 1996.14(10):2682-2687.

34. Greco FA, Figlin R, York M, et al. Phase III randomized study to compare interferon alfa-2a in combination with fluorouracil versus fluorouracil alone in patients with advanced colorectal cancer. *J Clin Oncol.* 1996;14(10):2674-2681.

35. Hansen RM, Ryan L, Anderson T, et al. Phase III study of bolus versus infusion fluorouracil with or without cisplatin in advanced colorectal cancer. *J Natl Cancer Inst.* 1996;88(10):668-674.

36. Efficacy of intravenous continuous infusion of fluorouracil compared with bolus administration in advanced colorectal cancer. Meta-analysis Group in Cancer. *J Clin Oncol.* 1998;16(1):301-308.

37. Hoff PM, Royce M, Medgyesy D, et al. Oral fluoropyrimidines. *Semin Oncol.* 1999;26(6):640-646.

38. Leichman CG, Fleming TR, Muggia FM, et al. Phase II study of fluorouracil and its modulation in advanced colorectal cancer: a Southwest Oncology Group study. *J Clin Oncol.* 1995;13(6):1303-1311.

39. Twelves C, Boyer M, Findlay M, et al. Capecitabine (Xeloda) improves medical resource use compared with 5-fluorouracil plus leucovorin in a phase III trial conducted in patients with advanced colorectal carcinoma. *Eur J Cancer.* 2001; 37(5):597-604.

40. Toxicity of fluorouracil in patients with advanced colorectal cancer: effect of administration schedule and prognostic factors. Meta-Analysis Group in Cancer. *J Clin Oncol.* 1998;16(11):3537-3541.

41. Gamelin E, Boisdron-Celle M, Guérin-Meyer V, et al. Correlation between uracil and dihydrouracil plasma ratio, fluorouracil (5-FU) pharmacokinetic parameters, and tolerance in patients with advanced colorectal cancer: A potential interest for predicting 5-FU toxicity and determining optimal 5-FU dosage. *J Clin Oncol.* 1999;17(4): 1105.

42. Morrison GB, Bastian A, Dela Rosa T, et al. Dihydropyrimidine dehydrogenase deficiency: a pharmacogenetic defect causing severe adverse reactions to 5-fluorouracil-based chemotherapy. *Oncol Nurs Forum.* 1997 Jan-Feb;24(1):83-88.

43. Diasio RB. Clinical implications of dihydropyrimidine dehydrogenase inhibition. *Oncology.* (Huntingt). 1999:13 (7 Suppl 3):17-21.

44. Rothenberg ML, Eckardt JR, Kuhn JG, et al. Phase II trial of irinotecan in patients with progressive or rapidly recurrent colorectal cancer. *J Clin Oncol.* 1996;14(4):1128-1235.

45. Conti JA, Kemeny NE, Saltz LB, et al. Irinotecan is an active agent in untreated patients with metastatic colorectal cancer. *J Clin Oncol.* 1996;14(3):709-715.

46. Cunningham D, Pyrhonen S, James RD, et al. A phase III multicenter randomized study of CPT-11 versus supportive care (SC) alone in patients (Pts) with 5FU-resistant metastatic colorectal cancer (MCRC).

[Abstract] *Proceedings of the American Society of Clinical Oncology.* 1998;17:A-1, 1a.

47. Rougier P, Van Cutsem E, Bajetta E, et al. Randomised trial of irinotecan versus fluorouracil by continuous infusion after fluorouracil failure in patients with metastatic colorectal cancer. *Lancet.* 1998;352(9138):1407-1412.

48. Cunningham D, Pyrhönen S, James RD, et al. Randomised trial of irinotecan plus supportive care versus supportive care alone after fluorouracil failure for patients with metastatic colorectal cancer. *Lancet.* 1998; 352(9138):1413-1418.

49. Saltz LB, Cox JV, Blanke C, et al. Irinotecan plus fluorouracil and leucovorin for metastatic colorectal cancer. Irinotecan Study Group. *N Engl J Med.* 2000;343(13): 905-914.

50. Douillard JY, Cunningham D, Roth AD, et al. Irinotecan combined with fluorouracil compared with fluorouracil alone as first-line treatment for metastatic colorectal cancer: a multicentre randomised trial. *Lancet.* 2000;355 (9209):1041-1047.

51. Saltz LB, Douillard J, Pirotta N, et al. Combined analysis of two phase III randomized trials comparing irinotecan (C), fluorouracil (F), leucovorin (L) vs F alone as first-line therapy of previously untreated metastatic colorectal cancer (MCRC). [Abstract] *Proceedings of the American Society of Clinical Oncology.* 2000;19:A-938, 242a.

52. Cunningham D. Mature results from three large controlled studies with raltitrexed ('Tomudex'). *Br J Cancer.* 1998;77(Suppl 2):15-21.

53. Cocconi G, Cunningham D, Van Cutsem E, et al. Open, randomized, multicenter trial of raltitrexed versus fluorouracil plus high-dose leucovorin in patients with advanced colorectal cancer. Tomudex Colorectal Cancer Study Group. *J Clin Oncol.* 1998;16(9):2943-2952.

54. Von Hoff DD. Promising new agents for treatment of patients with colorectal cancer. *Semin Oncol.* 1998;25(5 Suppl 11):47-52.

55. de Gramont A, Vignoud J, Tournigand C, et al. Oxaliplatin with high-dose leucovorin and 5-fluorouracil 48-hour continuous infusion in pretreated metastatic colorectal cancer. *Eur J Cancer.* 1997;33(2):214-219.

56. Bleiberg H, de Gramont A. Oxaliplatin plus 5-fluorouracil: clinical experience in patients with advanced colorectal cancer. *Semin Oncol.* 1998;25(2 Suppl 5):32-39.

57. Cvitkovic E, Bekradda M. Oxaliplatin: a new therapeutic option in colorectal cancer. *Semin Oncol.* 1999;26(6): 647-662.

58. André T, Bensmaine MA, Louvet C, et al. Multicenter phase II study of bimonthly high-dose leucovorin, fluorouracil infusion, and oxaliplatin for metastatic colorectal cancer resistant to the same leucovorin and fluorouracil regimen. *J Clin Oncol.* 1999;17(11):3560-3568.

59. Sargent DJ, Niedzwiecki D, O'Connell MJ, et al. Recommendation for caution with irinotecan, fluorouracil, and leucovorin for colorectal cancer. *N Engl J Med.* 2001; 345(2):144-145; discussion 146.

60. Wanebo HJ, Koness RJ, Vezeridis MP, et al. Pelvic resection of recurrent rectal cancer. *Ann Surg.* 1994;220(4):586-595; discussion 595-597.

61. Adson MA, van Heerden JA, Adson MH, et al. Resection of hepatic metastases from colorectal cancer. *Arch Surg.* 1984; 119(6):647-651.

62. Coppa GF, Eng K, Ranson JH, et al. Hepatic resection for metastatic colon and rectal cancer. An evaluation of preoperative and postoperative factors. *Ann Surg.* 1985;202 (2):203-208.

63. Taylor M, Forster J, Langer B, et al. A study of prognostic factors for hepatic resection for colorectal metastases. *Am J Surg.* 1997;173(6):467-471.

64. Jaeck D, Bachellier P, Guiguet M, et al. Long-term survival following resection of colorectal hepatic metastases. Association Française de Chirurgie. *Br J Surg.* 1997;84 (7):977-980.

65. Wong CS, Cummings BJ, Brierley JD, et al. Treatment of locally recurrent rectal carcinoma—results and prognostic factors. *Int J Radiat Oncol Biol Phys.* 1998;40(2):427-435.

66. Crane CH, Janjan NA, Abbruzzese JL, et al. Effective pelvic symptom control using initial chemoradiation without colostomy in metastatic rectal cancer. *Int J Radiat Oncol Biol Phys.* 2001;49(1):107-116.

RECURRENT RECTAL CANCER

[Note: Some citations in the text of this section are followed by a level of evidence. The PDQ editorial boards use a formal ranking system to help the reader judge the strength of evidence linked to the reported results of a therapeutic strategy. (Refer to the PDQ summary on *Levels of Evidence* for more information.)]

Locally recurrent rectal cancer may be resectable, particularly if an inadequate prior operation was performed. For patients with local recurrence alone following initial attempted curative resection, aggressive local therapy with repeat low anterior resection and coloanal anastomosis, abdominoperineal resection, or posterior or total pelvic exenteration can lead to long-term disease-free survival.[1] The use of induction chemoradiation for previously nonirradiated patients with locally advanced (pelvic side-wall, sacral, and/or adjacent organ involvement) pelvic recurrence may increase resectability and allow for sphincter preservation.[2,3] Intraoperative radiation therapy in patients who received previous external beam radiation may improve local control in patients with locally recurrent disease with acceptable morbidity.[4] The presence of hydronephrosis associated with recurrence appears to be a contraindication to surgery with curative intent.[5] Patients with limited pulmonary metastases and patients with both pulmonary and hepatic metastases may also be considered for surgical resection, with five-year survival possible in highly selected patients.[6-8]

In stage IV and recurrent rectal cancer, chemotherapy has been used for palliation with fluorouracil (5-FU)-based treatment and is considered to be standard therapy.[9,10] 5-FU has been shown to be more cytotoxic, with increased response rates but with variable effects on survival, when modulated by leucovorin,[11-17] methotrexate,[18] or other agents.[19-23] Interferon alfa appears to add toxic effects but no clinical benefit to 5-FU therapy.[24,25] Continuous-infusion 5-FU regimens have also resulted in increased response rates in some studies, with a modest benefit in median survival.[26] The benefits of continuous-infusion 5-FU compared to bolus regimens have been summarized in a meta-analysis.[27] Oral regimens using prodrugs of 5-FU or inhibitors of DPD pharmacologically simulate continuous infusion and are under clinical evaluation.[28] The choice of a 5-FU-based chemotherapy regimen for an individual patient should be based on known response rates and toxic effects profile of the chosen regimen, as well as cost and quality-of-life issues.[29,30] Innovative ways of altering toxic effects patterns, and potentially improving clinical benefit, include chronomodulated therapy, in which drug doses are varied throughout the day to allow for greater dose intensity without increased toxic effects.[31,32] In a meta-analysis of 1,219 patients in randomized trials where patients were assigned to receive 5-FU with or without leucovorin via either continuous infusion or bolus, neutropenia was noted in 4% of patients who received continuous infusion versus 31% of patients who received bolus and hand-foot syndrome was found in 34% of patients who received continuous infusion versus 13% of patients who received bolus. All other toxic effects were noted with similar frequency and severity, regardless of continuous infusion or bolus administration.[33]

Irinotecan (CPT-11) is a topoisomerase-I inhibitor with a 10% to 20% partial response rate in patients with metastatic rectal cancer, in patients who have received no prior chemotherapy, and in patients progressing on 5-FU therapy.[34,35] Irinotecan is now considered standard therapy for patients with stage IV disease who do not respond to or progress on 5-FU.[36]

CPT-11 has been compared to either retreatment with 5-FU or best supportive care in a pair of randomized European trials of patients with colorectal cancer refractory to 5-FU.[37,38] [Level of evidence: 1iiA,1iiC]

Two phase III prospective randomized, controlled trials were designed to evaluate the combination of 5-FU, leucovorin, and CPT-11 to 5-FU and leucovorin alone. The first of these trials compared the bolus 5-FU, leucovorin, and CPT-11 to bolus 5-FU and leucovorin alone and to CPT-11; the primary endpoint was progression-free survival.[39] The trial demonstrated significant benefit in terms of confirmed response rates, time-to-tumor progression, and overall survival.[39] [Level of evidence: 1iiA] The combination treatment showed confirmed responses in 39% of patients, compared with 21% in patients treated with 5-FU and leucovorin alone and 18% in patients treated with CPT-11. This benefit was highly significant in favor of the combination. In addition, time-to-tumor progression was significantly prolonged with the combination (7.0 vs. 4.3 months, $P=.004$). Median survival was also improved with the combination; median survival was 14.8 months for patients on the combination arm and 12.6 months for patients on the 5-FU and leucovorin arm ($P=.042$).

The second pivotal trial of combination chemotherapy with CPT-11 compared two different regimens of infusional 5-FU and folinic acid (either the AIO [Arbeitsgemeinschaft Internische Onkologie] or the deGramont regimen).[40] Either weekly or biweekly CPT-11 was administered according to the schedule of the infusional 5-FU. This trial also demonstrated improvements in response rate, time-to-tumor progression, and median survival. For the most important endpoint, median survival, the combination arm was associated with a median survival of 17.4 months, compared with 14.1 months for the 5-FU and folinic acid arm ($P=.032$).[40] [Level of evidence: 1iiA] A combined analysis of the survival advantages seen in these two trials was presented at the 2000 American Society of Clinical Oncology meeting.[41] The combined survival for the combination of CPT-11, 5-FU, and leucovorin was 15.9 months, compared to 13.3 months for the non-CPT-11 regimen ($P=.003$). This represents a survival hazard ratio of 0.79.

Another drug, raltitrexed (Tomudex), is a specific thymidylate synthase inhibitor which has demonstrated activity similar to that of bolus 5-FU and leucovorin.[42] [Level of evidence: 1iiA][43] A number of other drugs are undergoing evaluation for the treatment of rectal cancer.[44]

Oxaliplatin, alone or combined with 5-FU and leucovorin, has shown promising activity in previously treated and untreated patients with metastatic colorectal cancer and in patients with 5-FU refractory disease.[45-47] One multicenter trial reported a response rate of 21%, a median progression-free survival of five months, and a median survival of 11 months.[48] Overall survival from the start of first-line chemotherapy was 19 months. In this trial, oxaliplatin was given first, followed by 48-hour infusion of 5-FU, with short leucovorin infusion.

The data and safety monitoring committees of the cooperative groups conducting studies comparing the value of 5-FU/leucovorin/CPT-11 to 5-FU/leucovorin in the adjuvant setting, and comparing the value to 5-FU/leucovorin/oxaliplatin or oxaliplatin/CPT-11 in the advanced disease setting have suspended accrual to these trials because of an unexpectedly high death rate on the 5-FU/leucovorin/CPT-11 arms.[49] This three-drug regimen appears to be more toxic than initially reported. The majority of deaths in both studies were observed in the first 60 days, usually during the first chemotherapy cycle. This may imply increased sensitivity in a minority of patients, possibly based on genetic differences in key steps in the metabolic activation/deactivation of irinotecan, 5-FU, or both agents. Additional analyses may provide guidance in dose adjustment for the initial cycle and/or in patient selection. For the present, the use of this regimen should be accompanied by careful attention to early signs of diarrhea, dehydration, neutropenia, or other toxic effects, especially during the first chemotherapy cycle.

Standard treatment options:

1. Resection of locally recurrent rectal cancer may be palliative or curative in selected patients.[50]
2. Resection of liver metastases in selected patients (five-year cure rate with resection of solitary metastases exceeds 20%).[37,51-56]
3. Resection of isolated pulmonary or ovarian metastases.
4. Palliative radiation therapy.[4,38]
5. Palliative chemotherapy.[11-15,19,57]

6. Palliative chemoradiation.
7. Palliative endoscopic-placed stents to relieve obstruction.[58]

REFERENCES

1. Ogunbiyi OA, McKenna K, Birnbaum EH, et al. Aggressive surgical management of recurrent rectal cancer—is it worthwhile? *Dis Colon Rectum.* 1997;40(2):150-155.
2. Lowy AM, Rich TA, Skibber JM, et al. Preoperative infusional chemoradiation, selective intraoperative radiation, and resection for locally advanced pelvic recurrence of colorectal adenocarcinoma. *Ann Surg.* 1996;223(2):177-185.
3. Valentini V, Morganti AG, De Franco A, et al. Chemoradiation with or without intraoperative radiation therapy in patients with locally recurrent rectal carcinoma: prognostic factors and long term outcome. *Cancer.* 1999;86(12):2612-2624.
4. Haddock MG, Gunderson LL, Nelson H, et al. Intraoperative irradiation for locally recurrent colorectal cancer in previously irradiated patients. *Int J Radiat Oncol Biol Phys.* 2001;49(5):1267-1274.
5. Rodriguez-Bigas MA, Herrera L, Petrelli NJ. Surgery for recurrent rectal adenocarcinoma in the presence of hydronephrosis. *Am J Surg.* 1992;164(1):18-21.
6. McAfee MK, Allen MS, Trastek VF, et al. Colorectal lung metastases: results of surgical excision. *Ann Thorac Surg.* 1992;53(5):780-785; discussion 785-786.
7. Girard P, Ducreux M, Baldeyrou P, et al. Surgery for lung metastases from colorectal cancer: analysis of prognostic factors. *J Clin Oncol.* 1996;14(7):2047-2053.
8. Headrick JR, Miller DL, Nagorney DM, et al. Surgical treatment of hepatic and pulmonary metastases from colon cancer. *Ann Thorac Surg.* 2001;71(3):975-979; discussion 979-780.
9. Moertel CG. Chemotherapy for colorectal cancer. *N Engl J Med.* 1994;330(16):1136-1142.
10. Schmoll HJ, Büchele T, Grothey A, et al. Where do we stand with 5-fluorouracil? *Semin Oncol.* 1999;26(6):589-605.
11. Valone FH, Friedman MA, Wittlinger PS, et al. Treatment of patients with advanced colorectal carcinomas with fluorouracil alone, high-dose leucovorin plus fluorouracil, or sequential methotrexate, fluorouracil, and leucovorin: a randomized trial of the Northern California Oncology Group. *J Clin Oncol.* 1989;7(10):1427-1436.
12. Petrelli N, Douglass HO Jr, Herrera L, et al. The modulation of fluorouracil with leucovorin in metastatic colorectal adenocarcinoma: a prospective randomized phase III trial. Gastrointestinal Tumor Study Group. *J Clin Oncol.* 1989;7(10):1419-1426.
13. Erlichman C, Fine S, Wong A, et al. A randomized trial of fluorouracil and folinic acid in patients with metastatic colorectal carcinoma. *J Clin Oncol.* 1988;6(3):469-475.
14. Doroshow JH, Multhauf P, Leong L, et al. Prospective randomized comparison of fluorouracil versus fluorouracil and high-dose continuous infusion leucovorin calcium for the treatment of advanced measurable colorectal cancer in patients previously unexposed to chemotherapy. *J Clin Oncol.* 1990;8(3):491-501.
15. Poon MA, O'Connell MJ, Wieand HS, et al. Biochemical modulation of fluorouracil with leucovorin: confirmatory evidence of improved therapeutic efficacy in advanced colorectal cancer. *J Clin Oncol.* 1991;9(11):1967-1972.
16. Buroker TR, O'Connell MJ, Wieand HS, et al. Randomized comparison of two schedules of fluorouracil and leucovorin in the treatment of advanced colorectal cancer. *J Clin Oncol.* 1994;12(1):14-20.
17. Jäger E, Heike M, Bernhard H, et al. Weekly high-dose leucovorin versus low-dose leucovorin combined with fluorouracil in advanced colorectal cancer: results of a randomized multicenter trial.Study Group for Palliative Treatment of Metastatic Colorectal Cancer Study Protocol 1. *J Clin Oncol.* 1996;14(8):2274-2279.
18. Meta-analysis of randomized trials testing the biochemical modulation of fluorouracil by methotrexate in

metastatic colorectal cancer. Advanced Colorectal Cancer Meta-Analysis Project. *J Clin Oncol.* 1994;12(5):960-969.

19. Wadler S, Lembersky B, Atkins M, et al. Phase II trial of fluorouracil and recombinant interferon alfa-2a in patients with advanced colorectal carcinoma: an Eastern Cooperative Oncology Group study. *J Clin Oncol.* 1991;9(10):1806-1810.

20. Kemeny N, Younes A, Seiter K, et al. Interferon alpha-2a and 5-fluorouracil for advanced colorectal carcinoma. Assessment of activity and toxicity. *Cancer.* 1990;66(12):2470-2475.

21. Pazdur R, Ajani JA, Patt YZ, et al. Phase II study of fluorouracil and recombinant interferon alfa-2a in previously untreated advanced colorectal carcinoma. *J Clin Oncol.* 1990;8(12):2027-2031.

22. Phase III randomized study of two fluorouracil combinations with either interferon alfa-2a or leucovorin for advanced colorectal cancer. Corfu-A Study Group. *J Clin Oncol.* 1995;13(4):921-928.

23. Hill M, Norman A, Cunningham D, et al. Royal Marsden phase III trial of fluorouracil with or without interferon alfa-2b in advanced colorectal cancer. *J Clin Oncol.* 1995;13(6):1297-1302.

24. Kosmidis PA, Tsavaris N, Skarlos D, et al. Fluorouracil and leucovorin with or without interferon alfa-2b in advanced colorectal cancer: analysis of a prospective randomized phase III trial. Hellenic Cooperative Oncology Group. *J Clin Oncol.* 1996;14(10):2682-2687.

25. Greco FA, Figlin R, York M, et al. Phase III randomized study to compare interferon alfa-2a in combination with fluorouracil versus fluorouracil alone in patients with advanced colorectal cancer. *J Clin Oncol.* 1996;14(10):2674-2681.

26. Hansen RM, Ryan L, Anderson T, et al. Phase III study of bolus versus infusion fluorouracil with or without cisplatin in advanced colorectal cancer. *J Natl Cancer Inst.* 1996;88(10):668-674.

27. Efficacy of intravenous continuous infusion of fluorouracil compared with bolus administration in advanced colorectal cancer. Meta-analysis Group in Cancer. *J Clin Oncol.* 1998;16(1):301-308.

28. Hoff PM, Royce M, Medgyesy D, et al. Oral fluoropoyrimidines. *Semin Oncol.* 1999;26(6):640-646.

29. Leichman CG, Fleming TR, Muggia FM, et al. Phase II study of fluorouracil and its modulation in advanced colorectal cancer: a Southwest Oncology Group study. *J Clin Oncol.* 1995;13(6):1303-1311.

30. Twelves C, Boyer M, Findlay M, et al. Capecitabine (Xeloda) improves medical resource use compared with 5-fluorouracil plus leucovorin in a phase III trial conducted in patients with advanced colorectal carcinoma. *Eur J Cancer.* 2001;37(5):597-604.

31. Lévi FA, Zidani R, Vannetzel JM, et al. Chronomodulated versus fixed-infusion-rate delivery of ambulatory chemotherapy with oxaliplatin, fluorouracil, and folinic acid (leucovorin) in patients with colorectal cancer metastases: a randomized multi-institutional trial. *J Natl Cancer Inst.* 1994;86(21):1608-1617.

32. Bertheault-Cvitkovic F, Jami A, Ithzaki M, et al. Biweekly intensified ambulatory chronomodulated chemotherapy with oxaliplatin, fluorouracil, and leucovorin in patients with metastatic colorectal cancer. *J Clin Oncol.* 1996;14(11):2950-2958.

33. Toxicity of fluorouracil in patients with advanced colorectal cancer: effect of administration schedule and prognostic factors. Meta-Analysis Group in Cancer. *J Clin Oncol.* 1998;16(11):3537-3541.

34. Rothenberg ML, Eckardt JR, Kuhn JG, et al. Phase II trial of irinotecan in patients with progressive or rapidly recurrent colorectal cancer. *J Clin Oncol.* 1996;14(4):1128-1135.

35. Conti JA, Kemeny NE, Saltz LB, et al. Irinotecan is an active agent in untreated patients with metastatic colorectal cancer. *J Clin Oncol.* 1996;14(3):709-715.

36. Cunningham D, Pyrhonen S, James RD, et al. A phase III multicenter randomized study of CPT-11 versus supportive care (SC) alone in patients (Pts) with 5FU-resistant metastatic colorectal cancer (MCRC). [Abstract] *Proceedings of the American Society of Clinical Oncology.* 1998;17:A-1,1a.

37. Rougier P, Van Cutsem E, Bajetta E, et al. Randomised trial of irinotecan versus fluorouracil by continuous infusion after fluorouracil failure in patients with metastatic colorectal cancer. *Lancet.* 1998;352(9138):1407-1412.

38. Cunningham D, Pyrhönen S, James RD, et al. Randomised trial of irinotecan plus supportive care versus supportive care alone after fluorouracil failure for patients with metastatic colorectal cancer. *Lancet.* 1998;352(9138):1413-1418.

39. Saltz LB, Cox JV, Blanke C, et al. Irinotecan plus fluorouracil and leucovorin for metastatic colorectal cancer. Irinotecan Study Group. *N Engl J Med.* 2000;343(13):905-914.

40. Douillard JY, Cunningham D, Roth AD, et al. Irinotecan combined with fluorouracil compared with fluorouracil alone as first-line treatment for metastatic colorectal cancer: a multicentre randomised trial. *Lancet.* 2000;355(9209):1041-1047.

41. Saltz LB, Douillard J, Pirotta N, et al. Combined analysis of two phase III randomized trials comparing irinotecan (C), fluorouracil (F), leucovorin (L) vs F alone as first-line therapy of previously untreated metastatic colorectal cancer (MCRC). [Abstract] *Proceedings of the American Society of Clinical Oncology.* 2000;19:A-938, 242a.

42. Cunningham D. Mature results from three large controlled studies with raltitrexed ('Tomudex'). *Br J Cancer.* 1998;77(Suppl 2):15-21.

43. Cocconi G, Cunningham D, Van Cutsem E, et al. Open, randomized, multicenter trial of raltitrexed versus fluorouracil plus high-dose leucovorin in patients with advanced colorectal cancer. Tomudex Colorectal Cancer Study Group. *J Clin Oncol.* 1998;16(9):2943-2952.

44. Von Hoff DD. Promising new agents for treatment of patients with colorectal cancer. *Semin Oncol.* 1998;25(5 Suppl 11):47-52.

45. de Gramont A, Vignoud J, Tournigand C, et al. Oxaliplatin with high-dose leucovorin and 5-fluorouracil 48-hour continuous infusion in pretreated metastatic colorectal cancer. *Eur J Cancer.* 1997;33(2):214-219.

46. Bleiberg H, de Gramont A. Oxaliplatin plus 5-fluorouracil: clinical experience in patients with advanced colorectal cancer. *Semin Oncol.* 1998;25(2 Suppl 5):32-39.

47. Cvitkovic E, Bekradda M. Oxaliplatin: a new therapeutic option in colorectal cancer. *Semin Oncol.* 1999;26(6):647-662.

48. André T, Bensmaine MA, Louvet C, et al. Multicenter phase II study of bimonthly high-dose leucovorin, fluorouracil infusion, and oxaliplatin for metastatic colorectal cancer resistant to the same leucovorin and fluorouracil regimen. *J Clin Oncol.* 1999;17(11):3560-3568.

49. Sargent DJ, Niedzwiecki D, O'Connell MJ, et al. Recommendation for caution with irinotecan, fluorouracil, and leucovorin for colorectal cancer. *N Engl J Med.* 2001;345(2):144-145; discussion 146.

50. Wanebo HJ, Koness RJ, Vezeridis MP, et al. Pelvic resection of recurrent rectal cancer. *Ann Surg.* 1994;220(4):586-595; discussion 595-597.

51. Scheele J, Stangl R, Altendorf-Hofmann A. Hepatic metastases from colorectal carcinoma: impact of surgical resection on the natural history. *Br J Surg.* 1990;77(11):1241-1246.

52. Adson MA, van Heerden JA, Adson MH, et al. Resection of hepatic metastases from colorectal cancer. *Arch Surg.* 1984;119(6):647-651.

53. Coppa GF, Eng K, Ranson JH, et al. Hepatic resection for metastatic colon and rectal cancer. An evaluation of preoperative and postoperative factors. *Ann Surg.* 1985;202(2):203-208.

54. Gayowski TJ, Iwatsuki S, Madariaga JR, et al. Experience in hepatic resection for metastatic colorectal cancer: analysis of clinical and pathologic risk factors. *Surgery.* 1994;116(4):703-710; discussion 710-711.

55. Fernández-Trigo V, Shamsa F, Sugarbaker PH. Repeat liver resections from colorectal metastasis. Repeat Hepatic Metastases Registry. *Surgery.* 1995;117(3):296-304.

56. Taylor M, Forster J, Langer B, et al. A study of prognostic factors for hepatic resection for colorectal metastases. *Am J Surg.* 1997;173(6):467-471.

57. Grem JL, Jordan E, Robson ME, et al. Phase II study of fluorouracil, leucovorin, and interferon alfa-2a in metastatic colorectal carcinoma. *J Clin Oncol.* 1993;11(9):1737-1745.

58. Baron TH. Expandable metal stents for the treatment of cancerous obstruction of the gastrointestinal tract. *N Engl J Med.* 2001;344(22):1681-1687.

SECTION III
PRODUCT INFORMATION

AVASTIN™ ℞
[ā'văs-tin]
(bevacizumab)
For Intravenous Use

WARNINGS

Gastrointestinal Perforations/Wound Healing Complications

AVASTIN administration can result in the development of gastrointestinal perforation and wound dehiscence, in some instances resulting in fatality. Gastrointestinal perforation, sometimes associated with intra-abdominal abscess, occurred throughout treatment with AVASTIN (i.e., was not correlated to duration of exposure). The incidence of gastrointestinal perforation in patients receiving bolus-IFL with AVASTIN was 2%. The typical presentation was reported as abdominal pain associated with symptoms such as constipation and vomiting. Gastrointestinal perforation should be included in the differential diagnosis of patients presenting with abdominal pain on AVASTIN. AVASTIN therapy should be permanently discontinued in patients with gastrointestinal perforation or wound dehiscence requiring medical intervention. The appropriate interval between termination of AVASTIN and subsequent elective surgery required to avoid the risks of impaired wound healing/wound dehiscence has not been determined. (See **WARNINGS: Gastrointestinal Perforations/Wound Healing Complications** and **DOSAGE AND ADMINISTRATION: Dose Modifications**.)

Hemorrhage

Serious, and in some cases fatal, hemoptysis has occurred in patients with non–small cell lung cancer treated with chemotherapy and AVASTIN. In a small study, the incidence of serious or fatal hemoptysis was 31% in patients with squamous histology and 4% in patients with adenocarcinoma receiving AVASTIN as compared to no cases in patients treated with chemotherapy alone. Patients with recent hemoptysis should not receive AVASTIN. (See **WARNINGS: Hemorrhage** and **DOSAGE AND ADMINISTRATION: Dose Modifications**.)

DESCRIPTION

AVASTIN™ (Bevacizumab) is a recombinant humanized monoclonal IgG1 antibody that binds to and inhibits the biologic activity of human vascular endothelial growth factor (VEGF) in in vitro and in vivo assay systems. Bevacizumab contains human framework regions and the complementarity-determining regions of a murine antibody that binds to VEGF (1). Bevacizumab is produced in a Chinese Hamster Ovary mammalian cell expression system in a nutrient medium containing the antibiotic gentamicin and has a molecular weight of approximately 149 kilodaltons. AVASTIN is a clear to slightly opalescent, colorless to pale brown, sterile, pH 6.2 solution for intravenous (IV) infusion. AVASTIN is supplied in 100 mg and 400 mg preservative-free, single-use vials to deliver 4 mL or 16 mL of AVASTIN (25 mg/mL). The 100 mg product is formulated in 240 mg α,α-trehalose dihydrate, 23.2 mg sodium phosphate (monobasic, monohydrate), 4.8 mg sodium phosphate (dibasic, anhydrous), 1.6 mg polysorbate 20, and Water for Injection, USP. The 400 mg product is formulated in 960 mg α,α-trehalose dihydrate, 92.8 mg sodium phosphate (monobasic, monohydrate), 19.2 mg sodium phosphate (dibasic, anhydrous), 6.4 mg polysorbate 20, and Water for Injection, USP.

CLINICAL PHARMACOLOGY

Mechanism of Action

Bevacizumab binds VEGF and prevents the interaction of VEGF to its receptors (Flt-1 and KDR) on the surface of endothelial cells. The interaction of VEGF with its receptors leads to endothelial cell proliferation and new blood vessel formation in in vitro models of angiogenesis. Administration of Bevacizumab to xenotransplant models of colon cancer in nude (athymic) mice caused reduction of microvascular growth and inhibition of metastatic disease progression.

Pharmacokinetics

The pharmacokinetic profile of Bevacizumab was assessed using an assay that measures total serum Bevacizumab concentrations (i.e., the assay did not distinguish between free Bevacizumab and Bevacizumab bound to VEGF ligand). Based on a population pharmacokinetic analysis of 491 patients who received 1 to 20 mg/kg of AVASTIN weekly, every 2 weeks, or every 3 weeks, the estimated half-life of Bevacizumab was approximately 20 days (range 11–50 days). The predicted time to reach steady state was 100 days. The accumulation ratio following a dose of 10 mg/kg of Bevacizumab every 2 weeks was 2.8.

The clearance of Bevacizumab varied by body weight, by gender, and by tumor burden. After correcting for body weight, males had a higher Bevacizumab clearance (0.262 L/day vs. 0.207 L/day) and a larger V_c (3.25 L vs. 2.66 L) than females. Patients with higher tumor burden (at or above median value of tumor surface area) had a higher Bevacizumab clearance (0.249 L/day vs. 0.199 L/day) than patients with tumor burdens below the median. In a randomized study of 813 patients (Study 1), there was no evidence of lesser efficacy (hazard ratio for overall survival) in males or patients with higher tumor burden treated with AVASTIN as compared to females and patients with low tumor burden. The relationship between Bevacizumab exposure and clinical outcomes has not been explored.

Special Populations

Analyses of demographic data suggest that no dose adjustments are necessary for age or sex.

Patients with renal impairment. No studies have been conducted to examine the pharmacokinetics of Bevacizumab in patients with renal impairment.

Patients with hepatic dysfunction. No studies have been conducted to examine the pharmacokinetics of Bevacizumab in patients with hepatic impairment.

CLINICAL STUDIES

The safety and efficacy of AVASTIN in the initial treatment of patients with metastatic carcinoma of the colon or rectum were studied in two randomized, controlled clinical trials in combination with intravenous 5-fluorouracil–based chemotherapy.

AVASTIN in Combination with Bolus-IFL

Study 1 was a randomized, double-blind, active-controlled clinical trial evaluating AVASTIN as first-line treatment of metastatic carcinoma of the colon or rectum. Patients were randomized to bolus-IFL (irinotecan 125 mg/m² IV, 5-fluorouracil 500 mg/m² IV, and leucovorin 20 mg/m² IV given once weekly for 4 weeks every 6 weeks) plus placebo (Arm 1), bolus-IFL plus AVASTIN (5 mg/kg every 2 weeks) (Arm 2), or 5-FU/LV plus AVASTIN (5 mg/kg every 2 weeks) (Arm 3). Enrollment in Arm 3 was discontinued, as pre-specified, when the toxicity of AVASTIN in combination with the bolus-IFL regimen was deemed acceptable.

Of the 813 patients randomized to Arms 1 and 2, the median age was 60, 40% were female, and 79% were Caucasian. Fifty-seven percent had an ECOG performance status of 0. Twenty-one percent had a rectal primary and 28% received prior adjuvant chemotherapy. In the majority of patients, 56%, the dominant site of disease was extra-abdominal, while the liver was the dominant site in 38% of patients. The patient characteristics were similar across the study arms. The primary endpoint of this trial was overall survival. Results are presented in Table 1 and Figure 1.

Table 1
Study 1 Efficacy Results

	IFL + Placebo	IFL + AVASTIN 5 mg/kg q 2 wks
Number of Patients	411	402
Overall Survival[a]		
Median (months)	15.6	20.3

Hazard ratio		0.66
Progression-Free Survival[a]		
Median (months)	6.2	10.6
Hazard ratio		0.54
Overall Response Rate[b]		
Rate (percent)	35%	45%
Duration of Response		
Median (months)	7.1	10.4

[a] p<0.001 by stratified logrank test.
[b] p<0.01 by χ² test.

Figure 1
Duration of Survival in Study 1

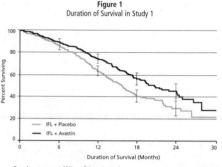

Error bars represent 95% confidence intervals.

The clinical benefit of AVASTIN, as measured by survival in the two principal arms, was seen in all subgroups tested. The subgroups examined were based on age, sex, race, ECOG performance status, location of primary tumor, prior adjuvant therapy, number of metastatic sites, and tumor burden.

Among the 110 patients enrolled in Arm 3, median overall survival was 18.3 months, median progression-free survival was 8.8 months, overall response rate was 39%, and median duration of response was 8.5 months.

AVASTIN in Combination with 5-FU/LV Chemotherapy
Study 2 was a randomized, active-controlled clinical trial testing AVASTIN in combination with 5-FU/LV as first-line treatment of metastatic colorectal cancer. Patients were randomized to receive 5-FU/LV (5-fluorouracil 500 mg/m², leucovorin 500 mg/m² weekly for 6 weeks every 8 weeks) or 5-FU/LV plus AVASTIN (5 mg/kg every 2 weeks) or 5-FU/LV plus AVASTIN (10 mg/kg every 2 weeks). Patients were treated until disease progression. The primary endpoints of the trial were objective response rate and progression-free survival. Results are presented in Table 2.

Table 2
Study 2 Efficacy Results

	5-FU/LV	5-FU/LV + AVASTIN 5 mg/kg	5-FU/LV + AVASTIN 10 mg/kg
Number of Patients	36	35	33
Overall Survival			
Median (months)	13.6	17.7	15.2
Progression-Free Survival			
Median (months)	5.2	9.0	7.2
Overall Response Rate			
Rate (percent)	17	40	24

Progression-free survival was significantly better in patients receiving 5-FU/LV plus AVASTIN at 5 mg/kg when compared to those not receiving AVASTIN. However, overall survival and overall response rate were not significantly different. Outcomes for patients receiving 5-FU/LV plus AVASTIN at 10 mg/kg were not significantly different than for patients who did not receive AVASTIN.

AVASTIN as a Single Agent
The efficacy of AVASTIN as a single agent in colorectal cancer has not been established. However, in an ongoing, ran-domized study of patients with metastatic colorectal cancer that had progressed following a 5-fluorouracil and irinote-can–based regimen, the arm in which patients were treated with single-agent AVASTIN was closed early due to evidence of an inferior survival in that arm as compared with pa-tients treated with the FOLFOX regimen of 5-fluorouracil, leucovorin, and oxaliplatin.

INDICATIONS AND USAGE
AVASTIN, used in combination with intravenous 5-fluoro-uracil–based chemotherapy, is indicated for first-line treat-ment of patients with metastatic carcinoma of the colon or rectum.

CONTRAINDICATIONS
There are no known contraindications to the use of AVASTIN.

WARNINGS
Gastrointestinal Perforations/Wound Healing Complica-tions (See DOSAGE AND ADMINISTRATION: Dose Modifications)
Gastrointestinal perforation and wound dehiscence, compli-cated by intra-abdominal abscesses, occurred at an in-creased incidence in patients receiving AVASTIN as com-pared to controls. AVASTIN has also been shown to impair wound healing in pre-clinical animal models.
In Study 1, one of 396 (0.3%) patients receiving bolus-IFL plus placebo, six of 392 (2%) patients receiving bolus-IFL plus AVASTIN, and four of 109 (4%) patients receiving 5-FU/LV plus AVASTIN developed gastrointestinal perfora-tion, in some instances with fatal outcome. These episodes occurred with or without intra-abdominal abscesses and at various time points during treatment. The typical presenta-tion was reported as abdominal pain associated with symp-toms such as constipation and vomiting.
In addition, two of 396 (0.5%) patients receiving bolus-IFL plus placebo, four of 392 (1%) patients receiving bolus-IFL plus AVASTIN, and one of 109 (1%) patients receiving 5-FU/LV plus AVASTIN developed a wound dehiscence dur-ing study treatment.
The appropriate interval between surgery and subsequent initiation of AVASTIN required to avoid the risks of im-paired wound healing has not been determined. In Study 1, the clinical protocol did not permit initiation of AVASTIN for at least 28 days following surgery. There was one patient (among 501 patients receiving AVASTIN on Study 1) in whom an anastomotic dehiscence occurred when AVASTIN was initiated per protocol. In this patient, the interval be-tween surgery and initiation of AVASTIN was greater than 2 months.
Similarly, the appropriate interval between termination of AVASTIN and subsequent elective surgery required to avoid the risks of impaired wound healing has not been deter-mined. In Study 1, 39 patients who were receiving bolus-IFL plus AVASTIN underwent surgery following AVASTIN therapy and, of these patients, six (15%) had wound heal-ing/bleeding complications. In the same study, 25 patients in the bolus-IFL arm underwent surgery and, of these pa-tients, one of 25 (4%) had wound healing/bleeding complica-tions. The longest interval between last dose of study drug and dehiscence was 56 days; this occurred in a patient on the bolus-IFL plus AVASTIN arm. The interval between ter-mination of AVASTIN and subsequent elective surgery should take into consideration the calculated half-life of AVASTIN (approximately 20 days).
AVASTIN therapy should be discontinued in patients with gastrointestinal perforation or wound dehiscence requiring medical intervention.
Hemorrhage (See DOSAGE AND ADMINISTRATION: Dose Modifications)
Two distinct patterns of bleeding have occurred in patients receiving AVASTIN. The first is minor hemorrhage, most commonly Grade 1 epistaxis. The second is serious, and in some cases fatal, hemorrhagic events. Serious hemorrhagic events occurred primarily in patients with non–small cell lung cancer, an indication for which AVASTIN is not ap-proved. In a randomized study in patients with non–small

ll lung cancer receiving chemotherapy with or without VASTIN, four of 13 (31%) AVASTIN-treated patients with quamous cell histology and two of 53 (4%) AVASTIN-reated patients with non-squamous histology experienced fe-threatening or fatal pulmonary hemorrhage as compared to none of the 32 (0%) patients receiving chemotherpy alone. Of the patients experiencing events of life-threatening pulmonary hemorrhage, many had cavitation nd/or necrosis of the tumor, either pre-existing or developg during AVASTIN therapy. These serious hemorrhagic vents occurred suddenly and presented as major or masve hemoptysis.

he risk of central nervous system (CNS) bleeding in paents with CNS metastases receiving AVASTIN has not een evaluated because these patients were excluded from enetech-sponsored studies following development of CNS emorrhage in a patient with a CNS metastasis in Phase 1 tudies.

ther serious bleeding events reported in patients receiving VASTIN were uncommon and included gastrointestinal emorrhage, subarachnoid hemorrhage, and hemorrhagic troke.

atients with serious hemorrhage i.e., requiring medical inervention, should have AVASTIN treatment discontinued nd receive aggressive medical management. Patients with ecent hemoptysis should not receive AVASTIN.

Arterial Thromboembolic Events (see DOSAGE AND ADMINISTRATION: Dose Modifications, and PRECAU-TIONS: Geriatric Use)

Arterial thromboembolic events occurred at a higher incience in patients receiving AVASTIN in combination with hemotherapy as compared to those receiving chemotherapy lone. Arterial thromboembolic events included cerebral inarction, transient ischemic attacks (TIAs), myocardial inarction (MI), angina, and a variety of other arterial thrompoembolic events. These events were fatal in some nstances.

n an exploratory analysis pooling the data from five randomized, controlled, clinical trials involving 1745 patients, he overall incidence of arterial thromboembolic events was ncreased (4.4% vs. 1.9%) among the 963 patients treated vith AVASTIN in combination with chemotherapy as compared to 782 patients treated with chemotherapy alone. Fatal outcomes from arterial thromboembolic events occurred n 7 of 963 patients (0.7%) who were treated with AVASTIN n combination with chemotherapy, compared to 3 of 782 patients (0.4%) who were treated with chemotherapy alone. The incidences of both cerebrovascular arterial events (1.9% s. 0.5%) and cardiovascular arterial events (2.1% vs. 1.0%) vere increased in patients receiving AVASTIN. In addition, here was a correlation between age (65 years and over) and he increase in risk of thromboembolic events (See PRECAUTIONS: Geriatric Use).

The safety of resumption of AVASTIN therapy after resoluion of an arterial thromboembolic event has not been studed. AVASTIN therapy should be permanently discontinued n patients who experience a severe arterial thromboembolic event during treatment.

Hypertension (See DOSAGE AND ADMINISTRATION: Dose Modifications)

The incidence of hypertension and severe hypertension was ncreased in patients receiving AVASTIN in Study 1 (see Table 3).

Table 3
Incidence of Hypertension and Severe
Hypertension in Study 1

	Arm 1 IFL + Placebo (n = 394)	Arm 2 IFL + AVASTIN (n = 392)	Arm 3 5-FU/LV + AVASTIN (n = 109)
Hypertension[a] (>150/100 mmHg)	43%	60%	67%
Severe Hypertension[a] (>200/110 mmHg)	2%	7%	10%

[a] This includes patients with either a systolic or diastolic reading greater than the cutoff value on one or more occasions.

Among patients with severe hypertension in the AVASTIN arms, slightly over half the patients (51%) had a diastolic reading greater than 110 associated with a systolic reading less than 200.

Medication classes used for management of patients with Grade 3 hypertension receiving AVASTIN included angiotensin-converting enzyme inhibitors, beta blockers, diuretics, and calcium channel blockers. Four months after discontinuation of therapy, persistent hypertension was present in 18 of 26 patients that received bolus-IFL plus AVASTIN and 8 of 10 patients that received bolus-IFL plus placebo.

Across pooled clinical studies (n=1032), development or worsening of hypertension resulted in hospitalization or discontinuation of AVASTIN in 17 patients. Four of these 17 patients developed hypertensive encephalopathy. Severe hypertension was complicated by subarachnoid hemorrhage in one patient.

In the post-marketing experience, acute increases in blood pressure associated with initial or subsequent infusions of AVASTIN have been reported (see PRECAUTIONS, Infusion Reactions). Some cases were serious and associated with clinical sequelae.

AVASTIN should be permanently discontinued in patients with hypertensive crisis. Temporary suspension is recommended in patients with severe hypertension that is not controlled with medical management.

Proteinuria (See DOSAGE AND ADMINISTRATION: Dose Modifications)

In Study 1, both the incidence and severity of proteinuria (defined as a urine dipstick reading of 1+ or greater) was increased in patients receiving AVASTIN as compared to those receiving bolus-IFL plus placebo. Urinary dipstick readings of 2+ or greater occurred in 14% of patients receiving bolus-IFL plus placebo, 17% receiving bolus-IFL plus AVASTIN, and in 28% of patients receiving 5-FU/LV plus AVASTIN. Twenty-four–hour urine collections were obtained in patients with new onset or worsening proteinuria. None of the 118 patients receiving bolus-IFL plus placebo, three of 158 patients (2%) receiving bolus-IFL plus AVASTIN, and two of 50 (4%) patients receiving 5-FU/LV plus AVASTIN who had a 24-hour collection experienced NCI-CTC Grade 3 proteinuria (>3.5 gm protein/24 hours).

In a dose-ranging, placebo-controlled, randomized study of AVASTIN in patients with metastatic renal cell carcinoma, an indication for which AVASTIN is not approved, 24-hour urine collections were obtained in approximately half the patients enrolled. Among patients in whom 24-hour urine collections were obtained, four of 19 (21%) patients receiving AVASTIN at 10 mg/kg every two weeks, two of 14 (14%) receiving AVASTIN at 3 mg/kg every two weeks, and none of the 15 placebo patients experienced NCI-CTC Grade 3 proteinuria (>3.5 gm protein/24 hours).

Nephrotic syndrome occurred in five of 1032 (0.5%) patients receiving AVASTIN in Genentech-sponsored studies. One patient died and one required dialysis. In three patients, proteinuria decreased in severity several months after discontinuation of AVASTIN. No patient had normalization of urinary protein levels (by 24-hour urine) following discontinuation of AVASTIN.

AVASTIN should be discontinued in patients with nephrotic syndrome. The safety of continued AVASTIN treatment in patients with moderate to severe proteinuria has not been evaluated. In most clinical studies, AVASTIN was interrupted for ≥2 grams of proteinuria/24 hours and resumed when proteinuria was <2 gm/24 hours. Patients with moderate to severe proteinuria based on 24-hour collections should be monitored regularly until improvement and/or resolution is observed.

Congestive Heart Failure

Congestive heart failure (CHF), defined as NCI-CTC Grade 2–4 left ventricular dysfunction, was reported in 22 of 1032 (2%) patients receiving AVASTIN in Genentech-sponsored studies. Congestive heart failure occurred in six of 44 (14%) patients receiving AVASTIN and concurrent anthracyclines. Congestive heart failure occurred in 13 of 299 (4%) patients who received prior anthracyclines and/or left chest wall irradiation. In a controlled study, the incidence was higher in patients receiving AVASTIN plus chemotherapy as compared to patients receiving chemotherapy alone. The safety of continuation or resumption of AVASTIN in patients with cardiac dysfunction has not been studied.

PRECAUTIONS

General

AVASTIN should be used with caution in patients with known hypersensitivity to AVASTIN or any component of this drug product.

Infusion Reactions

In clinical studies, infusion reactions with the first dose of AVASTIN were uncommon (<3%) and severe reactions occurred in 0.2% of patients. Infusion reactions reported in the clinical trials and postmarketing experience include hypertension, hypertensive crises associated with neurologic signs and symptoms, wheezing, oxygen desaturation, Grade 3 hypersensitivity, chest pain, headaches, rigors, and diaphoresis. Adequate information on rechallenge is not available. AVASTIN infusion should be interrupted in all patients with severe infusion reactions and appropriate medical therapy administered.

There are no data regarding the most appropriate method of identification of patients who may safely be retreated with AVASTIN after experiencing a severe infusion reaction.

Surgery

AVASTIN therapy should not be initiated for at least 28 days following major surgery. The surgical incision should be fully healed prior to initiation of AVASTIN. Because of the potential for impaired wound healing, AVASTIN should be suspended prior to elective surgery. The appropriate interval between the last dose of AVASTIN and elective surgery is unknown; however, the half-life of AVASTIN is estimated to be 20 days (see **CLINICAL PHARMACOLOGY: Pharmacokinetics**) and the interval chosen should take into consideration the half-life of the drug. (See **WARNINGS: Gastrointestinal Perforations/Wound Healing Complications.**)

Cardiovascular Disease

Patients were excluded from participation in AVASTIN clinical trials if, in the previous year, they had experienced clinically significant cardiovascular disease. In an exploratory analysis pooling the data from five randomized, placebo-controlled, clinical trials conducted in patients without a recent history of clinically significant cardiovascular disease, the overall incidence of arterial thromboembolic events, the incidence of fatal arterial thromboembolic events, and the incidence of cardiovascular thromboembolic events were increased in patients receiving AVASTIN plus chemotherapy as compared to chemotherapy alone.

Immunogenicity

As with all therapeutic proteins, there is a potential for immunogenicity. The incidence of antibody development in patients receiving AVASTIN has not been adequately determined because the assay sensitivity was inadequate to reliably detect lower titers. Enzyme-linked immunosorbent assays (ELISAs) were performed on sera from approximately 500 patients treated with AVASTIN, primarily in combination with chemotherapy. High titer human anti-AVASTIN antibodies were not detected.

Immunogenicity data are highly dependent on the sensitivity and specificity of the assay. Additionally, the observed incidence of antibody positivity in an assay may be influenced by several factors, including sample handling, timing of sample collection, concomitant medications, and underlying disease. For these reasons, comparison of the incidence of antibodies to AVASTIN with the incidence of antibodies to other products may be misleading.

Laboratory Tests

Blood pressure monitoring should be conducted every two to three weeks during treatment with AVASTIN. Patients who develop hypertension on AVASTIN may require blood pressure monitoring at more frequent intervals. Patients with AVASTIN-induced or -exacerbated hypertension who discontinue AVASTIN should continue to have their blood pressure monitored at regular intervals.

Patients receiving AVASTIN should be monitored for the development or worsening of proteinuria with serial urinalyses. Patients with a 2+ or greater urine dipstick reading should undergo further assessment, e.g., a 24-hour urine collection. (See **WARNINGS: Proteinuria** and **DOSAGE AND ADMINISTRATION: Dose Modifications.**)

Drug Interactions

No formal drug interaction studies with anti-neoplastic agents have been conducted. In Study 1, patients with colorectal cancer were given irinotecan/5-FU/leucovorin (bolus-IFL) with or without AVASTIN. Irinotecan concentrations were similar in patients receiving bolus-IFL alone and in combination with AVASTIN. The concentrations of SN38, the active metabolite of irinotecan, were on average 33% higher in patients receiving bolus-IFL in combination with AVASTIN when compared with bolus-IFL alone. In Study 1, patients receiving bolus-IFL plus AVASTIN had a higher incidence of Grade 3–4 diarrhea and neutropenia. Due to high inter-patient variability and limited sampling, the extent of the increase in SN38 levels in patients receiving concurrent irinotecan and AVASTIN is uncertain.

Carcinogenesis, Mutagenesis, Impairment of Fertility

No carcinogenicity data are available for AVASTIN in animals or humans.

AVASTIN may impair fertility. Dose-related decreases in ovarian and uterine weights, endometrial proliferation, number of menstrual cycles, and arrested follicular development or absent corpora lutea were observed in female cynomolgus monkeys treated with 10 or 50 mg/kg of AVASTIN for 13 or 26 weeks. Following a 4- or 12-week recovery period, which examined only the high–dose group, trends suggestive of reversibility were noted in the two females for each regimen that were assigned to recover. After the 12-week recovery period, follicular maturation arrest was no longer observed, but ovarian weights were still moderately decreased. Reduced endometrial proliferation was no longer observed at the 12-week recovery time point, but uterine weight decreases were still notable, corpora lutea were absent in 1 out of 2 animals, and the number of menstrual cycles remained reduced (67%).

Pregnancy Category C

AVASTIN has been shown to be teratogenic in rabbits when administered in doses that are two-fold greater than the recommended human dose on a mg/kg basis. Observed effects included decreases in maternal and fetal body weights, an increased number of fetal resorptions, and an increased incidence of specific gross and skeletal fetal alterations. Adverse fetal outcomes were observed at all doses tested. Angiogenesis is critical to fetal development and the inhibition of angiogenesis following administration of AVASTIN is likely to result in adverse effects on pregnancy. There are no adequate and well-controlled studies in pregnant women. AVASTIN should be used during pregnancy or in any woman not employing adequate contraception only if the potential benefit justifies the potential risk to the fetus. All patients should be counseled regarding the potential risk of AVASTIN to the developing fetus prior to initiation of therapy. If the patient becomes pregnant while receiving AVASTIN, she should be apprised of the potential hazard to the fetus and/or the potential risk of loss of pregnancy. Patients who discontinue AVASTIN should also be counseled concerning the prolonged exposure following discontinuation of therapy (half-life of approximately 20 days) and the possible effects of AVASTIN on fetal development.

Nursing Mothers

It is not known whether AVASTIN is secreted in human milk. Because human IgG1 is secreted into human milk, the potential for absorption and harm to the infant after ingestion is unknown. Women should be advised to discontinue

Table 4
NCI-CTC Grade 3 and 4 Adverse Events in Study 1
(Occurring at Higher Incidence (≥2%) in AVASTIN vs. Control)

	Arm 1 IFL + Placebo (n = 396)	Arm 2 IFL + AVASTIN (n = 392)
Grade 3–4 Events	295 (74%)	340 (87%)
Body as a Whole		
Asthenia	28 (7%)	38 (10%)
Abdominal Pain	20 (5%)	32 (8%)
Pain	21 (5%)	30 (8%)
Cardiovascular		
Deep Vein Thrombosis	19 (5%)	34 (9%)
Hypertension	10 (2%)	46 (12%)
Intra-Abdominal Thrombosis	5 (1%)	13 (3%)
Syncope	4 (1%)	11 (3%)
Digestive		
Diarrhea	99 (25%)	133 (34%)
Constipation	9 (2%)	14 (4%)
Hemic/Lymphatic		
Leukopenia	122 (31%)	145 (37%)
Neutropenia[a]	41 (14%)	58 (21%)

[a] Central laboratories were collected on Days 1 and 21 of each cycle. Neutrophil counts are available in 303 patients in Arm 1 and 276 in Arm 2.

nursing during treatment with AVASTIN and for a prolonged period following the use of AVASTIN, taking into account the half-life of the product, approximately 20 days [range 11-50 days]. (See **CLINICAL PHARMACOLOGY: Pharmacokinetics.**)

Pediatric Use
The safety and effectiveness of AVASTIN in pediatric patients has not been studied. However, physeal dysplasia was observed in juvenile cynomolgus monkeys with open growth plates treated for four weeks with doses that were less than the recommended human dose based on mg/kg and exposure. The incidence and severity of physeal dysplasia were dose-related and were at least partially reversible upon cessation of treatment.

Geriatric Use
In Study 1, NCI-CTC Grade 3–4 adverse events were collected in all patients receiving study drug (396 bolus-IFL plus placebo; 392 bolus-IFL plus AVASTIN; 109 5-FU/LV plus AVASTIN), while NCI-CTC Grade 1 and 2 adverse events were collected in a subset of 309 patients. There were insufficient numbers of patients 65 years and older in the subset in which Grade 1–4 adverse events were collected to determine whether the overall adverse event profile was different in the elderly as compared to younger patients. Among the 392 patients receiving bolus-IFL plus AVASTIN, 126 were at least 65 years of age. Severe adverse events that occurred at a higher incidence (≥2%) in the elderly when compared to those less than 65 years were asthenia, sepsis, deep thrombophlebitis, hypertension, hypotension, myocardial infarction, congestive heart failure, diarrhea, constipation, anorexia, leukopenia, anemia, dehydration, hypokalemia, and hyponatremia. The effect of AVASTIN on overall survival was similar in elderly patients as compared to younger patients.
Of the 742 patients enrolled in Genentech-sponsored clinical studies in which all adverse events were captured, 212 (29%) were age 65 or older and 43 (6%) were age 75 or older. Adverse events of any severity that occurred at a higher incidence in the elderly as compared to younger patients, in addition to those described above, were dyspepsia, gastrointestinal hemorrhage, edema, epistaxis, increased cough, and vomiting alteration.
In an exploratory, pooled analysis of 1745 patients treated in five randomized, controlled studies, there were 618 (35%)

patients age 65 or older and 1127 patients less than 65 years of age. The overall incidence of arterial thromboembolic events was increased in all patients receiving AVASTIN with chemotherapy as compared to those receiving chemotherapy alone, regardless of age. However, the increase in arterial thromboembolic events incidence was greater in patients 65 and over (8.5% vs. 2.9%) as compared to those less than 65 (2.1% vs. 1.4%). (See **WARNINGS: Arterial Thromboembolic Events**)

ADVERSE EVENTS
The most serious adverse events associated with AVASTIN were:
• Gastrointestinal Perforations/Wound Healing Complications (see **WARNINGS**)
• Hemorrhage (see **WARNINGS**)
• Arterial Thromboembolic Events (see **WARNINGS**)
• Hypertensive Crises (see **WARNINGS; Hypertension**)
• Nephrotic Syndrome (see **WARNINGS; Proteinuria**)
• Congestive Heart Failure (see **WARNINGS**)
The most common severe (NCI-CTC Grade 3–4) adverse events among 1032 patients receiving AVASTIN in Genentech-sponsored studies were asthenia, pain, hypertension, diarrhea, and leukopenia.
The most common adverse events of any severity among 742 patients receiving AVASTIN in Genentech-sponsored studies were asthenia, pain, abdominal pain, headache, hypertension, diarrhea, nausea, vomiting, anorexia, stomatitis, constipation, upper respiratory infection, epistaxis, dyspnea, exfoliative dermatitis, and proteinuria.
Because clinical trials are conducted under widely varying conditions, adverse reaction rates observed in the clinical trials of a drug cannot be directly compared to rates in the clinical trials of another drug and may not reflect the rates observed in practice. The adverse reaction information from clinical trials does, however, provide a basis for identifying the adverse events that appear to be related to drug use and for approximating their rates.
In pooled safety data, 1032 patients with metastatic colorectal cancer (n=568) and with other cancers (n=464) received AVASTIN either as a single agent (n=157) or in combination with chemotherapy (n=875) in Genentech-sponsored clinical trials. All adverse events were collected in 742 of the 1032 patients; for the remaining 290, all NCI-CTC Grade 3 and 4

Table 5
NCI-CTC Grade 1–4 Adverse Events in Study 1 Subset
(Occurring at Higher Incidence (≥5%) in AVASTIN vs. Control)

	Arm 1 IFL + Placebo (n = 98)	Arm 2 IFL + AVASTIN (n = 102)	Arm 3 5-FU/LV + AVASTIN (n = 109)
Body as a Whole			
Asthenia	68 (70%)	75 (74%)	80 (73%)
Pain	54 (55%)	62 (61%)	67 (62%)
Abdominal Pain	54 (55%)	62 (61%)	55 (50%)
Headache	19 (19%)	27 (26%)	30 (26%)
Cardiovascular			
Hypertension	14 (14%)	23 (23%)	37 (34%)
Hypotension	7 (7%)	15 (15%)	8 (7%)
Deep Vein Thrombosis	3 (3%)	9 (9%)	6 (6%)
Digestive			
Vomiting	46 (47%)	53 (52%)	51 (47%)
Anorexia	29 (30%)	44 (43%)	38 (35%)
Constipation	28 (29%)	41 (40%)	32 (29%)
Stomatitis	18 (18%)	33 (32%)	33 (30%)
Dyspepsia	15 (15%)	25 (24%)	19 (17%)
Weight Loss	10 (10%)	15 (15%)	18 (16%)
Flatulence	10 (10%)	11 (11%)	21 (19%)
GI Hemorrhage	6 (6%)	25 (24%)	21 (19%)
Dry Mouth	2 (2%)	7 (7%)	4 (4%)
Colitis	1 (1%)	6 (6%)	1 (1%)
Hemic/Lymphatic			
Thrombocytopenia	0	5 (5%)	5 (5%)
Metabolic/Nutrition			
Hypokalemia	11 (11%)	12 (12%)	18 (16%)
Bilirubinemia	0	1 (1%)	7 (6%)
Musculoskeletal			
Myalgia	7 (7%)	8 (8%)	16 (15%)
Nervous			
Dizziness	20 (20%)	27 (26%)	21 (19%)
Confusion	1 (1%)	1 (1%)	6 (6%)
Abnormal Gait	0	1 (1%)	5 (5%)
Respiratory			
Upper Respiratory Infection	38 (39%)	48 (47%)	44 (40%)
Dyspnea	15 (15%)	26 (26%)	27 (25%)
Epistaxis	10 (10%)	36 (35%)	35 (32%)
Voice Alteration	2 (2%)	9 (9%)	6 (6%)
Skin/Appendages			
Alopecia	25 (26%)	33 (32%)	6 (6%)
Dry Skin	7 (7%)	7 (7%)	22 (20%)
Exfoliative Dermatitis	3 (3%)	3 (3%)	21 (19%)
Nail Disorder	3 (3%)	2 (2%)	9 (8%)
Skin Discoloration	3 (3%)	2 (2%)	17 (16%)
Skin Ulcer	1 (1%)	6 (6%)	7 (6%)
Special Senses			
Taste Disorder	9 (9%)	14 (14%)	23 (21%)
Excess Lacrimation	2 (2%)	6 (6%)	20 (18%)
Urogenital			
Proteinuria	24 (24%)	37 (36%)	39 (36%)
Urinary Frequency/Urgency	1 (1%)	3 (3%)	6 (6%)

adverse events and only selected Grade 1 and 2 adverse events (hypertension, proteinuria, thromboembolic events) were collected. Adverse events across all Genentech-sponsored studies were used to further characterize specific adverse events. (See **WARNINGS: Hemorrhage, Arterial Thromboembolic Events, Hypertension, Proteinuria, Congestive Heart Failure** and **PRECAUTIONS: Geriatric Use**.) Comparative data on adverse experiences, except where indicated, are limited to Study 1, a randomized, active-controlled study in 897 patients receiving initial treatment for metastatic colorectal cancer. All NCI-CTC Grade 3 and 4 adverse events and selected Grade 1 and 2 adverse events (hypertension, proteinuria, thromboembolic events) were reported for the overall study population. In Study 1, the median age was 60, 60% were male, 78% had colon primary lesion, and 29% had prior adjuvant or neoadjuvant chemotherapy. The median duration of exposure to AVASTIN in Study 1 was 8 months in Arm 2 and 7 months in Arm 3. All adverse events, including all NCI-CTC Grade 1 and 2 events, were reported in a subset of 309 patients. The base-ne entry characteristics in the 309 patient safety subset ere similar to the overall study population and ell-balanced across the three study arms.

evere and life-threatening (NCI-CTC Grade 3 and 4) adrse events, which occurred at a higher incidence (≥2%) in atients receiving bolus-IFL plus AVASTIN as compared to olus-IFL plus placebo, are presented in Table 4.

See table 4 at top of page 305]

dverse events of any severity, which occurred at a higher cidence (≥5%) in the initial phase of the study in patients ceiving AVASTIN (bolus-IFL plus AVASTIN or 5-FU/LV lus AVASTIN) as compared to the bolus-IFL plus placebo rm, are presented in Table 5.

See table 5 at top of previous page]

lucocutaneous Hemorrhage

n Study 1, both serious and non-serious hemorrhagic vents occurred at a higher incidence in patients receiving VASTIN. (See **WARNINGS: Hemorrhage**.) In the 309 patents in which Grade 1–4 events were collected, epistaxis as common and reported in 35% of patients receiving olus-IFL plus AVASTIN compared with 10% of patients reeiving bolus-IFL plus placebo. These events were generally ild in severity (NCI–CTC Grade 1) and resolved without edical intervention. Other mild to moderate hemorrhagic vents reported more frequently in patients receiving bolus-FL plus AVASTIN when compared to those receiving bolus-FL plus placebo included gastrointestinal hemorrhage 24% vs. 6%), minor gum bleeding (2% vs. 0), and vaginal emorrhage (4% vs. 2%).

enous Thromboembolic Events

n Study 1, 15.1% of patients receiving bolus-IFL plus VASTIN and 13.6% of patients receiving bolus-IFL plus lacebo experienced a Grade 3–4 venous thromboembolic vent. The incidence of the following Grade 3 and 4 venous hromboembolic events was higher in patients receiving olus-IFL plus AVASTIN as compared to patients receiving olus-IFL plus placebo: deep venous thrombosis (34 vs. 19 atients) and intra-abdominal venous thrombosis (10 vs. 5 atients). The incidence of pulmonary embolism was higher n patients receiving bolus-IFL plus placebo (16 vs. 20 atients).

n Study 1, 53 of 392 (14%) patients who received bolus-IFL lus AVASTIN and 30 of 396 (8%) patients who received olus-IFL plus placebo had a thromboembolic event and reeived full-dose warfarin. Two patients in each treatment rm (four total) developed bleeding complications. In the wo patients treated with full-dose warfarin and AVASTIN, hese events were associated with marked elevations in heir INR. Eleven of 53 (21%) patients receiving bolus-IFL lus AVASTIN and one of 30 (3%) patients receiving bolus-FL developed an additional thromboembolic event.

)ther Serious Adverse Events

The following other serious adverse events are considered nusual in cancer patients receiving cytotoxic chemotherpy and occurred in at least one subject treated with VASTIN in clinical studies.

Body as a Whole: *polyserositis*
Digestive: *intestinal obstruction, intestinal necrosis, mesenteric venous occlusion, anastomotic ulceration*
Hemic and lymphatic: *pancytopenia*
Metabolic and nutritional disorders: *hyponatremia.*
Urogenital: *ureteral stricture*

OVERDOSAGE

The maximum tolerated dose of AVASTIN has not been determined. The highest dose tested in humans (20 mg/kg IV) was associated with headache in nine of 16 patients and with severe headache in three of 16 patients.

DOSAGE AND ADMINISTRATION

The recommended dose of AVASTIN is 5 mg/kg given once every 14 days as an IV infusion until disease progression is detected.

AVASTIN therapy should not be initiated for at least 28 days following major surgery. The surgical incision should be fully healed prior to initiation of AVASTIN.

Dose Modifications

There are no recommended dose reductions for the use of AVASTIN. If needed, AVASTIN should be either discontinued or temporarily suspended as described below.

AVASTIN should be permanently discontinued in patients who develop gastrointestinal perforation, wound dehiscence requiring medical intervention, serious bleeding, a severe arterial thromboembolic event, nephrotic syndrome, or hypertensive crisis.

Temporary suspension of AVASTIN is recommended in patients with evidence of moderate to severe proteinuria pending further evaluation and in patients with severe hypertension that is not controlled with medical management. The risk of continuation or temporary suspension of AVASTIN in patients with moderate to severe proteinuria is unknown.

AVASTIN should be suspended at least several weeks prior to elective surgery. (See **WARNINGS: Gastrointestinal Perforation/Wound Healing Complications** and **PRECAUTIONS: Surgery.**) AVASTIN should not be resumed until the surgical incision is fully healed.

Preparation for Administration

AVASTIN should be diluted for infusion by a healthcare professional using aseptic technique. Withdraw the necessary amount of AVASTIN for a dose of 5 mg/kg and dilute in a total volume of 100 mL of 0.9% Sodium Chloride Injection, USP. Discard any unused portion left in a vial, as the product contains no preservatives. Parenteral drug products should be inspected visually for particulate matter and discoloration prior to administration.

Diluted AVASTIN solutions for infusion may be stored at 2–8°C (36–46°F) for up to 8 hours. No incompatibilities between AVASTIN and polyvinylchloride or polyolefin bags have been observed.

AVASTIN infusions should not be administered or mixed with dextrose solutions.

Administration

DO NOT ADMINISTER AS AN IV PUSH OR BOLUS. The initial AVASTIN dose should be delivered over 90 minutes as an IV infusion following chemotherapy. If the first infusion is well tolerated, the second infusion may be administered over 60 minutes. If the 60-minute infusion is well tolerated, all subsequent infusions may be administered over 30 minutes.

Stability and Storage

AVASTIN vials must be refrigerated at 2–8°C (36–46°F). AVASTIN vials should be protected from light. Store in the original carton until time of use. **DO NOT FREEZE. DO NOT SHAKE.**

HOW SUPPLIED

AVASTIN is supplied as 4 mL and 16 mL of a sterile solution in single–use glass vials to deliver 100 and 400 mg of Bevacizumab per vial, respectively.

Single unit 100 mg carton: Contains one 4 mL vial of AVASTIN (25 mg/mL). NDC 50242-060-01

Single unit 400 mg carton: Contains one 16 mL vial of AVASTIN (25 mg/mL). NDC 50242-061-01

REFERENCES

1. Presta LG, Chen H, O'Connor SJ, Chisholm V, Meng YG, Krummen L, et al. Humanization of an anti-vascular endothelial growth factor monoclonal antibody for the therapy of solid tumors and other disorders. Cancer Res 1997;57:4593-9.

Genentech
BIOONCOLOGY™

AVASTIN™
(Bevacizumab)
For Intravenous Use 7455303
Manufactured by: 4829004
Genentech, Inc. FDA Approval Date: December 2004
1 DNA Way Code Revision Date: January 2005
South San Francisco, CA 94080-4990
©2004 Genentech, Inc.

CAMPTOSAR®   ℞
irinotecan hydrochloride injection
For Intravenous Use Only

WARNINGS

CAMPTOSAR Injection should be administered only under the supervision of a physician who is experienced in the use of cancer chemotherapeutic agents. Appropriate management of complications is possible only when adequate diagnostic and treatment facilities are readily available. CAMPTOSAR can induce both early and late forms of diarrhea that appear to be mediated by different mechanisms. Both forms of diarrhea may be severe. Early diarrhea (occurring during or shortly after infusion of CAMPTOSAR) may be accompanied by cholinergic symptoms of rhinitis, increased salivation, miosis, lacrimation, diaphoresis, flushing, and intestinal hyperperistalsis that can cause abdominal cramping. Early diarrhea and other cholinergic symptoms may be prevented or ameliorated by atropine (see PRECAUTIONS, General). Late diarrhea (generally occurring more than 24 hours after administration of CAMPTOSAR) can be life threatening since it may be prolonged and may lead to dehydration, electrolyte imbalance, or sepsis. Late diarrhea should be treated promptly with loperamide. Patients with diarrhea should be carefully monitored and given fluid and electrolyte replacement if they become dehydrated or antibiotic therapy if they develop ileus, fever, or severe neutropenia (see WARNINGS). Administration of CAMPTOSAR should be interrupted and subsequent doses reduced if severe diarrhea occurs (see DOSAGE AND ADMINISTRATION).

Severe myelosuppression may occur (see WARNINGS).

DESCRIPTION

CAMPTOSAR Injection (irinotecan hydrochloride injection) is an antineoplastic agent of the topoisomerase I inhibitor class. Irinotecan hydrochloride was clinically investigated as CPT-11.

CAMPTOSAR is supplied as a sterile, pale yellow, clear, aqueous solution. It is available in two single-dose sizes: 2 mL-fill vials contain 40 mg irinotecan hydrochloride and 5 mL-fill vials contain 100 mg irinotecan hydrochloride. Each milliliter of solution contains 20 mg of irinotecan hydrochloride (on the basis of the trihydrate salt), 45 mg of sorbitol NF powder, and 0.9 mg of lactic acid, USP. The pH of the solution has been adjusted to 3.5 (range, 3.0 to 3.8) with sodium hydroxide or hydrochloric acid. CAMPTOSAR is intended for dilution with 5% Dextrose Injection, USP (D5W), or 0.9% Sodium Chloride Injection, USP, prior to intravenous infusion. The preferred diluent is 5% Dextrose Injection, USP.

Irinotecan hydrochloride is a semisynthetic derivative of camptothecin, an alkaloid extract from plants such as *Camptotheca acuminata*. The chemical name is (*S*)-4,11-diethyl-3,4,12,14-tetrahydro-4-hydroxy-3,14-dioxo1*H*-pyrano[3′,4′:6,7]-indolizino[1,2-b]quinolin-9-yl-[1,4′-bipiperidine]-1′-carboxylate, monohydrochloride, trihydrate. Its structural formula is as follows:

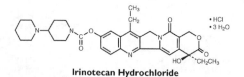

Irinotecan Hydrochloride

Irinotecan hydrochloride is a pale yellow to yellow crystalline powder, with the empirical formula $C_{33}H_{38}N_4O_6 \cdot HCl \cdot 3H_2O$ and a molecular weight of 677.19. It is slightly soluble in water and organic solvents.

CLINICAL PHARMACOLOGY

Irinotecan is a derivative of camptothecin. Camptothecin interact specifically with the enzyme topoisomerase I which relieves torsional strain in DNA by inducing reversible single-strand breaks. Irinotecan and its active metabolite SN-38 bind to the topoisomerase I-DNA complex and prevent religation of these single-strand breaks. Current research suggests that the cytotoxicity of irinotecan is due to double-strand DNA damage produced during DNA synthesis when replication enzymes interact with the ternary complex formed by topoisomerase I, DNA, and either irinotecan or SN-38. Mammalian cells cannot efficiently repair these double-strand breaks.

Irinotecan serves as a water-soluble precursor of the lipophilic metabolite SN-38. SN-38 is formed from irinotecan by carboxylesterase-mediated cleavage of the carbamate bond between the camptothecin moiety and the dipiperidino side chain. SN-38 is approximately 1000 times as potent as irinotecan as an inhibitor of topoisomerase I purified from human and rodent tumor cell lines. In vitro cytotoxicity assays show that the potency of SN-38 relative to irinotecan varies from 2- to 2000-fold. However, the plasma area under the concentration versus time curve (AUC) values for SN-38 are 2% to 8% of irinotecan and SN-38 is 95% bound to plasma proteins compared to approximately 50% bound to plasma proteins for irinotecan (see Pharmacokinetics). The precise contribution of SN-38 to the activity of CAMPTOSAR is thus unknown. Both irinotecan and SN-38 exist in an active lactone form and an inactive hydroxy acid anion form. A pH-dependent equilibrium exists between the two forms such that an acid pH promotes the formation of the lactone, while a more basic pH favors the hydroxy acid anion form.

Administration of irinotecan has resulted in antitumor activity in mice bearing cancers of rodent origin and in human carcinoma xenografts of various histological types.

Pharmacokinetics

After intravenous infusion of irinotecan in humans, irinotecan plasma concentrations decline in a multiexponential manner, with a mean terminal elimination half-life of about 6 to 12 hours. The mean terminal elimination half-life of the active metabolite SN-38 is about 10 to 20 hours. The half-lives of the lactone (active) forms of irinotecan and SN-38 are similar to those of total irinotecan and SN-38, as the lactone and hydroxy acid forms are in equilibrium.

Over the recommended dose range of 50 to 350 mg/m², the AUC of irinotecan increases linearly with dose; the AUC of SN-38 increases less than proportionally with dose. Maximum concentrations of the active metabolite SN-38 are generally seen within 1 hour following the end of a 90-minute infusion of irinotecan. Pharmacokinetic parameters for irinotecan and SN-38 following a 90-minute infusion of irinotecan at dose levels of 125 and 340 mg/m² determined in two clinical studies in patients with solid tumors are summarized in Table 1:

[See table 1 at top of next page]

Irinotecan exhibits moderate plasma protein binding (30% to 68% bound). SN-38 is highly bound to human plasma proteins (approximately 95% bound). The plasma protein to which irinotecan and SN-38 predominantly binds is albumin.

Metabolism and Excretion: The metabolic conversion of irinotecan to the active metabolite SN-38 is mediated by carboxylesterase enzymes and primarily occurs in the liver. SN-38 is subsequently conjugated predominantly by the enzyme UDP-glucuronosyl transferase 1A1 (UGT1A1) to form a glucuronide metabolite. UGT1A1 activity is reduced in individuals with genetic polymorphisms that lead to reduced enzyme activity such as the UGT1A1*28 polymorphism. Approximately 10% of the North American population is homozygous for the UGT1A1*28 allele. In a prospective study, in which irinotecan was administered as a single-agent on a once-every-3-week schedule, patients who were homozygous for UGT1A1*28 had a higher exposure to SN-38 than patients with the wild-type UGT1A1 allele (See WARNINGS and DOSAGE AND ADMINISTRATION). SN-38 glucuro-

Table 1. Summary of Mean (±Standard Deviation)
Irinotecan and SN-38 Pharmacokinetic
Parameters in Patients with Solid Tumors

Dose (mg/m^2)	Irinotecan					SN-38		
	C_{max} (ng/mL)	AUC_{0-24} (ng·h/mL)	$t_{1/2}$ (h)	V_z (L/m^2)	CL (L/h/m^2)	C_{max} (ng/mL)	AUC_{0-24} (ng·h/mL)	$t_{1/2}$ (h)
125 (N=64)	1,660 ±797	10,200 ±3,270	5.8[a] ±0.7	110 ±48.5	13.3 ±6.01	26.3 ±11.9	229 ±108	10.4[a] ±3.1
340 (N=6)	3,392 ±874	20,604 ±6,027	11.7[b] ±1.0	234 ±69.6	13.9 ±4.0	56.0 ±28.2	474 ±245	21.0[b] ±4.3

C_{max} - Maximum plasma concentration
AUC_{0-24} - Area under the plasma concentration-time curve from time 0 to 24 hours after the end of the 90-minute infusion
$t_{1/2}$ - Terminal elimination half-life
V_z - Volume of distribution of terminal elimination phase
CL - Total systemic clearance
[a] Plasma specimens collected for 24 hours following the end of the 90-minute infusion.
[b] Plasma specimens collected for 48 hours following the end of the 90-minute infusion. Because of the longer collection period, these values provide a more accurate reflection of the terminal elimination half-lives of irinotecan and SN-38.

nide had 1/50 to 1/100 the activity of SN-38 in cytotoxicity assays using two cell lines in vitro. The disposition of irinotecan has not been fully elucidated in humans. The urinary excretion of irinotecan is 11% to 20%; SN-38, <1%; and SN-38 glucuronide, 3%. The cumulative biliary and urinary excretion of irinotecan and its metabolites (SN-38 and SN-38 glucuronide) over a period of 48 hours following administration of irinotecan in two patients ranged from approximately 25% (100 mg/m^2) to 50% (300 mg/m^2).

Pharmacokinetics in Special Populations
Geriatric: In studies using the weekly schedule, the terminal half-life of irinotecan was 6.0 hours in patients who were 65 years or older and 5.5 hours in patients younger than 65 years. Dose-normalized AUC_{0-24} for SN-38 in patients who were at least 65 years of age was 11% higher than in patients younger than 65 years. No change in the starting dose is recommended for geriatric patients receiving the weekly dosage schedule of irinotecan. The pharmacokinetics of irinotecan given once every 3 weeks has not been studied in the geriatric population; a lower starting dose is recommended in patients 70 years or older based on clinical toxicity experience with this schedule (see DOSAGE AND ADMINISTRATION).
Pediatric: See **Pediatric Use** under **PRECAUTIONS**.
Gender: The pharmacokinetics of irinotecan do not appear to be influenced by gender.
Race: The influence of race on the pharmacokinetics of irinotecan has not been evaluated.
Hepatic Insufficiency: Irinotecan clearance is diminished in patients with hepatic dysfunction while exposure to the active metabolite SN-38 is increased relative to that in patients with normal hepatic function. The magnitude of these effects is proportional to the degree of liver impairment as measured by elevations in total bilirubin and transaminase concentrations. However, the tolerability of irinotecan in patients with hepatic dysfunction (bilirubin greater than 2 mg/dl) has not been assessed sufficiently, and no recommendations for dosing can be made (see DOSAGE AND ADMINISTRATION and PRECAUTIONS: Patients at Particular Risk Sections).
Renal Insufficiency: The influence of renal insufficiency on the pharmacokinetics of irinotecan has not been evaluated.

Drug-Drug Interactions
5-fluorouracil (5-FU) and leucovorin (LV): In a phase 1 clinical study involving irinotecan, 5-fluorouracil (5-FU), and leucovorin (LV) in 26 patients with solid tumors, the disposition of irinotecan was not substantially altered when the drugs were co-administered. Although the C_{max} and AUC_{0-24} of SN-38, the active metabolite, were reduced (by 14% and 8%, respectively) when irinotecan was followed by 5-FU and LV administration compared with when irinotecan was given alone, this sequence of administration was used in the combination trials and is recommended (see

DOSAGE AND ADMINISTRATION). Formal in vivo or in vitro drug interaction studies to evaluate the influence of irinotecan on the disposition of 5-FU and LV have not been conducted.
Anticonvulsants: Exposure to irinotecan and its active metabolite SN-38 is substantially reduced in adult and pediatric patients concomitantly receiving the CYP3A4 enzyme-inducing anticonvulsants phenytoin, phenobarbital or carbamazepine. The appropriate starting dose for patients taking these medications has not been formally defined. The following drugs are also CYP3A4 inducers: rifampin, rifabutin. For patients requiring anticonvulsant treatment, consideration should be given to substituting non-enzyme inducing anticonvulsants at least 2 weeks prior to initiation of irinotecan therapy. Dexamethasone does not appear to alter the pharmacokinetics of irinotecan.
St. John's Wort: St. John's Wort is an inducer of CYP3A4 enzymes. Exposure to the active metabolite SN-38 is reduced in patients receiving concomitant St. John's Wort. St. John's Wort should be discontinued at least 2 weeks prior to the first cycle of irinotecan, and St. John's Wort is contraindicated during irinotecan therapy.
Ketoconazole: Ketoconazole is a strong inhibitor of CYP3A4 enzymes. Patients receiving concomitant ketoconazole have increased exposure to irinotecan and its active metabolite SN-38. Patients should discontinue ketoconazole at least 1 week prior to starting irinotecan therapy and ketoconazole is contraindicated during irinotecan therapy.

CLINICAL STUDIES
Irinotecan has been studied in clinical trials in combination with 5-fluorouracil (5-FU) and leucovorin (LV) and as a single agent (see DOSAGE AND ADMINISTRATION). When given as a component of combination-agent treatment, irinotecan was either given with a weekly schedule of bolus 5-FU/LV or with an every-2-week schedule of infusional 5-FU/LV. Weekly and a once-every-3-week dosage schedules were used for the single-agent irinotecan studies. Clinical studies of combination and single-agent use are described below.

First-Line Therapy in Combination with 5-FU/LV for the Treatment of Metastatic Colorectal Cancer
Two phase 3, randomized, controlled, multinational clinical trials support the use of CAMPTOSAR Injection as first-line treatment of patients with metastatic carcinoma of the colon or rectum. In each study, combinations of irinotecan with 5-FU and LV were compared with 5-FU and LV alone. Study 1 compared combination irinotecan/bolus 5-FU/LV therapy given weekly with a standard bolus regimen of 5-FU/LV alone given daily for 5 days every 4 weeks; an irinotecan-alone treatment arm given on a weekly schedule was also included. Study 2 evaluated two different methods of administering infusional 5-FU/LV, with or without irinotecan. In both studies, concomitant medications such

Table 2. Combination Dosage Schedule: Study Results

	Study 1			Study 2	
	Irinotecan + Bolus 5-FU/LV weekly×4 q 6 weeks	Bolus 5-FU/LV daily×5 q 4 weeks	Irinotecan weekly×4 q 6 weeks	Irinotecan + Infusional 5-FU/LV	Infusional 5-FU/LV
Number of Patients	231	226	226	198	187
Demographics and Treatment Administration					
Female/Male (%)	34/65	45/54	35/64	33/67	47/53
Median Age in years (range)	62 (25–85)	61 (19–85)	61 (30–87)	62 (27–75)	59 (24–75)
Performance Status (%)					
0	39	41	46	51	51
1	46	45	46	42	41
2	15	13	8	7	8
Primary Tumor (%)					
Colon	81	85	84	55	65
Rectum	17	14	15	45	35
Median Time from Diagnosis to Randomization (months, range)	1.9 (0–161)	1.7 (0–203)	1.8 (0.1–185)	4.5 (0–88)	2.7 (0–104)
Prior Adjuvant 5-FU Therapy (%)					
No	89	92	90	74	76
Yes	11	8	10	26	24
Median Duration of Study Treatment[a] (months)	5.5	4.1	3.9	5.6	4.5
Median Relative Dose Intensity (%)[a]					
Irinotecan	72	—	75	87	—
5-FU	71	86	—	86	93
Efficacy Results					
Confirmed Objective Tumor Response Rate[b] (%)	39	21 ($p<0.0001$)[c]	18	35	22 ($p<0.005$)[c]
Median Time to Tumor Progression[d] (months)	7.0	4.3 ($p=0.004$)[d]	4.2	6.7	4.4 ($p<0.001$)[d]
Median Survival (months)	14.8	12.6 ($p<0.05$)[d]	12.0	17.4	14.1 ($p<0.05$)[d]

[a] Study 1: N=225 (irinotecan/5-FU/LV), N=219 (5-FU/LV), N=223 (irinotecan)
Study 2: N=199 (irinotecan/5-FU/LV), N=186 (5-FU/LV)
[b] Confirmed ≥ 4 to 6 weeks after first evidence of objective response
[c] Chi-square test
[d] Log-rank test

as antiemetics, atropine, and loperamide were given to patients for prophylaxis and/or management of symptoms from treatment. In Study 2, a 7-day course of fluoroquinolone antibiotic prophylaxis was given in patients whose diarrhea persisted for greater than 24 hours despite loperamide or if they developed a fever in addition to diarrhea. Treatment with oral fluoroquinolone was also initiated in patients who developed an absolute neutrophil count (ANC) <500/mm[3], even in the absence of fever or diarrhea. Patients in both studies also received treatment with intravenous antibiotics if they had persistent diarrhea or fever or if ileus developed.

In both studies, the combination of irinotecan/5-FU/LV therapy resulted in significant improvements in objective tumor response rates, time to tumor progression, and survival when compared with 5-FU/LV alone. These differences in survival were observed in spite of second-line therapy in a majority of patients on both arms, including crossover to irinotecan-containing regimens in the control arm. Patient characteristics and major efficacy results are shown in Table 2.

[See table 2 above]
Improvement was noted with irinotecan-based combination therapy relative to 5-FU/LV when response rates and time to tumor progression were examined across the following demographic and disease-related subgroups (age, gender, ethnic origin, performance status, extent of organ involvement with cancer, time from diagnosis of cancer, prior adjuvant therapy, and baseline laboratory abnormalities). Figures 1 and 2 illustrate the Kaplan-Meier survival curves for the comparison of irinotecan/5-FU/LV versus 5-FU/LV in Studies 1 and 2, respectively.
[See figure 1 at top of next column]
[See figure 2 at top of next column]

Second-Line Treatment for Recurrent or Progressive Metastatic Colorectal Cancer After 5-FU-Based Treatment
Weekly Dosage Schedule
Data from three open-label, single-agent, clinical studies, involving a total of 304 patients in 59 centers, support the use of CAMPTOSAR in the treatment of patients with metastatic cancer of the colon or rectum that has recurred

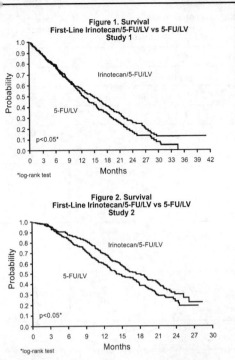

Figure 1. Survival
First-Line Irinotecan/5-FU/LV vs 5-FU/LV
Study 1

Irinotecan/5-FU/LV

5-FU/LV

p<0.05*

*log-rank test

Months

Figure 2. Survival
First-Line Irinotecan/5-FU/LV vs 5-FU/LV
Study 2

Irinotecan/5-FU/LV

5-FU/LV

p<0.05*

*log-rank test

Months

or progressed following treatment with 5-FU-based therapy. These studies were designed to evaluate tumor response rate and do not provide information on actual clinical benefit, such as effects on survival and disease-related symptoms. In each study, CAMPTOSAR was administered in repeated 6-week cycles consisting of a 90-minute intravenous infusion once weekly for 4 weeks, followed by a 2-week rest period. Starting doses of CAMPTOSAR in these trials were 100, 125, or 150 mg/m^2, but the 150-mg/m^2 dose was poorly tolerated (due to unacceptably high rates of grade 4 late diarrhea and febrile neutropenia). Study 1 enrolled 48 patients and was conducted by a single investigator at several regional hospitals. Study 2 was a multicenter study conducted by the North Central Cancer Treatment Group. All 90 patients enrolled in Study 2 received a starting dose of 125 mg/m^2. Study 3 was a multicenter study that enrolled 166 patients from 30 institutions. The initial dose in Study 3 was 125 mg/m^2 but was reduced to 100 mg/m^2 because the toxicity seen at the 125-mg/m^2 dose was perceived to be greater than that seen in previous studies. All patients in these studies had metastatic colorectal cancer, and the majority had disease that recurred or progressed following a 5-FU-based regimen administered for metastatic disease. The results of the individual studies are shown in Table 3. [See table 3 at top of next page]
In the intent-to-treat analysis of the pooled data across all three studies, 193 of the 304 patients began therapy at the recommended starting dose of 125 mg/m^2. Among these 193 patients, 2 complete and 27 partial responses were observed, for an overall response rate of 15.0% (95% Confidence Interval [CI], 10.0% to 20.1%) at this starting dose. A considerably lower response rate was seen with a starting dose of 100 mg/m^2. The majority of responses were observed within the first two cycles of therapy, but responses did occur in later cycles of treatment (one response was observed after the eighth cycle). The median response duration for patients beginning therapy at 125 mg/m^2 was 5.8 months (range, 2.6 to 15.1 months). Of the 304 patients treated in the three studies, response rates to CAMPTOSAR were similar in males and females and among patients older and younger than 65 years. Rates were also similar in patients with cancer of the colon or cancer of the rectum and in patients with single and multiple metastatic sites. The response rate was 18.5% in patients with a performance status of 0 and 8.2% in patients with a performance status of 1 or 2. Patients with a performance status of 3 or 4 have not been studied. Over half of the patients responding to CAMPTOSAR had not responded to prior 5-FU. Patients who had received previous irradiation to the pelvis responded to CAMPTOSAR at approximately the same rate as those who had not previously received irradiation.

Once-Every-3-Week Dosage Schedule
Single-Arm Studies: Data from an open-label, single-agent, single-arm, multicenter, clinical study involving a total of 132 patients support a once every-3-week dosage schedule of irinotecan in the treatment of patients with metastatic cancer of the colon or rectum that recurred or progressed following treatment with 5-FU. Patients received a starting dose of 350 mg/m^2 given by 30-minute intravenous infusion once every 3 weeks. Among the 132 previously treated patients in this trial, the intent-to-treat response rate was 12.1% (95% CI, 7.0% to 18.1%).
Randomized Trials: Two multicenter, randomized, clinical studies further support the use of irinotecan given by the once-every-3-week dosage schedule in patients with metastatic colorectal cancer whose disease has recurred or progressed following prior 5-FU therapy. In the first study, second-line irinotecan therapy plus best supportive care was compared with best supportive care alone. In the second study, second-line irinotecan therapy was compared with infusional 5-FU-based therapy. In both studies, irinotecan was administered intravenously at a starting dose of 350 mg/m^2 over 90 minutes once every 3 weeks. The starting dose was 300 mg/m^2 for patients who were 70 years and older or who had a performance status of 2. The highest total dose permitted was 700 mg. Dose reductions and/or administration delays were permitted in the event of severe hematologic and/or nonhematologic toxicities while on treatment. Best supportive care was provided to patients in both arms of Study 1 and included antibiotics, analgesics, corticosteroids, transfusions, psychotherapy, or any other symptomatic therapy as clinically indicated. In both studies, concomitant medications such as antiemetics, atropine, and loperamide were given to patients for prophylaxis and/or management of symptoms from treatment. If late diarrhea persisted for greater than 24 hours despite loperamide, a 7-day course of fluoroquinolone antibiotic prophylaxis was given. Patients in the control arm of the second study received one of the following 5-FU regimens: (1) LV, 200 mg/m^2 IV over 2 hours; followed by 5-FU, 400 mg/m^2 IV bolus; followed by 5-FU, 600 mg/m^2 continuous IV infusion over 22 hours on days 1 and 2 every 2 weeks; (2) 5-FU, 250 to 300 mg/m^2/day protracted continuous IV infusion until toxicity; (3) 5-FU, 2.6 to 3 g/m^2 IV over 24 hours every week for 6 weeks with or without LV, 20 to 500 mg/m^2/day every week IV for 6 weeks with 2-week rest between cycles. Patients were to be followed every 3 to 6 weeks for 1 year.
A total of 535 patients were randomized in the two studies at 94 centers. The primary endpoint in both studies was survival. The studies demonstrated a significant overall survival advantage for irinotecan compared with best supportive care (p=0.0001) and infusional 5-FU-based therapy (p=0.035) as shown in Figures 3 and 4. In Study 1, median survival for patients treated with irinotecan was 9.2 months compared with 6.5 months for patients receiving best supportive care. In Study 2, median survival for patients treated with irinotecan was 10.8 months compared with 8.5 months for patients receiving infusional 5-FU-based therapy. Multiple regression analyses determined that patients' baseline characteristics also had a significant effect on survival. When adjusted for performance status and other baseline prognostic factors, survival among patients treated with irinotecan remained significantly longer than in the control populations (p=0.001 for Study 1 and p=0.017 for Study 2). Measurements of pain, performance status, and weight loss were collected prospectively in the two studies; however, the plan for the analysis of these data was defined retrospectively. When comparing irinotecan with best supportive care in Study 1, this analysis showed a statistically

Table 3. Weekly Dosage Schedule: Study Results

	Study		
	1	2	3
Number of Patients	48	90	64	102
Starting Dose (mg/m^2/wk × 4)	125[a]	125	125	100
Demographics and Treatment Administration				
Female/Male (%)	46/54	36/64	50/50	51/49
Median Age in years (range)	63 (29–78)	63 (32–81)	61 (42–84)	64 (25–84)
Ethnic Origin (%)				
White	79	96	81	91
African American	12	4	11	5
Hispanic	8	0	8	2
Oriental/Asian	0	0	0	2
Performance Status (%)				
0	60	38	59	44
1	38	48	33	51
2	2	14	8	5
Primary Tumor (%)				
Colon	100	71	89	87
Rectum	0	29	11	8
Unknown	0	0	0	5
Prior 5-FU Therapy (%)				
For Metastatic Disease	81	66	73	68
≤ 6 months after Adjuvant	15	7	27	28
> 6 months after Adjuvant	2	16	0	2
Classification Unknown	2	12	0	3
Prior Pelvic/Abdominal Irradiation (%)				
Yes	3	29	0	0
Other	0	9	2	4
None	97	62	98	96
Duration of Treatment with CAMPTOSAR (median, months)	5	4	4	3
Relative Dose Intensity[b] (median %)	74	67	73	81
Efficacy				
Confirmed Objective Response Rate (%)[c] (95% CI)	21 (9.3–32.3)	13 (6.3–20.4)	14 (5.5–22.6)	9 (3.3–14.3)
Time to Response (median, months)	2.6	1.5	2.8	2.8
Response Duration (median, months)	6.4	5.9	5.6	6.4
Survival (median, months)	10.4	8.1	10.7	9.3
1-Year Survival (%)	46	31	45	43

[a] Nine patients received 150 mg/m^2 as a starting dose; two (22.2%) responded to CAMPTOSAR.
[b] Relative dose intensity for CAMPTOSAR based on planned dose intensity of 100, 83.3, and 66.7 mg/m^2/wk corresponding with 150, 125, and 100 mg/m^2 starting doses, respectively.
[c] Confirmed ≥ 4 to 6 weeks after first evidence of objective response.

significant advantage for irinotecan, with longer time to development of pain (6.9 months versus 2.0 months), time to performance status deterioration (5.7 months versus 3.3 months), and time to > 5% weight loss (6.4 months versus 4.2 months). Additionally, 33.3% (33/99) of patients with a baseline performance status of 1 or 2 showed an improvement in performance status when treated with irinotecan versus 11.3% (7/62) of patients receiving best supportive care (p=0.002). Because of the inclusion of patients with non-measurable disease, intent-to-treat response rates could not be assessed.
[See figure 3 at top of page 313]

[See figure 4 at top of next column]
In the two randomized studies, the EORTC QLQ-C30 instrument was utilized. At the start of each cycle of therapy, patients completed a questionnaire consisting of 30 questions, such as "Did pain interfere with daily activities?" (1 = Not at All, to 4 = Very Much) and "Do you have any trouble taking a long walk?" (Yes or No). The answers from the 30 questions were converted into 15 subscales, that were scored from 0 to 100, and the global health status subscale that was derived from two questions about the patient's sense of general well being in the past week. In addition to the global health status subscale, there were five functional

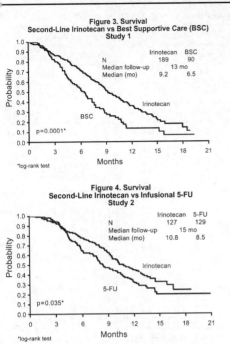

Figure 3. Survival
Second-Line Irinotecan vs Best Supportive Care (BSC)
Study 1

	Irinotecan	BSC
N	189	90
Median follow-up	13 mo	
Median (mo)	9.2	6.5

p=0.0001*

*log-rank test

Figure 4. Survival
Second-Line Irinotecan vs Infusional 5-FU
Study 2

	Irinotecan	5-FU
N	127	129
Median follow-up	15 mo	
Median (mo)	10.8	8.5

p=0.035*

*log-rank test

i.e., cognitive, emotional, social, physical, role) and nine symptom (i.e., fatigue, appetite loss, pain assessment, insomnia, constipation, dyspnea, nausea/vomiting, financial impact, diarrhea) subscales. The results as summarized in Table 5 are based on patients' worst post-baseline scores. In Study 1, a multivariate analysis and univariate analyses of the individual subscales were performed and corrected for multivariate testing. Patients receiving irinotecan reported significantly better results for the global health status, on two of five functional subscales, and on four of nine symptom subscales. As expected, patients receiving irinotecan noted significantly more diarrhea than those receiving best supportive care. In Study 2, the multivariate analysis on all 15 subscales did not indicate a statistically significant difference between irinotecan and infusional 5-FU.
[See table 4 at top of next page]
[See table 5 at top of page 315]

INDICATIONS AND USAGE

CAMPTOSAR Injection is indicated as a component of first-line therapy in combination with 5-fluorouracil and leucovorin for patients with metastatic carcinoma of the colon or rectum. CAMPTOSAR is also indicated for patients with metastatic carcinoma of the colon or rectum whose disease has recurred or progressed following initial fluorouracil-based therapy.

CONTRAINDICATIONS

CAMPTOSAR Injection is contraindicated in patients with a known hypersensitivity to the drug.

WARNINGS

General

Outside of a well-designed clinical study, CAMPTOSAR Injection should not be used in combination with the "Mayo Clinic" regimen of 5-FU/LV (administration for 4–5 consecutive days every 4 weeks) because of reports of increased toxicity, including toxic deaths. CAMPTOSAR should be used as recommended (see DOSAGE AND ADMINISTRATION, Table 10).
In patients receiving either irinotecan/5-FU/LV or 5-FU/LV in the clinical trials, higher rates of hospitalization, neutropenic fever, thromboembolism, first-cycle treatment discontinuation, and early deaths were observed in patients with a baseline performance status of 2 than in patients with a baseline performance status of 0 or 1.

Diarrhea

CAMPTOSAR can induce both early and late forms of diarrhea that appear to be mediated by different mechanisms. Early diarrhea (occurring during or shortly after infusion of CAMPTOSAR) is cholinergic in nature. It is usually transient and only infrequently is severe. It may be accompanied by symptoms of rhinitis, increased salivation, miosis, lacrimation, diaphoresis, flushing, and intestinal hyperperistalsis that can cause abdominal cramping. Early diarrhea and other cholinergic symptoms may be prevented or ameliorated by administration of atropine (see PRECAUTIONS, General, for dosing recommendations for atropine).
Late diarrhea (generally occurring more than 24 hours after administration of CAMPTOSAR) can be life threatening since it may be prolonged and may lead to dehydration, electrolyte imbalance, or sepsis. Late diarrhea should be treated promptly with loperamide (see PRECAUTIONS, Information for Patients, for dosing recommendations for loperamide). Patients with diarrhea should be carefully monitored, should be given fluid and electrolyte replacement if they become dehydrated, and should be given antibiotic support if they develop ileus, fever, or severe neutropenia. After the first treatment, subsequent weekly chemotherapy treatments should be delayed in patients until return of pretreatment bowel function for at least 24 hours without need for antidiarrhea medication. If grade 2, 3, or 4 late diarrhea occurs subsequent doses of CAMPTOSAR should be decreased within the current cycle (see DOSAGE AND ADMINISTRATION).

Neutropenia

Deaths due to sepsis following severe neutropenia have been reported in patients treated with CAMPTOSAR. Neutropenic complications should be managed promptly with antibiotic support (see PRECAUTIONS). Therapy with CAMPTOSAR should be temporarily omitted during a cycle of therapy if neutropenic fever occurs or if the absolute neutrophil count drops <1000/mm^3. After the patient recovers to an absolute neutrophil count ≥1000/mm^3, subsequent doses of CAMPTOSAR should be reduced depending upon the level of neutropenia observed (see DOSAGE AND ADMINISTRATION).
Routine administration of a colony-stimulating factor (CSF) is not necessary, but physicians may wish to consider CSF use in individual patients experiencing significant neutropenia.

Patients with Reduced UGT1A1 Activity

Individuals who are homozygous for the UGT1A1*28 allele are at increased risk for neutropenia following initiation of CAMPTOSAR treatment. A reduced initial dose should be considered for patients known to be homozygous for the UGT1A1*28 allele (see DOSAGE AND ADMINISTRATION). Heterozygous patients (carriers of one variant allele and one wild-type allele which results in intermediate UGT1A1 activity) may be at increased risk for neutropenia; however, clinical results have been variable and such patients have been shown to tolerate normal starting doses.

Hypersensitivity

Hypersensitivity reactions including severe anaphylactic or anaphylactoid reactions have been observed.

Colitis/Ileus

Cases of colitis complicated by ulceration, bleeding, ileus, and infection have been observed. Patients experiencing ileus should receive prompt antibiotic support (see PRECAUTIONS).

Renal Impairment/Renal Failure

Rare cases of renal impairment and acute renal failure have been identified, usually in patients who became volume depleted from severe vomiting and/or diarrhea.

Thromboembolism

Thromboembolic events have been observed in patients receiving irinotecan-containing regimens; the specific cause of these events has not been determined.

Table 4. Once-Every-3-Week Dosage Schedule: Study Results

	Study 1		Study 2	
	Irinotecan	BSC[a]	Irinotecan	5-FU
Number of Patients	189	90	127	129
Demographics and Treatment Administration				
Female/Male (%)	32/68	42/58	43/57	35/65
Median Age in years (range)	59 (22–75)	62 (34–75)	58 (30–75)	58 (25–75)
Performance Status (%)				
0	47	31	58	54
1	39	46	35	43
2	14	23	8	3
Primary Tumor (%)				
Colon	55	52	57	62
Rectum	45	48	43	38
Prior 5-FU Therapy (%)				
For Metastatic Disease	70	63	58	68
As Adjuvant Treatment	30	37	42	32
Prior Irradiation (%)	26	27	18	20
Duration of Study Treatment (median, months) (Log-rank test)	4.1	—	4.2 (p=0.02)	2.8
Relative Dose Intensity (median %)[b]	94	—	95	81–99
Survival				
Survival (median, months) (Log-rank test)	9.2 (p=0.0001)	6.5	10.8 (p=0.035)	8.5

[a]BSC = best supportive care
[b]Relative dose intensity for irinotecan based on planned dose intensity of 116.7 and 100 mg/m^2/wk corresponding with 350 and 300 mg/m^2 starting doses, respectively.

Pregnancy
CAMPTOSAR may cause fetal harm when administered to a pregnant woman. Radioactivity related to ^{14}C-irinotecan crosses the placenta of rats following intravenous administration of 10 mg/kg (which in separate studies produced an irinotecan C_{max} and AUC about 3 and 0.5 times, respectively, the corresponding values in patients administered 125 mg/m^2). Administration of 6 mg/kg/day intravenous irinotecan to rats (which in separate studies produced an irinotecan C_{max} and AUC about 2 and 0.2 times, respectively, the corresponding values in patients administered 125 mg/m^2) and rabbits (about one-half the recommended human weekly starting dose on a mg/m^2 basis) during the period of organogenesis, is embryotoxic as characterized by increased post-implantation loss and decreased numbers of live fetuses. Irinotecan was teratogenic in rats at doses greater than 1.2 mg/kg/day (which in separate studies produced an irinotecan C_{max} and AUC about 2/3 and 1/40th, respectively, of the corresponding values in patients administered 125 mg/m^2) and in rabbits at 6.0 mg/kg/day (about one-half the recommended human starting dose on a mg/m^2 basis). Teratogenic effects included a variety of external, visceral, and skeletal abnormalities. Irinotecan administered to rat dams for the period following organogenesis through weaning at doses of 6 mg/kg/day caused decreased learning ability and decreased female body weights in the offspring. There are no adequate and well-controlled studies of irinotecan in pregnant women. If the drug is used during pregnancy, or if the patient becomes pregnant while receiving this drug, the patient should be apprised of the potential hazard to the fetus. Women of childbearing potential should be advised to avoid becoming pregnant while receiving treatment with CAMPTOSAR.

PRECAUTIONS
General
Care of Intravenous Site: CAMPTOSAR Injection is administered by intravenous infusion. Care should be taken to avoid extravasation, and the infusion site should be monitored for signs of inflammation. Should extravasation occur, flushing the site with sterile water and applications of ice are recommended.
Premedication with Antiemetics: Irinotecan is emetigenic. It is recommended that patients receive premedication with antiemetic agents. In clinical studies of the weekly dosage schedule, the majority of patients received 10 mg of dexamethasone given in conjunction with another type of antiemetic agent, such as a 5-HT^3 blocker (e.g., ondansetron or granisetron). Antiemetic agents should be given on the day of treatment, starting at least 30 minutes before administration of CAMPTOSAR. Physicians should also consider providing patients with an antiemetic regimen (e.g., prochlorperazine) for subsequent use as needed.
Treatment of Cholinergic Symptoms: Prophylactic or therapeutic administration of 0.25 to 1 mg of intravenous or subcutaneous atropine should be considered (unless clinically contraindicated) in patients experiencing rhinitis, increased salivation, miosis, lacrimation, diaphoresis, flushing, abdominal cramping, or diarrhea (occurring during or shortly after infusion of CAMPTOSAR). These symptoms are expected to occur more frequently with higher irinotecan doses.
Patients at Particular Risk: In patients receiving either irinotecan/5-FU/LV or 5-FU/LV in the clinical trials, higher rates of hospitalization, neutropenic fever, thromboembolism, first-cycle treatment discontinuation, and early deaths were observed in patients with a baseline performance status of 2 than in patients with a baseline performance status of 0 or 1. Patients who had previously received pelvic/ab-

Table 5. EORTC QLQ-C30: Mean Worst Post-Baseline Score[a]

QLQ-C30 Subscale	Study 1			Study 2		
	Irinotecan	BSC	p-value	Irinotecan	5-FU	p-value
Global Health Status	47	37	0.03	53	52	0.9
Functional Scales						
Cognitive	77	68	0.07	79	83	0.9
Emotional	68	64	0.4	64	68	0.9
Social	58	47	0.06	65	67	0.9
Physical	60	40	0.0003	66	66	0.9
Role	53	35	0.02	54	57	0.9
Symptom Scales						
Fatigue	51	63	0.03	47	46	0.9
Appetite Loss	37	57	0.0007	35	38	0.9
Pain Assessment	41	56	0.009	38	34	0.9
Insomnia	39	47	0.3	39	33	0.9
Constipation	28	41	0.03	25	19	0.9
Dyspnea	31	40	0.2	25	24	0.9
Nausea/Vomiting	27	29	0.5	25	16	0.09
Financial Impact	22	26	0.5	24	15	0.3
Diarrhea	32	19	0.01	32	22	0.2

[a]For the five functional subscales and global health status subscale, higher scores imply better functioning, whereas, on the nine symptom subscales, higher scores imply more severe symptoms. The subscale scores of each patient were collected at each visit until the patient dropped out of the study.

dominal radiation and elderly patients with comorbid conditions should be closely monitored.

The use of CAMPTOSAR in patients with significant hepatic dysfunction has not been established. In clinical trials of either dosing schedule, irinotecan was not administered to patients with serum bilirubin >2.0 mg/dL, or transaminase >3 times the upper limit of normal if no liver metastasis, or transaminase >5 times the upper limit of normal with liver metastasis. In clinical trials of the weekly dosage schedule, patients with modestly elevated baseline serum total bilirubin levels (1.0 to 2.0 mg/dL) had a significantly greater likelihood of experiencing first-cycle, grade 3 or 4 neutropenia than those with bilirubin levels that were less than 1.0 mg/dL (50% [19/38] versus 18% [47/226]; p<0.001). (Also see CLINICAL PHARMACOLOGY: Pharmacokinetics in Special Populations: *Hepatic Insufficiency*). Patients with deficient glucuronidation of bilirubin, such as those with Gilbert's syndrome, may be at greater risk of myelosuppression when receiving therapy with CAMPTOSAR.

Ketoconazole, enzyme-inducing anticonvulsants and St. John's Wort are known to have drug-drug interactions with irinotecan therapy. (See Drug-Drug Interactions sub-section under CLINICAL PHARMACOLOGY)

Information for Patients

Patients and patients' caregivers should be informed of the expected toxic effects of CAMPTOSAR, particularly of its gastrointestinal complications, such as nausea, vomiting, abdominal cramping, diarrhea, and infection. Each patient should be instructed to have loperamide readily available and to begin treatment for late diarrhea (generally occurring more than 24 hours after administration of CAMPTOSAR) at the first episode of poorly formed or loose stools or the earliest onset of bowel movements more frequent than normally expected for the patient. One dosage regimen for loperamide used in clinical trials consisted of the following (Note: This dosage regimen exceeds the usual dosage recommendations for loperamide.): 4 mg at the first onset of late diarrhea and then 2 mg every 2 hours until the patient is diarrhea-free for at least 12 hours. During the night, the patient may take 4 mg of loperamide every 4 hours. Premedication with loperamide is not recommended. The use of drugs with laxative properties should be avoided because of the potential for exacerbation of diarrhea. Patients should be advised to contact their physician to discuss any laxative use.

Patients should be instructed to contact their physician or nurse if any of the following occur: diarrhea for the first time during treatment; black or bloody stools; symptoms of dehydration such as lightheadedness, dizziness, or faintness; inability to take fluids by mouth due to nausea or vomiting; inability to get diarrhea under control within 24 hours; or fever or evidence of infection.

Patients should be alerted to the possibility of alopecia.

Laboratory Tests

Careful monitoring of the white blood cell count with differential, hemoglobin, and platelet count is recommended before each dose of CAMPTOSAR.

Drug Interactions

The adverse effects of CAMPTOSAR, such as myelosuppression and diarrhea, would be expected to be exacerbated by other antineoplastic agents having similar adverse effects. Patients who have previously received pelvic/abdominal irradiation are at increased risk of severe myelosuppression following the administration of CAMPTOSAR. The concurrent administration of CAMPTOSAR with irradiation has not been adequately studied and is not recommended.

Lymphocytopenia has been reported in patients receiving CAMPTOSAR, and it is possible that the administration of dexamethasone as antiemetic prophylaxis may have enhanced the likelihood of this effect. However, serious opportunistic infections have not been observed, and no complications have specifically been attributed to lymphocytopenia.

Hyperglycemia has also been reported in patients receiving CAMPTOSAR. Usually, this has been observed in patients with a history of diabetes mellitus or evidence of glucose intolerance prior to administration of CAMPTOSAR. It is probable that dexamethasone, given as antiemetic prophylaxis, contributed to hyperglycemia in some patients.

The incidence of akathisia in clinical trials of the weekly dosage schedule was greater (8.5%, 4/47 patients) when prochlorperazine was administered on the same day as CAMPTOSAR than when these drugs were given on separate days (1.3%, 1/80 patients). The 8.5% incidence of akathisia, however, is within the range reported for use of prochlorperazine when given as a premedication for other chemotherapies.

It would be expected that laxative use during therapy with CAMPTOSAR would worsen the incidence or severity of diarrhea, but this has not been studied.

In view of the potential risk of dehydration secondary to vomiting and/or diarrhea induced by CAMPTOSAR, the physician may wish to withhold diuretics during dosing with CAMPTOSAR and, certainly, during periods of active vomiting or diarrhea.

Drug-Laboratory Test Interactions

There are no known interactions between CAMPTOSAR and laboratory tests.

Carcinogenesis, Mutagenesis & Impairment of Fertility

Long-term carcinogenicity studies with irinotecan were not conducted. Rats were, however, administered intravenous doses of 2 mg/kg or 25 mg/kg irinotecan once per week for 13 weeks (in separate studies, the 25 mg/kg dose produced an irinotecan C_{max} and AUC that were about 7.0 times and 1.3 times the respective values in patients administered 125 mg/m^2 weekly) and were then allowed to recover for 91 weeks. Under these conditions, there was a significant linear trend with dose for the incidence of combined uterine horn endometrial stromal polyps and endometrial stromal sarcomas. Neither irinotecan nor SN-38 was mutagenic in the in vitro Ames assay. Irinotecan was clastogenic both in vitro (chromosome aberrations in Chinese hamster ovary cells) and in vivo (micronucleus test in mice). No significant adverse effects on fertility and general reproductive performance were observed after intravenous administration of irinotecan in doses of up to 6 mg/kg/day to rats and rabbits. However, atrophy of male reproductive organs was observed after multiple daily irinotecan doses both in rodents at 20 mg/kg (which in separate studies produced an irinotecan C_{max} and AUC about 5 and 1 times, respectively, the corresponding values in patients administered 125 mg/m^2 weekly) and dogs at 0.4 mg/kg (which in separate studies produced an irinotecan C_{max} and AUC about one-half and 1/15th, respectively, the corresponding values in patients administered 125 mg/m^2 weekly).

Pregnancy

Pregnancy Category D—see WARNINGS.

Nursing Mothers

Radioactivity appeared in rat milk within 5 minutes of intravenous administration of radiolabeled irinotecan and was concentrated up to 65-fold at 4 hours after administration relative to plasma concentrations. Because many drugs are excreted in human milk and because of the potential for serious adverse reactions in nursing infants, it is recommended that nursing be discontinued when receiving therapy with CAMPTOSAR.

Pediatric Use

The effectiveness of irinotecan in pediatric patients has not been established. Results from two open-label, single arm studies were evaluated. One hundred and seventy children with refractory solid tumors were enrolled in one phase 2 trial in which 50 mg/m^2 of irinotecan was infused for 5 consecutive days every 3 weeks. Grade 3–4 neutropenia was experienced by 54 (31.8%) patients. Neutropenia was complicated by fever in 15 (8.8%) patients. Grade 3–4 diarrhea was observed in 35 (20.6%) patients. This adverse event profile was comparable to that observed in adults. In the second phase 2 trial of 21 children with previously untreated rhabdomyosarcoma, 20 mg/m^2 of irinotecan was infused for 5 consecutive days on weeks 0, 1, 3 and 4. This single agent therapy was followed by multimodal therapy. Accrual to the single agent irinotecan phase was halted due to the high rate (28.6%) of progressive disease and the early deaths (14%). The adverse event profile was different in this study from that observed in adults; the most significant grade 3 or 4 adverse events were dehydration experienced by 6 patients (28.6%) associated with severe hypokalemia in 5 patients (23.8%) and hyponatremia in 3 patients (14.3%); in addition Grade 3-4 infection was reported in 5 patients (23.8%) (across all courses of therapy and irrespective of causal relationship).

Pharmacokinetic parameters for irinotecan and SN-38 were determined in 2 pediatric solid-tumor trials at dose levels of 50 mg/m^2 (60-min infusion, n=48) and 125 mg/m^2 (90-min infusion, n=6). Irinotecan clearance (mean ± S.D.) was 17.3 ± 6.7 L/h/m^2 for the 50mg/m^2 dose and 16.2 ± 4.6 L/h/m^2 for the 125 mg/m^2 dose, which is comparable to that in adults. Dose-normalized SN-38 AUC values were comparable between adults and children. Minimal accumulation of irinotecan and SN-38 was observed in children on daily dosing regimens [daily × 5 every 3 weeks or (daily × 5) × 2 weeks every 3 weeks].

Geriatric Use

Patients greater than 65 years of age should be closely monitored because of a greater risk of late diarrhea in this population (see CLINICAL PHARMACOLOGY, Pharmacokinetics in Special Populations and ADVERSE REACTIONS, Overview of Adverse Events). The starting dose of CAMPTOSAR in patients 70 years and older for the once-every-3-week-dosage schedule should be 300 mg/m^2 (see DOSAGE AND ADMINISTRATION).

ADVERSE REACTIONS

First-Line Combination Therapy

A total of 955 patients with metastatic colorectal cancer received the recommended regimens of irinotecan in combination with 5-FU/LV, 5-FU/LV alone, or irinotecan alone. In the two phase 3 studies, 370 patients received irinotecan in combination with 5-FU/LV, 362 patients received 5-FU/LV alone, and 223 patients received irinotecan alone. (See Table 10 in DOSAGE AND ADMINISTRATION for recommended combination-agent regimens.)

In Study 1, 49 (7.3%) patients died within 30 days of last study treatment: 21 (9.3%) received irinotecan in combination with 5-FU/LV, 15 (6.8%) received 5-FU/LV alone, and 13 (5.8%) received irinotecan alone. Deaths potentially related to treatment occurred in 2 (0.9%) patients who received irinotecan in combination with 5-FU/LV (2 neutropenic fever/sepsis), 3 (1.4%) patients who received 5-FU/LV alone (1 neutropenic fever/sepsis, 1 CNS bleeding during thrombocytopenia, 1 unknown) and 2 (0.9%) patients who received irinotecan alone (2 neutropenic fever). Deaths from any cause within 60 days of first study treatment were reported for 15 (6.7%) patients who received irinotecan in combination with 5-FU/LV, 16 (7.3%) patients who received 5-FU/LV alone, and 15 (6.7%) patients who received irinotecan alone. Discontinuations due to adverse events were reported for 17 (7.6%) patients who received irinotecan in combination with 5FU/LV, 14 (6.4%) patients who received 5-FU/LV alone, and 26 (11.7%) patients who received irinotecan alone.

In Study 2, 10 (3.5%) patients died within 30 days of last study treatment: 6 (4.1%) received irinotecan in combination with 5-FU/LV and 4 (2.8%) received 5-FU/LV alone. There was one potentially treatment-related death, which occurred in a patient who received irinotecan in combination with 5-FU/LV (0.7%, neutropenic sepsis). Deaths from any cause within 60 days of first study treatment were reported for 3 (2.1%) patients who received irinotecan in combination with 5-FU/LV and 2 (1.4%) patients who received 5-FU/LV alone. Discontinuations due to adverse events

Table 6. Study 1: Percent (%) of Patients Experiencing Clinically Relevant Adverse Events in Combination Therapies[a]

Adverse Event	Study 1					
	Irinotecan + Bolus 5-FU/LV weekly × 4 q 6 weeks N=225		Bolus 5-FU/LV daily × 5 q 4 weeks N=219		Irinotecan weekly × 4 q 6 weeks N=223	
	Grade 1–4	Grade 3&4	Grade 1–4	Grade 3&4	Grade 1–4	Grade 3&4
TOTAL Adverse Events	100	53.3	100	45.7	99.6	45.7
GASTROINTESTINAL						
Diarrhea						
late	84.9	22.7	69.4	13.2	83.0	31.0
grade 3	—	15.1	—	5.9	—	18.4
grade 4	—	7.6	—	7.3	—	12.6
early	45.8	4.9	31.5	1.4	43.0	6.7
Nausea	79.1	15.6	67.6	8.2	81.6	16.1
Abdominal pain	63.1	14.6	50.2	11.5	67.7	13.0
Vomiting	60.4	9.7	46.1	4.1	62.8	12.1
Anorexia	34.2	5.8	42.0	3.7	43.9	7.2
Constipation	41.3	3.1	31.5	1.8	32.3	0.4
Mucositis	32.4	2.2	76.3	16.9	29.6	2.2
HEMATOLOGIC						
Neutropenia	96.9	53.8	98.6	66.7	96.4	31.4
grade 3	—	29.8	—	23.7	—	19.3
grade 4	—	24.0	—	42.5	—	12.1
Leukopenia	96.9	37.8	98.6	23.3	96.4	21.5
Anemia	96.9	8.4	98.6	5.5	96.9	4.5
Neutropenic fever	—	7.1	—	14.6	—	5.8
Thrombocytopenia	96.0	2.6	98.6	2.7	96.0	1.7
Neutropenic infection	—	1.8	—	0	—	2.2
BODY AS A WHOLE						
Asthenia	70.2	19.5	64.4	11.9	69.1	13.9
Pain	30.7	3.1	26.9	3.6	22.9	2.2
Fever	42.2	1.7	32.4	3.6	43.5	0.4
Infection	22.2	0	16.0	1.4	13.9	0.4
METABOLIC & NUTRITIONAL						
↑ Bilirubin	87.6	7.1	92.2	8.2	83.9	7.2
DERMATOLOGIC						
Exfoliative dermatitis	0.9	0	3.2	0.5	0	0
Rash	19.1	0	26.5	0.9	14.3	0.4
Alopecia[b]	43.1	—	26.5	—	46.1	—
RESPIRATORY						
Dyspnea	27.6	6.3	16.0	0.5	22.0	2.2
Cough	26.7	1.3	18.3	0	20.2	0.4
Pneumonia	6.2	2.7	1.4	1.0	3.6	1.3
NEUROLOGIC						
Dizziness	23.1	1.3	16.4	0	21.1	1.8
Somnolence	12.4	1.8	4.6	1.8	9.4	1.3
Confusion	7.1	1.8	4.1	0	2.7	0
CARDIOVASCULAR						
Vasodilatation	9.3	0.9	5.0	0	9.0	0
Hypotension	5.8	1.3	2.3	0.5	5.8	1.7
Thromboembolic events[c]	9.3	—	11.4	—	5.4	—

[a]Severity of adverse events based on NCI CTC (version 1.0)
[b]Complete hair loss = Grade 2
[c]Includes angina pectoris, arterial thrombosis, cerebral infarct, cerebrovascular accident, deep thrombophlebitis, embolus lower extremity, heart arrest, myocardial infarct, myocardial ischemia, peripheral vascular disorder, pulmonary embolus, sudden death, thrombophlebitis, thrombosis, vascular disorder.

were reported for 9 (6.2%) patients who received irinotecan in combination with 5FU/LV and 1 (0.7%) patient who received 5-FU/LV alone.

The most clinically significant adverse events for patients receiving irinotecan-based therapy were diarrhea, nausea, vomiting, neutropenia, and alopecia. The most clinically significant adverse events for patients receiving 5-FU/LV therapy were diarrhea, neutropenia, neutropenic fever, and mucositis. In Study 1, grade 4 neutropenia, neutropenic fever (defined as grade 2 fever and grade 4 neutropenia), and mucositis were observed less often with weekly irinotecan/5-FU/LV than with monthly administration of 5-FU/LV.

Tables 6 and 7 list the clinically relevant adverse events reported in Studies 1 and 2, respectively.
[See table 6 at top of previous page]
[See table 7 below]

Second-Line Single-Agent Therapy

Weekly Dosage Schedule

In three clinical studies evaluating the weekly dosage schedule, 304 patients with metastatic carcinoma of the colon or rectum that had recurred or progressed following 5-FU-based therapy were treated with CAMPTOSAR. Seventeen of the patients died within 30 days of the adminis-

tration of CAMPTOSAR; in five cases (1.6%, 5/304), the deaths were potentially drug-related. These five patients experienced a constellation of medical events that included known effects of CAMPTOSAR. One of these patients died of neutropenic sepsis without fever. Neutropenic fever occurred in nine (3.0%) other patients; these patients recovered with supportive care.

One hundred nineteen (39.1%) of the 304 patients were hospitalized a total of 156 times because of adverse events; 81 (26.6%) patients were hospitalized for events judged to be related to administration of CAMPTOSAR. The primary

Table 7. Study 2: Percent (%) of Patients Experiencing Clinically Relevant Adverse Events in Combination Therapies[a]

Adverse Event	Study 2			
	Irinotecan + 5-FU/LV infusional d 1&2 q 2 weeks N=145		5-FU/LV infusional d 1&2 q 2 weeks N=143	
	Grade 1–4	Grade 3&4	Grade 1–4	Grade 3&4
TOTAL Adverse Events	100	72.4	100	39.2
GASTROINTESTINAL				
Diarrhea				
late	72.4	14.4	44.8	6.3
grade 3	—	10.3	—	4.2
grade 4	—	4.1	—	2.1
Cholinergic syndrome[b]	28.3	1.4	0.7	0
Nausea	66.9	2.1	55.2	3.5
Abdominal pain	17.2	2.1	16.8	0.7
Vomiting	44.8	3.5	32.2	2.8
Anorexia	35.2	2.1	18.9	0.7
Constipation	30.3	0.7	25.2	1.4
Mucositis	40.0	4.1	28.7	2.8
HEMATOLOGIC				
Neutropenia	82.5	46.2	47.9	13.4
grade 3	—	36.4	—	12.7
grade 4	—	9.8	—	0.7
Leukopenia	81.3	17.4	42.0	3.5
Anemia	97.2	2.1	90.9	2.1
Neutropenic fever	—	3.4	—	0.7
Thrombocytopenia	32.6	0	32.2	0
Neutropenic infection	—	2.1	—	0
BODY AS A WHOLE				
Asthenia	57.9	9.0	48.3	4.2
Pain	64.1	9.7	61.5	8.4
Fever	22.1	0.7	25.9	0.7
Infection	35.9	7.6	33.6	3.5
METABOLIC & NUTRITIONAL				
↑ Bilirubin	19.1	3.5	35.9	10.6
DERMATOLOGIC				
Hand & foot syndrome	10.3	0.7	12.6	0.7
Cutaneous signs	17.2	0.7	20.3	0
Alopecia[c]	56.6	—	16.8	—
RESPIRATORY				
Dyspnea	9.7	1.4	4.9	0
CARDIOVASCULAR				
Hypotension	3.4	1.4	0.7	0
Thromboembolic events[d]	11.7	—	5.6	—

[a]Severity of adverse events based on NCI CTC (version 1.0)
[b]Includes rhinitis, increased salivation, miosis, lacrimation, diaphoresis, flushing, abdominal cramping or diarrhea (occurring during or shortly after infusion of irinotecan)
[c]Complete hair loss = Grade 2
[d]Includes angina pectoris, arterial thrombosis, cerebral infarct, cerebrovascular accident, deep thrombophlebitis, embolus lower extremity, heart arrest, myocardial infarct, myocardial ischemia, peripheral vascular disorder, pulmonary embolus, sudden death, thrombophlebitis, thrombosis, vascular disorder.

reasons for drug-related hospitalization were diarrhea, with or without nausea and/or vomiting (18.4%); neutropenia/leukopenia, with or without diarrhea and/or fever (8.2%); and nausea and/or vomiting (4.9%).

Adjustments in the dose of CAMPTOSAR were made during the cycle of treatment and for subsequent cycles based on individual patient tolerance. The first dose of at least one cycle of CAMPTOSAR was reduced for 67% of patients who began the studies at the 125-mg/m^2 starting dose. Within-cycle dose reductions were required for 32% of the cycles initiated at the 125-mg/m^2 dose level. The most common reasons for dose reduction were late diarrhea, neutropenia, and leukopenia. Thirteen (4.3%) patients discontinued treatment with CAMPTOSAR because of adverse events. The adverse events in Table 8 are based on the experience of the 304 patients enrolled in the three studies described in the CLINICAL STUDIES, Studies Evaluating the Weekly Dosage Schedule, section.

Table 8. Adverse Events Occurring in >10% of 304 Previously Treated Patients with Metastatic Carcinoma of the Colon or Rectum[a]

Body System & Event	% of Patients Reporting	
	NCI Grades 1–4	NCI Grades 3 & 4
GASTROINTESTINAL		
Diarrhea (late)[b]	88	31
7–9 stools/day (grade 3)	—	(16)
≥10 stools/day (grade 4)	—	(14)
Nausea	86	17
Vomiting	67	12
Anorexia	55	6
Diarrhea (early)[c]	51	8
Constipation	30	2
Flatulence	12	0
Stomatitis	12	1
Dyspepsia	10	0
HEMATOLOGIC		
Leukopenia	63	28
Anemia	60	7
Neutropenia	54	26
500 to <1000/mm^3 (grade 3)	—	(15)
<500/mm^3 (grade 4)	—	(12)
BODY AS A WHOLE		
Asthenia	76	12
Abdominal cramping/pain	57	16
Fever	45	1
Pain	24	2
Headache	17	1
Back pain	14	2
Chills	14	0
Minor infection[d]	14	0
Edema	10	1
Abdominal enlargement	10	0
METABOLIC & NUTRITIONAL		
↓ Body weight	30	1
Dehydration	15	4
↑ Alkaline phosphatase	13	4
↑ SGOT	10	1
DERMATOLOGIC		
Alopecia	60	NA[e]
Sweating	16	0
Rash	13	1
RESPIRATORY		
Dyspnea	22	4
↑ Coughing	17	0
Rhinitis	16	0

NEUROLOGIC		
Insomnia	19	0
Dizziness	15	0
CARDIOVASCULAR		
Vasodilation (flushing)	11	0

[a] Severity of adverse events based on NCI CTC (version 1.0)
[b] Occurring >24 hours after administration of CAMPTOSAR
[c] Occurring ≤24 hours after administration of CAMPTOSAR
[d] Primarily upper respiratory infections
[e] Not applicable; complete hair loss = NCI grade 2

Once-Every-3-Week Dosage Schedule

A total of 535 patients with metastatic colorectal cancer whose disease had recurred or progressed following prior 5-FU therapy participated in the two phase 3 studies: 316 received irinotecan, 129 received 5-FU, and 90 received best supportive care. Eleven (3.5%) patients treated with irinotecan died within 30 days of treatment. In three cases (1%, 3/316), the deaths were potentially related to irinotecan treatment and were attributed to neutropenic infection, grade 4 diarrhea, and asthenia, respectively. One (0.8%, 1/129) patient treated with 5-FU died within 30 days of treatment; this death was attributed to grade 4 diarrhea. Hospitalizations due to serious adverse events (whether or not related to study treatment) occurred at least once in 60% (188/316) of patients who received irinotecan, 63% (57/90) who received best supportive care, and 39% (50/129) who received 5-FU-based therapy. Eight percent of patients treated with irinotecan and 7% treated with 5-FU-based therapy discontinued treatment due to adverse events.

Of the 316 patients treated with irinotecan, the most clinically significant adverse events (all grades, 1–4) were diarrhea (84%), alopecia (72%), nausea (70%), vomiting (62%), cholinergic symptoms (47%), and neutropenia (30%). Table 9 lists the grade 3 and 4 adverse events reported in the patients enrolled to all treatment arms of the two studies described in the CLINICAL STUDIES, Studies Evaluating the Once-Every-3-Week Dosage Schedule, section.

Table 9. Percent Of Patients Experiencing Grade 3 & 4 Adverse Events In Comparative Studies Of Once-Every-3-Week Irinotecan Therapy[a]

Adverse Event	Study 1		Study 2	
	Irinotecan N=189	BSC[b] N=90	Irinotecan N=127	5-FU N=129
TOTAL Grade 3/4 Adverse Events	79	67	69	54
GASTROINTESTINAL				
Diarrhea	22	6	22	11
Vomiting	14	8	14	5
Nausea	14	3	11	4
Abdominal pain	14	16	9	8
Constipation	10	8	8	6
Anorexia	5	7	6	4
Mucositis	2	1	2	5
HEMATOLOGIC				
Leukopenia/ Neutropenia	22	0	14	2
Anemia	7	6	6	3
Hemorrhage	5	3	1	3
Thrombocytopenia	1	0	4	2
Infection				
without grade 3/4 neutropenia	8	3	1	4
with grade 3/4 neutropenia	1	0	2	0

Fever				
without grade 3/4 neutropenia	2	1	2	0
with grade 3/4 neutropenia	2	0	4	2
BODY AS A WHOLE				
Pain	19	22	17	13
Asthenia	15	19	13	12
METABOLIC & NUTRITIONAL				
Hepatic[c]	9	7	9	6
DERMATOLOGIC				
Hand & foot syndrome	0	0	0	5
Cutaneous signs[d]	2	0	1	3
RESPIRATORY[e]	10	8	5	7
NEUROLOGIC[f]	12	13	9	4
CARDIOVASCULAR[g]	9	3	4	2
OTHER[h]	32	28	12	14

[a] Severity of adverse events based on NCI CTC (version 1.0)
[b] BSC = best supportive care
[c] Hepatic includes events such as ascites and jaundice
[d] Cutaneous signs include events such as rash
[e] Respiratory includes events such as dyspnea and cough
[f] Neurologic includes events such as somnolence
[g] Cardiovascular includes events such as dysrhythmias, ischemia, and mechanical cardiac dysfunction
[h] Other includes events such as accidental injury, hepatomegaly, syncope, vertigo, and weight loss

Overview of Adverse Events

Gastrointestinal: Nausea, vomiting, and diarrhea are common adverse events following treatment with CAMPTOSAR and can be severe. When observed, nausea and vomiting usually occur during or shortly after infusion of CAMPTOSAR. In the clinical studies testing the every 3-week-dosage schedule, the median time to the onset of late diarrhea was 5 days after irinotecan infusion. In the clinical studies evaluating the weekly dosage schedule, the median time to onset of late diarrhea was 11 days following administration of CAMPTOSAR. For patients starting treatment at the 125-mg/m² weekly dose, the median duration of any grade of late diarrhea was 3 days. Among those patients treated at the 125-mg/m² weekly dose who experienced grade 3 or 4 late diarrhea, the median duration of the entire episode of diarrhea was 7 days. The frequency of grade 3 or 4 late diarrhea was somewhat greater in patients starting treatment at 125 mg/m² than in patients given a 100-mg/m² weekly starting dose (34% [65/193] versus 23% [24/102]; p=0.08). The frequency of grade 3 and 4 late diarrhea by age was significantly greater in patients ≥65 years than in patients <65 years (40% [53/133] versus 23% [40/171]; p=0.002). In one study of the weekly dosage treatment, the frequency of grade 3 and 4 late diarrhea was significantly greater in male than in female patients (43% [25/58] versus 16% [5/32]; p=0.01), but there were no gender differences in the frequency of grade 3 and 4 late diarrhea in the other two studies of the weekly dosage treatment schedule. Colonic ulceration, sometimes with gastrointestinal bleeding, has been observed in association with administration of CAMPTOSAR.

Hematology: CAMPTOSAR commonly causes neutropenia, leukopenia (including lymphocytopenia), and anemia. Serious thrombocytopenia is uncommon. When evaluated in the trials of weekly administration, the frequency of grade 3 and 4 neutropenia was significantly higher in patients who received previous pelvic/abdominal irradiation than in those who had not received such irradiation (48% [13/27] versus 24% [67/277]). In these same studies, patients with baseline serum total bilirubin levels of 1.0 mg/dL or more also had a significantly greater likelihood of experiencing first-cycle grade 3 or 4 neutropenia than those with bilirubin levels that were less than 1.0 mg/dL (50% [19/38] versus 18% [47/266]; p<0.001). There were no significant differences in the frequency of grade 3 and 4 neutropenia by age or gender. In the clinical studies evaluating the weekly dosage schedule, neutropenic fever (concurrent NCI grade 4 neutropenia and fever of grade 2 or greater) occurred in 3% of the patients; 6% of patients received G-CSF for the treatment of neutropenia. NCI grade 3 or 4 anemia was noted in 7% of the patients receiving weekly treatment; blood transfusions were given to 10% of the patients in these trials.

Table 10. Combination-Agent Dosage Regimens & Dose Modifications[a]

Regimen 1 6-wk cycle with bolus 5-FU/LV (next cycle begins on day 43)	CAMPTOSAR LV 5-FU	125 mg/m² IV over 90 min, d 1,8,15,22 20 mg/m² IV bolus, d 1,8,15,22 500 mg/m² IV bolus, d 1,8,15,22		
		Starting Dose & Modified Dose Levels (mg/m²)		
		Starting Dose	Dose Level −1	Dose Level −2
	CAMPTOSAR LV 5-FU	125 20 500	100 20 400	75 20 300
Regimen 2 6-wk cycle with infusional 5-FU/LV (next cycle begins on day 43)	CAMPTOSAR LV 5-FU Bolus 5-FU Infusion[b]	180 mg/m² IV over 90 min, d 1,15,29 200 mg/m² IV over 2 h, d 1,2,15,16,29,30 400 mg/m² IV bolus, d 1,2,15,16,29,30 600 mg/m² IV over 22 h, d 1,2,15,16,29,30		
		Starting Dose & Modified Dose Levels (mg/m²)		
		Starting Dose	Dose Level −1	Dose Level −2
	CAMPTOSAR LV 5-FU Bolus 5-FU Infusion[b]	180 200 400 600	150 200 320 480	120 200 240 360

[a] Dose reductions beyond dose level −2 by decrements of ≈20% may be warranted for patients continuing to experience toxicity. Provided intolerable toxicity does not develop, treatment with additional cycles may be continued indefinitely as long as patients continue to experience clinical benefit.
[b] Infusion follows bolus administration.

**Table 11. Recommended Dose Modifications for
CAMPTOSAR/5-Fluorouracil (5-FU)/Leucovorin (LV) Combination Schedules**

Patients should return to pre-treatment bowel function without requiring antidiarrhea medications for at least 24 hours before the next chemotherapy administration. A new cycle of therapy should not begin until the granulocyte count has recovered to $\geq 1500/mm^3$, and the platelet count has recovered to $\geq 100,000/mm^3$, and treatment-related diarrhea is fully resolved. Treatment should be delayed 1 to 2 weeks to allow for recovery from treatment-related toxicities. If the patient has not recovered after a 2-week delay, consideration should be given to discontinuing therapy.

Toxicity NCI CTC Grade[a] (Value)	During a Cycle of Therapy	At the Start of Subsequent Cycles of Therapy[b]
No toxicity	Maintain dose level	Maintain dose level
Neutropenia 1 (1500 to 1999/mm^3) 2 (1000 to 1499/mm^3) 3 (500 to 999/mm^3) 4 (<500/mm^3)	Maintain dose level ↓ 1 dose level Omit dose until resolved to ≤ grade 2, then ↓ 1 dose level Omit dose until resolved to ≤ grade 2, then ↓ 2 dose levels	Maintain dose level Maintain dose level ↓ 1 dose level ↓ 2 dose levels
Neutropenic fever	Omit dose until resolved, then ↓ 2 dose levels	
Other hematologic toxicities	Dose modifications for leukopenia or thrombocytopenia during a cycle of therapy and at the start of subsequent cycles of therapy are also based on NCI toxicity criteria and are the same as recommended for neutropenia above.	
Diarrhea 1 (2–3 stools/day > pretx[c]) 2 (4–6 stools/day > pretx) 3 (7–9 stools/day > pretx) 4 (≥10 stools/day > pretx)	Delay dose until resolved to baseline, then give same dose Omit dose until resolved to baseline, then ↓ 1 dose level Omit dose until resolved to baseline, then ↓ 1 dose level Omit dose until resolved to baseline, then ↓ 2 dose levels	Maintain dose level Maintain dose level ↓ 1 dose level ↓ 2 dose levels
Other nonhematologic toxicities[d] 1 2 3 4	Maintain dose level Omit dose until resolved to ≤ grade 1, then ↓ 1 dose level Omit dose until resolved to ≤ grade 2, then ↓ 1 dose level Omit dose until resolved to ≤ grade 2, then ↓ 2 dose levels *For mucositis/stomatitis decrease only 5-FU, not CAMPTOSAR*	Maintain dose level Maintain dose level ↓ 1 dose level ↓ 2 dose levels *For mucositis/stomatitis decrease only 5-FU, not CAMPTOSAR*

[a] National Cancer Institute Common Toxicity Criteria (version 1.0)
[b] Relative to the starting dose used in the previous cycle
[c] Pretreatment
[d] Excludes alopecia, anorexia, asthenia

Body as a Whole: Asthenia, fever, and abdominal pain are generally the most common events of this type.

Cholinergic Symptoms: Patients may have cholinergic symptoms of rhinitis, increased salivation, miosis, lacrimation, diaphoresis, flushing, and intestinal hyperperistalsis that can cause abdominal cramping and early diarrhea. If these symptoms occur, they manifest during or shortly after drug infusion. They are thought to be related to the anticholinesterase activity of the irinotecan parent compound and are expected to occur more frequently with higher irinotecan doses.

Hepatic: In the clinical studies evaluating the weekly dosage schedule, NCI grade 3 or 4 liver enzyme abnormalities were observed in fewer than 10% of patients. These events typically occur in patients with known hepatic metastases.

Dermatologic: Alopecia has been reported during treatment with CAMPTOSAR. Rashes have also been reported but did not result in discontinuation of treatment.

Respiratory: Severe pulmonary events are infrequent. In the clinical studies evaluating the weekly dosage schedule, NCI grade 3 or 4 dyspnea was reported in 4% of patients. Over half the patients with dyspnea had lung metastases; the extent to which malignant pulmonary involvement or other preexisting lung disease may have contributed to dyspnea in these patients is unknown.

Neurologic: Insomnia and dizziness can occur, but are not usually considered to be directly related to the administration of CAMPTOSAR. Dizziness may sometimes represent symptomatic evidence of orthostatic hypotension in patients with dehydration.

Cardiovascular: Vasodilation (flushing) may occur during administration of CAMPTOSAR. Bradycardia may also occur, but has not required intervention. These effects have been attributed to the cholinergic syndrome sometimes observed during or shortly after infusion of CAMPTOSAR. Thromboembolic events have been observed in patients receiving CAMPTOSAR; the specific cause of these events has not been determined.

Other Non-U.S. Clinical Trials

Irinotecan has been studied in over 1100 patients in Japan. Patients in these studies had a variety of tumor types, including cancer of the colon or rectum, and were treated with several different doses and schedules. In general, the types of toxicities observed were similar to those seen in U.S. trials with CAMPTOSAR. There is some information from Japanese trials that patients with considerable ascites or pleural effusions were at increased risk for neutropenia or diarrhea. A potentially life-threatening pulmonary syndrome, consisting of dyspnea, fever, and a reticulonodular pattern on chest x-ray, was observed in a small percentage of patients in early Japanese studies. The contribution of irinotecan to these preliminary events was difficult to assess because these patients also had lung tumors and some had preexisting nonmalignant pulmonary disease. As a result of these observations, however, clinical studies in the United States have enrolled few patients with compromised pulmonary function, significant ascites, or pleural effusions.

Post-Marketing Experience
The following events have been identified during post-marketing use of CAMPTOSAR in clinical practice. Cases of colitis complicated by ulceration, bleeding, ileus, or infection have been observed. There have been rare cases of renal impairment and acute renal failure, generally in patients who became infected and/or volume depleted from severe gastrointestinal toxicities (see WARNINGS). Rare cases of symptomatic pancreatitis or asymptomatic elevated pancreatic enzymes have been observed.
Hypersensitivity reactions including severe anaphylactic or anaphylactoid reactions have also been observed (see WARNINGS).

OVERDOSAGE
In U.S. phase 1 trials, single doses of up to 345 mg/m² of irinotecan were administered to patients with various cancers. Single doses of up to 750 mg/m² of irinotecan have been given in non-U.S. trials. The adverse events in these patients were similar to those reported with the recommended dosage and regimen. There is no known antidote for overdosage of CAMPTOSAR. Maximum supportive care should be instituted to prevent dehydration due to diarrhea and to treat any infectious complications.

DOSAGE AND ADMINISTRATION
Dosage in Patients with Reduced UGT1A1 Activity
When administered in combination with other agents, or as a single-agent, a reduction in the starting dose by at least one level of CAMPTOSAR should be considered for patients known to be homozygous for the UGT1A1*28 allele (see CLINICAL PHARMACOLOGY and WARNINGS). However, the precise dose reduction in this patient population is not known and subsequent dose modifications should be considered based on individual patient tolerance to treatment (see Tables 10–13).
Combination-Agent Dosage
Dosage Regimens
CAMPTOSAR Injection in Combination with 5-Fluorouracil (5-FU) and Leucovorin (LV)
CAMPTOSAR should be administered as an intravenous infusion over 90 minutes (see Preparation of Infusion Solution). For all regimens, the dose of LV should be administered immediately after CAMPTOSAR, with the administration of 5-FU to occur immediately after receipt of LV. CAMPTOSAR should be used as recommended; the currently recommended regimens are shown in Table 10.
[See table 10 at bottom of page 320]
Dosing for patients with bilirubin >2 mg/dL cannot be recommended because there is insufficient information to recommend a dose in these patients. It is recommended that patients receive premedication with antiemetic agents. Prophylactic or therapeutic administration of atropine should be considered in patients experiencing cholinergic symptoms. See PRECAUTIONS, General.

Dose Modifications
Patients should be carefully monitored for toxicity and assessed prior to each treatment. Doses of CAMPTOSAR and 5-FU should be modified as necessary to accommodate individual patient tolerance to treatment. Based on the recommended dose-levels described in Table 10, Combination-Agent Dosage Regimens & Dose Modifications, subsequent doses should be adjusted as suggested in Table 11, Recommended Dose Modifications for Combination Schedules. All dose modifications should be based on the worst preceding

toxicity. After the first treatment, patients with active diarrhea should return to pre-treatment bowel function without requiring anti-diarrhea medications for at least 24 hours before the next chemotherapy administration.
A new cycle of therapy should not begin until the toxicity has recovered to NCI grade 1 or less. Treatment maybe delayed 1 to 2 weeks to allow for recovery from treatment-related toxicity. If the patient has not recovered, consideration should be given to discontinuing therapy. Provided intolerable toxicity does not develop, treatment with additional cycles of CAMPTOSAR/5-FU/LV may be continued indefinitely as long as patients continue to experience clinical benefit.
[See table 11 at top of previous page]
Single-Agent Dosage Schedules
Dosage Regimens
CAMPTOSAR should be administered as an intravenous infusion over 90 minutes for both the weekly and once-every-3-week dosage schedules (see Preparation of Infusion Solution). Single-agent dosage regimens are shown in Table 12.

Table 12. Single-Agent Regimens of CAMPTOSAR and Dose Modifications

Weekly Regimen[a]	125 mg/m² IV over 90 min, d 1,8,15,22 then 2-wk rest

Starting Dose & Modified Dose Levels[c] (mg/m²)		
Starting Dose	Dose Level −1	Dose Level −2
125	100	75

Once-Every-3-Week Regimen[b]	350 mg/m² IV over 90 min, once every 3 wks[c]

Starting Dose & Modified Dose Levels (mg/m²)		
Starting Dose	Dose Level −1	Dose Level −2
350	300	250

[a] Subsequent doses may be adjusted as high as 150 mg/m² or to as low as 50 mg/m² in 25 to 50 mg/m² decrements depending upon individual patient tolerance.
[b] Subsequent doses may be adjusted as low as 200 mg/m² in 50 mg/m² decrements depending upon individual patient tolerance.
[c] Provided intolerable toxicity does not develop, treatment with additional cycles may be continued indefinitely as long as patients continue to experience clinical benefit.

A reduction in the starting dose by one dose level of CAMPTOSAR may be considered for patients with any of the following conditions: age ≥65 years, prior pelvic/abdominal radiotherapy, performance status of 2, or increased bilirubin levels. Dosing for patients with bilirubin >2 mg/dL cannot be recommended because there is insufficient information to recommend a dose in these patients. It is recommended that patients receive premedication with antiemetic agents. Prophylactic or therapeutic administration of atropine should be considered in patients experiencing cholinergic symptoms. See PRECAUTIONS, General.

Dose Modifications
Patients should be carefully monitored for toxicity and doses of CAMPTOSAR should be modified as necessary to accommodate individual patient tolerance to treatment. Based on recommended dose-levels described in Table 12, Single-Agent Regimens of CAMPTOSAR and Dose Modifications, subsequent doses should be adjusted as suggested in Table 13, Recommended Dose Modifications for Single-Agent Schedules. All dose modifications should be based on the worst preceding toxicity.

Table 13. Recommended Dose Modifications For Single-Agent Schedules[a]

A new cycle of therapy should not begin until the granulocyte count has recovered to ≥1500/mm³, and the platelet count has recovered to ≥100,000/mm³, and treatment-related diarrhea is fully resolved. Treatment should be delayed 1 to 2 weeks to allow for recovery from treatment-related toxicities. If the patient has not recovered after a 2-week delay, consideration should be given to discontinuing CAMPTOSAR.

Worst Toxicity NCI Grade[b] (Value)	During a Cycle of Therapy	At the Start of the Next Cycles of Therapy (After Adequate Recovery), Compared with the Starting Dose in the Previous Cycle[a]	
	Weekly	Weekly	Once Every 3 Weeks
No toxicity	Maintain dose level	↑ 25 mg/m² up to a maximum dose of 150 mg/m²	Maintain dose level
Neutropenia			
1 (1500 to 1999/mm³)	Maintain dose level	Maintain dose level	Maintain dose level
2 (1000 to 1499/mm³)	↓ 25 mg/m²	Maintain dose level	Maintain dose level
3 (500 to 999/mm³)	Omit dose until resolved to ≤ grade 2, then ↓ 25 mg/m²	↓ 25 mg/m²	↓ 50 mg/m²
4 (<500/mm³)	Omit dose until resolved to ≤ grade 2, then ↓ 50 mg/m²	↓ 50 mg/m²	↓ 50 mg/m²
Neutropenic fever	Omit dose until resolved, then ↓ 50 mg/m² when resolved	↓ 50 mg/m²	↓ 50 mg/m²
Other hematologic toxicities	Dose modifications for leukopenia, thrombocytopenia, and anemia during a cycle of therapy and at the start of subsequent cycles of therapy are also based on NCI toxicity criteria and are the same as recommended for neutropenia above.		
Diarrhea			
1 (2–3 stools/day > pretx[c])	Maintain dose level	Maintain dose level	Maintain dose level
2 (4–6 stools/day > pretx)	↓ 25 mg/m²	Maintain dose level	Maintain dose level
3 (7–9 stools/day > pretx)	Omit dose until resolved to ≤ grade 2, then ↓ 25 mg/m²	↓ 25 mg/m²	↓ 50 mg/m²
4 (≥10 stools/day > pretx)	Omit dose until resolved to ≤ grade 2, then ↓ 50 mg/m²	↓ 50 mg/m²	↓ 50 mg/m²
Other nonhematologic[d] toxicities			
1	Maintain dose level	Maintain dose level	Maintain dose level
2	↓ 25 mg/m²	↓ 25 mg/m²	↓ 50 mg/m²
3	Omit dose until resolved to ≤ grade 2, then ↓ 25 mg/m²	↓ 25 mg/m²	↓ 50 mg/m²
4	Omit dose until resolved to ≤ grade 2, then ↓ 50 mg/m²	↓ 50 mg/m²	↓ 50 mg/m²

[a] All dose modifications should be based on the worst preceding toxicity
[b] National Cancer Institute Common Toxicity Criteria (version 1.0)
[c] Pretreatment
[d] Excludes alopecia, anorexia, asthenia

A new cycle of therapy should not begin until the toxicity has recovered to NCI grade 1 or less. Treatment may be delayed 1 to 2 weeks to allow for recovery from treatment-related toxicity. If the patient has not recovered, consideration should be given to discontinuing this combination therapy. Provided intolerable toxicity does not develop, treatment with additional cycles of CAMPTOSAR may be continued indefinitely as long as patients continue to experience clinical benefit.
[See table 13 above]

Preparation & Administration Precautions
As with other potentially toxic anticancer agents, care should be exercised in the handling and preparation of infusion solutions prepared from CAMPTOSAR Injection. The use of gloves is recommended. If a solution of CAMPTOSAR contacts the skin, wash the skin immediately and thoroughly with soap and water. If CAMPTOSAR contacts the mucous membranes, flush thoroughly with water. Several published guidelines for handling and disposal of anticancer agents are available.[1–7]

Preparation of Infusion Solution
Inspect vial contents for particulate matter and repeat inspection when drug product is withdrawn from vial into syringe.
CAMPTOSAR Injection must be diluted prior to infusion. CAMPTOSAR should be diluted in 5% Dextrose Injection, USP, (preferred) or 0.9% Sodium Chloride Injection, USP, to a final concentration range of 0.12 to 2.8 mg/mL. In most clinical trials, CAMPTOSAR was administered in 250 mL to 500 mL of 5% Dextrose Injection, USP.
The solution is physically and chemically stable for up to 24 hours at room temperature (approximately 25°C) and in ambient fluorescent lighting. Solutions diluted in 5% Dextrose Injection, USP, and stored at refrigerated temperatures (approximately 2° to 8°C), and protected from light are physically and chemically stable for 48 hours. Refrigeration of admixtures using 0.9% Sodium Chloride Injection, USP, is not recommended due to a low and sporadic incidence of visible particulates. Freezing CAMPTOSAR and admixtures of CAMPTOSAR may result in precipitation of

the drug and should be avoided. Because of possible micro-bial contamination during dilution, it is advisable to use the admixture prepared with 5% Dextrose Injection, USP, within 24 hours if refrigerated (2° to 8°C, 36° to 46°F). In the case of admixtures prepared with 5% Dextrose Injection, USP, or Sodium Chloride Injection, USP, the solutions should be used within 6 hours if kept at room temperature (15° to 30°C, 59° to 86°F).
Other drugs should not be added to the infusion solution. Parenteral drug products should be inspected visually for particulate matter and discoloration prior to administration whenever solution and container permit.

HOW SUPPLIED

Each mL of CAMPTOSAR Injection contains 20 mg irinotecan (on the basis of the trihydrate salt); 45 mg sorbi-tol; and 0.9 mg lactic acid. When necessary, pH has been adjusted to 3.5 (range, 3.0 to 3.8) with sodium hydroxide or hydrochloric acid.
CAMPTOSAR Injection is available in single-dose amber glass vials in the following package sizes:

    2 mL   NDC 0009-7529-02
    5 mL   NDC 0009-7529-01

This is packaged in a backing/plastic blister to protect against inadvertent breakage and leakage. The vial should be inspected for damage and visible signs of leaks before re-moving the backing/plastic blister. If damaged, incinerate the unopened package.
Store at controlled room temperature 15° to 30°C (59° to 86°F). Protect from light. It is recommended that the vial (and backing/plastic blister) should remain in the carton un-til the time of use.
Rx only

REFERENCES

1. ONS Clinical Practice Committee. Cancer Chemotherapy Guidelines and Recommendations for Practice. Pitts-burgh, Pa: Oncology Nursing Society; 1999:32–41.
2. Recommendations for the safe handling of parenteral an-tineoplastic drugs. Washington, DC: Division of Safety, National Institutes of Health; 1983. US Dept of Health and Human Services, Public Health Service publication NIH 83-2621.
3. AMA Council on Scientific Affairs. Guidelines for han-dling parenteral antineoplastics. *JAMA*. 1985;253:1590–1592.
4. National Study Commission on Cytotoxic Exposure. Rec-ommendations for handling cytotoxic agents. 1987. Avail-able from Louis P. Jeffrey, Chairman, National Study Commission on Cytotoxic Exposure. Massachusetts Col-lege of Pharmacy and Allied Health Sciences, 179 Long-wood Avenue, Boston, MA 02115.
5. Clinical Oncological Society of Australia. Guidelines and recommendations for safe handling of antineoplastic agents. *Med J Australia*. 1983;1:426–428.
6. Jones RB, Frank R, Mass T. Safe handling of chemother-apeutic agents: a report from the Mount Sinai Medical Center. *CA-A Cancer J for Clin*. 1983;33:258–263.
7. American Society of Hospital Pharmacists. ASHP techni-cal assistance bulletin on handling cytotoxic and hazard-ous drugs. *Am J Hosp Pharm*. 1990;47:1033–1049.
8. Controlling Occupational Exposure to Hazardous Drugs. (OSHA Work-Practice Guidelines). *Am J Health-Syst Pharm*. 1996;53;1669–1685.

Camptosar brand of irinotecan hydrochloride injection
Distributed by Pharmacia & Upjohn Co
Division of Pfizer Inc, NY, NY 10017
Licensed from Yakult Honsha Co., LTD, Japan, and Daiichi Pharmaceutical Co., LTD, Japan
Revised July 2005
LAB-0134-9.0

ELOXATIN™ ℞
[ē-lŏks-ă-tĭn]
(oxaliplatin injection)

WARNING

ELOXATIN (oxaliplatin injection) should be administered under the supervision of a qualified physician experienced in the use of cancer chemotherapeutic agents. Appropriate management of therapy and complications is possible only when adequate diagnostic and treatment facilities are readily available.

Anaphylactic-like reactions to ELOXATIN have been reported, and may occur within minutes of ELOXATIN administration. Epinephrine, corticosteroids, and antihistamines have been employed to alleviate symptoms (see WARNINGS and ADVERSE REACTIONS).

DESCRIPTION

ELOXATIN™ (oxaliplatin injection) is an antineoplastic agent with the molecular formula $C_8H_{14}N_2O_4Pt$ and the chemical name of cis-[(1 R,2 R)-1,2-cyclohexanediamine-N,N'] [oxalato(2-)- O,O'] platinum. Oxaliplatin is an organoplatinum complex in which the platinum atom is complexed with 1,2-diaminocyclohexane (DACH) and with an oxalate ligand as a leaving group.

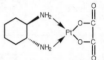

The molecular weight is 397.3. Oxaliplatin is slightly soluble in water at 6 mg/mL, very slightly soluble in methanol, and practically insoluble in ethanol and acetone.

CLINICAL PHARMACOLOGY

Mechanism of Action

Oxaliplatin undergoes nonenzymatic conversion in physiologic solutions to active derivatives via displacement of the labile oxalate ligand. Several transient reactive species are formed, including monoaquo and diaquo DACH platinum, which covalently bind with macromolecules. Both inter- and intrastrand Pt-DNA crosslinks are formed. Crosslinks are formed between the N7 positions of two adjacent guanines (GG), adjacent adenine-guanines (AG), and guanines separated by an intervening nucleotide (GNG). These crosslinks inhibit DNA replication and transcription. Cytotoxicity is cell-cycle nonspecific.

Pharmacology

In vivo studies have shown antitumor activity of oxaliplatin against colon carcinoma. In combination with 5-fluorouracil (5-FU), oxaliplatin exhibits in vitro and in vivo antiproliferative activity greater than either compound alone in several tumor models [HT29 (colon), GR (mammary), and L1210 (leukemia)].

Human Pharmacokinetics

The reactive oxaliplatin derivatives are present as a fraction of the unbound platinum in plasma ultrafiltrate. The decline of ultrafilterable platinum levels following oxaliplatin administration is triphasic, characterized by two relatively short distribution phases ($t_{1/2\alpha}$; 0.43 hours and $t_{1/2\beta}$; 16.8 hours) and a long terminal elimination phase ($t_{1/2\gamma}$; 391 hours). Pharmacokinetic parameters obtained after a single 2-hour IV infusion of ELOXATIN at a dose of 85 mg/m^2 expressed as ultrafilterable platinum were C_{max} of 0.814 µg/mL and volume of distribution of 440 L. Interpatient and intrapatient variability in ultrafilterable platinum exposure (AUC_{0-48hr}) assessed over 3 cycles was moderate to low (23% and 6%, respectively). A pharmacodynamic relationship between platinum ultrafiltrate levels and clinical safety and effectiveness has not been established.

Distribution

At the end of a 2-hour infusion of ELOXATIN, approximately 15% of the administered platinum is present in the systemic circulation. The remaining 85% is rapidly distributed into tissues or eliminated in the urine. In patients, plasma protein binding of platinum is irreversible and is greater than 90%. The main binding proteins are albumin and gammaglobulins. Platinum also binds irreversibly and accumulates (approximately 2-fold) in erythrocytes, where it appears to have no relevant activity. No platinum accumulation was observed in plasma ultrafiltrate following 85 mg/m^2 every two weeks.

Metabolism

Oxaliplatin undergoes rapid and extensive nonenzymatic biotransformation. There is no evidence of cytochrome P450-mediated metabolism in vitro.

Up to 17 platinum-containing derivatives have been observed in plasma ultrafiltrate samples from patients, including several cytotoxic species (monochloro DACH platinum, dichloro DACH platinum, and monoaquo and diaquo DACH platinum) and a number of noncytotoxic, conjugated species.

Elimination

The major route of platinum elimination is renal excretion. At five days after a single 2-hour infusion of ELOXATIN, urinary elimination accounted for about 54% of the platinum eliminated, with fecal excretion accounting for only about 2%. Platinum was cleared from plasma at a rate (10 - 17 L/h) that was similar to or exceeded the average human glomerular filtration rate (GFR; 7.5 L/h). There was no significant effect of gender on the clearance of ultrafilterable platinum. The renal clearance of ultrafilterable platinum is significantly correlated with GFR (see ADVERSE REACTIONS).

Pharmacokinetics in Special Populations

Renal Impairment

The AUC_{0-48hr} of platinum in the plasma ultrafiltrate increases as renal function decreases. The AUC_{0-48hr} of platinum in patients with mild (creatinine clearance, CL_{cr} 50 to 80 mL/min), moderate (CL_{cr} 30 to <50 mL/min) and severe renal (CL_{cr} <30 mL/min) impairment is increased by about 60, 140 and 190%, respectively, compared to patients with normal renal function (CL_{cr} >80 mL/min) (see PRECAUTIONS and ADVERSE REACTIONS).

Drug - Drug Interactions

No pharmacokinetic interaction between 85 mg/m^2 of ELOXATIN and infusional 5-FU has been observed in patients treated every 2 weeks, but increases of 5-FU plasma concentrations by approximately 20% have been observed with doses of 130 mg/m^2 of ELOXATIN administered every 3 weeks. In vitro, platinum was not displaced from plasma proteins by the following medications: erythromycin, salicylate, sodium valproate, granisetron, and paclitaxel. In vitro, oxaliplatin is not metabolized by, nor does it inhibit, human cytochrome P450 isoenzymes. No P450-mediated drug-drug interactions are therefore anticipated in patients.

Since platinum-containing species are eliminated primarily through the kidney, clearance of these products may be decreased by co-administration of potentially nephrotoxic compounds, although this has not been specifically studied.

CLINICAL STUDIES

Combination Adjuvant Therapy with ELOXATIN and Infusional 5-FU/LV in Patients with Stage II or III Colon Cancer

An international, multicenter, randomized study compared the efficacy and evaluated the safety of ELOXATIN in combination with an infusional schedule of 5-FU/LV alone, in patients with stage II (Dukes' B2) or III (Dukes' C) colon cancer who had undergone complete resection of the primary tumor. The primary objective of the study was to compare the 3-year disease-free survival (DFS) in patients receiving ELOXATIN and infusional 5-FU/LV to those receiving 5-FU/LV alone. Patients were to be treated for a total of 6 months (i.e., 12 cycles). A total of 2246 patients were randomized; 1123 patients per study arm. Patients in the study had to be between 18 and 75 years of age, have histologically proven stage II (T_3-T_4, N0, M0; Dukes' B2) or III (any T, N_{1-2} M0; Dukes' C) colon carcinoma (with the inferior pole of the tumor above the peritoneal reflec-

Table 1 – Dosing Regimens in Adjuvant Therapy Study

Treatment Arm	Dose	Regimen
ELOXATIN + 5-FU/LV FOLFOX4 (N=1123)	Day 1: ELOXATIN: 85 mg/m^2 (2-hour infusion) + LV: 200 mg/m^2 (2-hour infusion), followed by 5-FU: 400 mg/m^2 (bolus), 600 mg/m^2 (22-hour infusion) Day 2: LV: 200 mg/m^2 (2-hour infusion), followed by 5-FU: 400 mg/m^2 (bolus), 600 mg/m^2 (22-hour infusion)	q2w 12 cycles
5-FU/LV (N=1123)	Day 1: LV: 200 mg/m^2 (2-hour infusion), followed by 5-FU: 400 mg/m^2 (bolus), 600 mg/m^2 (22-hour infusion) Day 2: LV: 200 mg/m^2 (2-hour infusion), followed by 5-FU: 400 mg/m^2 (bolus), 600 mg/m^2 (22-hour infusion)	q2w 12 cycles

Table 2 – Patient Characteristics in Adjuvant Therapy Study

	ELOXATIN + infusional 5-FU/LV N=1123	Infusional 5-FU/LV N=1123
Sex: Male (%)	56.1	52.4
Female (%)	43.9	47.6
Median age (years)	61.0	60.0
<65 years of age (%)	64.4	66.2
≥65 years of age (%)	35.6	33.8
Karnofsky Performance Status (KPS) (%)		
100	29.7	30.5
90	52.2	53.9
80	4.4	3.3
70	13.2	11.9
≤60	0.6	0.4
Primary site (%)		
Colon including caecum	54.6	54.4
Sigmoid	31.9	33.8
Recto sigmoid	12.9	10.9
Other including rectum	0.6	0.9
Bowel obstruction (%)		
Yes	17.9	19.3
Perforation (%)		
Yes	6.9	6.9

(Table continued on next page)

tion, i.e., ≥15 cm from the anal margin) and undergone (within 7 weeks prior to randomization) complete resection of the primary tumor without gross or microscopic evidence of residual disease. Patients had to have had no prior chemotherapy, immunotherapy, or radiotherapy, and have an ECOG performance status of 0,1, or 2 (KPS ≥60%), absolute neutrophil count (ANC) >1.5×10^9/L, platelets ≥100×10^9/L, serum creatinine ≤1.25 × ULN total bilirubin <2 × ULN, AST/ALT <2 × ULN and carcinoembryogenic antigen (CEA) <10 ng/mL. Patients with preexisting peripheral neuropathy (NCI grade ≥1) were ineligible for this trial.
The following table shows the dosing regimens for the two arms of the study.

[See table 1 above]
The following tables show the baseline characteristics and dosing of the patient population entered into this study. The baseline characteristics were well balanced between arms.
[See table 2 above and on next page]
[See table 3 at top of next page]
The following table and figures summarize the disease-free survival (DFS) results in the overall randomized population and in patients with stage II and III disease based on an ITT analysis.
[See table 4 at top of page 328]
In the overall study population DFS was statistically significantly improved in the ELOXATIN combination arm com-

Table 2 *(cont.)* – Patient Characteristics in Adjuvant Therapy Study

	ELOXATIN + infusional 5-FU/LV N=1123	Infusional 5-FU/LV N=1123
Stage at randomization (%)		
II (T=3,4, N=0, M=0)	40.1	39.9
III (T=any, N=1,2, M=0)	59.6	59.3
IV (T=any, N=any, M=1)	0.4	0.8
Staging – T (%)		
T1	0.5	0.7
T2	4.5	4.8
T3	76.0	75.9
T4	19.0	18.5
Staging – N (%)		
N0	40.2	39.9
N1	39.4	39.4
N2	20.4	20.7
Staging – M (%)		
M1	0.4	0.8

Table 3 – Dosing in Adjuvant Therapy Study

	ELOXATIN + infusional 5-FU/LV (N=1108)	Infusional 5-FU/LV (N=1111)
Median relative dose intensity (%)		
5-FU	84.4	97.7
ELOXATIN	80.5	N/A
Median number of cycles	12	12
Median number of cycles with ELOXATIN	11	N/A

pared to infusional 5-FU/LV alone. A statistically significant improvement in DFS was noted in Stage III patients, but not in Stage II patients.

Figure 1 shows the Kaplan-Meier DFS curves for the comparison of ELOXATIN and infusional 5-FU/LV combination and infusional 5-FU/LV alone for the overall population (ITT analysis). Figure 2 shows the Kaplan-Meier DFS curves for the comparison of ELOXATIN and infusional 5-FU/LV combination and infusional 5-FU/LV alone for the Stage III Subgroup.

[See figure 1 at right]

[See figure 2 on next page]

Survival data were not mature at the time of the analysis with a median follow-up of 47 months. No statistically significant difference in overall survival [Hazard Ratio 0.89 (95% CI 0.72, 1.09) p=0.236] was shown between the two treatment arms in the entire population or in the Stage II [Hazard Ratio 0.98 (95% CI 0.63, 1.53) p=0.94] or Stage III [Hazard Ratio 0.86 (95% CI 0.68, 1.08) p=0.196] Subgroups. A descriptive subgroup analysis demonstrated that the improvement in DFS for the ELOXATIN combination arm compared to the infusional 5-FU/LV alone arm appeared to be maintained across genders. The effect of ELOXATIN on disease-free survival benefit in patients ≥65 years of age was not conclusive. Insufficient subgroup sizes prevented analysis by race.

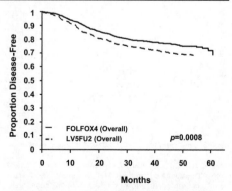

Figure 1 – Kaplan-Meier DFS curves by treatment arm for Overall Population

Combination Therapy with ELOXATIN and 5-FU/LV in Patients Previously Untreated for Advanced Colorectal Cancer
A North American, multicenter, open-label, randomized controlled study was sponsored by the National Cancer Insti-

Table 4 – Summary of DFS Analysis
[ITT Analysis (minimum follow-up of 41 months)]

Parameter	ELOXATIN + infusional 5-FU/LV	Infusional 5-FU/LV
Overall		
N	1123	1123
Median follow-up (months)*	47.7	47.4
Number of events – relapse or death (%)	267 (23.8)	332 (29.6)
4-year Disease-free survival % [95% CI]	75.9 [73.4, 78.5]	69.1 [66.3, 71.9]
Hazard ratio [95% CI]	0.76 [0.65, 0.90]	
Stratified Log-rank test	p=0.0008	
Stage III		
N	672	675
Number of events – relapse or death (%)	200 (29.8)	252 (37.3)
4-year Disease-free survival % [95% CI]	69.7 [66.2, 73.3]	61.0 [57.1, 64.8]
Hazard ratio [95% CI]	0.75 [0.62, 0.90]	
Log-rank test	p=0.002	
Stage II		
N	451	448
Number of events – relapse or death (%)	67 (14.9)	80 (17.9)
4-year Disease-free survival % [95% CI]	85.1 [81.7, 88.6]	81.3 [77.6, 85.1]
Hazard ratio [95% CI]	0.80 [0.58, 1.11]	
Log-rank test	p=0.179	

*For patients alive or lost to follow-up

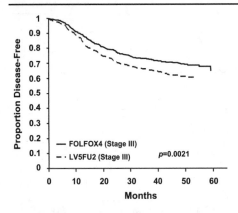

Figure 2 – Kaplan-Meier DFS curves by treatment arm for Stage III Subgroup

tute (NCI) as an intergroup study led by the North Central Cancer Treatment Group (NCCTG). The study had 7 arms at different times during its conduct, four of which were closed due to either changes in the standard of care, toxicity, or simplification. During the study, the control arm was changed to irinotecan plus 5-FU/LV. The results reported below compared the efficacy and safety of two experimental regimens, ELOXATIN in combination with infusional 5-FU/LV and a combination of ELOXATIN plus irinotecan, to an approved control regimen of irinotecan plus 5-FU/LV

in 795 concurrently randomized patients previously untreated for locally advanced or metastatic colorectal cancer. After completion of enrollment, the dose of irinotecan plus 5-FU/LV was decreased due to toxicity. Patients had to be at least 18 years of age, have known locally advanced, locally recurrent, or metastatic colorectal adenocarcinoma not curable by surgery or amenable to radiation therapy with curative intent, histologically proven colorectal adenocarcinoma, measurable or evaluable disease, with an ECOG performance status 0,1, or 2. Patients had to have granulocyte count $\geq 1.5 \times 10^9$/L, platelets $\geq 100 \times 10^9$/L, hemoglobin ≥ 9.0 g/dL, creatinine $\leq 1.5 \times$ ULN, total bilirubin ≤ 1.5 mg/dL, AST $\leq 5 \times$ ULN, and alkaline phosphatase $\leq 5 \times$ ULN. Patients may have received adjuvant therapy for resected Stage II or III disease without recurrence within 12 months. The patients were stratified for ECOG performance status (0, 1 vs. 2), prior adjuvant chemotherapy (yes vs. no), prior immunotherapy (yes vs. no), and age (<65 vs. ≥65 years). Although no post study treatment was specified in the protocol, 65 to 72% of patients received additional post study chemotherapy after study treatment discontinuation on all arms. Fifty-eight percent of patients on the ELOXATIN plus 5-FU/LV arm received an irinotecan-containing regimen and 23% of patients on the irinotecan plus 5-FU/LV arm received oxaliplatin-containing regimens. Oxaliplatin was not commercially available during the trial. The following table presents the dosing regimens of the three arms of the study.
[See table 5 on next page]
The following table presents the demographics and dosing of the patient population entered into this study.
[See table 6 at bottom of next page]

The length of a treatment cycle was 2 weeks for the ELOXATIN and 5-FU/LV regimen; 6 weeks for the irinotecan plus 5-FU/LV regimen; and 3 weeks for the ELOXATIN plus irinotecan regimen. The median number of cycles administered per patient was 10 (23.9 weeks) for the ELOXATIN and 5-FU/LV regimen, 4 (23.6 weeks) for the irinotecan plus 5-FU/LV regimen, and 7 (21.0 weeks) for the ELOXATIN plus irinotecan regimen. Patients treated with the ELOXATIN and 5-FU/LV combination had a significantly longer time to tumor progression based on investigator assessment, longer overall survival, and a significantly higher confirmed response rate based on investigator assessment compared to patients given irinotecan plus 5-FU/LV. The following table summarizes the efficacy results. [See table 7 at top of next page]

The numbers in the response rate and TTP analysis are based on unblinded investigator assessment.

Figure 3 illustrates the Kaplan-Meier survival curves for the comparison of ELOXATIN and 5-FU/LV combination and ELOXATIN plus irinotecan to irinotecan plus 5-FU/LV. [See figure at top of next column]

A descriptive subgroup analysis demonstrated that the improvement in survival for ELOXATIN plus 5-FU/LV compared to irinotecan plus 5-FU/LV appeared to be maintained across age groups, prior adjuvant therapy, and number of organs involved. An estimated survival advantage in ELOXATIN plus 5-FU/LV versus irinotecan plus 5-FU/LV was seen in both genders; however, it was greater among women than men. Insufficient subgroup sizes prevented analysis by race.

Combination Therapy with ELOXATIN and 5-FU/LV in Previously Treated Patients with Advanced Colorectal Cancer

A multicenter, open-label, randomized, three-arm controlled study was conducted in the US and Canada comparing the

Table 5 – Dosing Regimens in Patients Previously Untreated for Advanced Colorectal Cancer Clinical Trial

Treatment Arm	Dose	Regimen
ELOXATIN + 5-FU/LV FOLFOX4 (N=267)	Day 1: ELOXATIN: 85 mg/m^2 (2-hour infusion) + LV 200 mg/m^2 (2-hour infusion), followed by 5-FU: 400 mg/m^2 (bolus), 600 mg/m^2 (22-hour infusion) Day 2: LV 200 mg/m^2 (2-hour infusion), followed by 5-FU: 400 mg/m^2 (bolus), 600 mg/m^2 (22-hour infusion)	q2w
Irinotecan + 5-FU/LV IFL (N=264)	Day 1: irinotecan 125 mg/m^2 as a 90-min infusion + LV 20 mg/m^2 as a 15-min infusion or IV push, followed by 5-FU 500 mg/m^2 IV bolus weekly × 4	q6w
ELOXATIN + irinotecan IROX (N=264)	Day 1: ELOXATIN: 85 mg/m^2 IV (2-hour infusion) + irinotecan 200 mg/m^2 IV over 30 minutes	q3w

Table 6 – Patient Demographics and Dosing in Patients Previously Untreated for Advanced Colorectal Cancer Clinical Trial

	ELOXATIN + 5-FU/LV (N=267)	Irinotecan + 5-FU/LV (N=264)	ELOXATIN + irinotecan (N=264)
Sex: Male (%)	58.8	65.2	61.0
Female (%)	41.2	34.8	39.0
Median age (years)	61.0	61.0	61.0
>65 years of age (%)	61	62	63
≥65 years of age (%)	39	38	37
ECOG (%)			
0.1	94.4	95.5	94.7
2	5.6	4.5	5.3
Involved organs (%)			
Colon only	0.7	0.8	0.4
Liver only	39.3	44.3	39.0
Liver + other	41.2	38.6	40.9
Lung only	6.4	3.8	5.3
Other (including lymph nodes)	11.6	11.0	12.9
Not reported	0.7	1.5	1.5
Prior radiation (%)	3.0	1.5	3.0
Prior surgery (%)	74.5	79.2	81.8
Prior adjuvant (%)	15.7	14.8	15.2

Table 7 – Summary of Efficacy

	ELOXATIN + 5-FU/LV (N=267)	Irinotecan + 5-FU/LV (N=264)	ELOXATIN + irinotecan (N=264)
Survival (ITT)			
Number of deaths N (%)	155 (58.1)	192 (72.7)	175 (66.3)
Median survival (months)	19.4	14.6	17.6
Hazard Ratio and (95% confidence interval)	0.65 (0.53-0.80)*		
P-value	<0.0001*	–	–
TTP (ITT, investigator assessment)			
Percentage of progressors	82.8	81.8	89.4
Median TTP (months)	8.7	6.9	6.5
Hazard Ratio and (95% confidence interval)	0.74 (0.61-0.89)*		
P-value	0.0014*	–	–
Response Rate (investigator assessment)**			
Patients with measurable disease	210	212	215
Complete response N (%)	13 (6.2)	5 (2.4)	7 (3.3)
Partial response N (%)	82 (39.0)	64 (30.2)	67 (31.2)
Complete and partial response N (%)	95 (45.2)	69 (32.5)	74 (34.4)
95% confidence interval	(38.5-52.0)	(26.2-38.9)	(28.1-40.8)
P-value	0.0080*	–	–

*Compared to irinotecan plus 5-FU/LV (IFL) arm
**Based on all patients with measurable disease at baseline

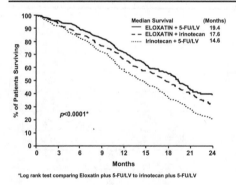

Median Survival	(Months)
ELOXATIN + 5-FU/LV	19.4
ELOXATIN + irinotecan	17.6
Irinotecan + 5-FU/LV	14.6

$p<0.0001*$

*Log rank test comparing Eloxatin plus 5-FU/LV to irinotecan plus 5-FU/LV

Figure 3 – Kaplan-Meier Overall Survival by treatment arm

efficacy and safety of ELOXATIN in combination with an infusional schedule of 5-FU/LV to the same dose and schedule of 5-FU/LV alone and to single agent oxaliplatin in patients with advanced colorectal cancer who had relapsed/progressed during or within 6 months of first-line therapy with bolus 5-FU/LV and irinotecan. The study was intended to be analyzed for response rate after 450 patients were enrolled. Survival will be subsequently assessed in all patients enrolled in the completed study. Accrual to this study is complete, with 821 patients enrolled. Patients in the study had to be at least 18 years of age, have unresectable, measurable, histologically proven colorectal adenocarcinoma, with a Karnofsky performance status >50%. Patients had to have SGOT(AST) and SGPT(ALT) ≤2× the institution's upper limit of normal (ULN), unless liver metastases were present

and documented at baseline by CT or MRI scan, in which case ≤5× ULN was permitted. Patients had to have alkaline phosphatase ≤2× the institution's ULN, unless liver metastases were present and documented at baseline by CT or MRI scan, in which cases ≤5× ULN was permitted. Prior radiotherapy was permitted if it had been completed at least 3 weeks before randomization.

The dosing regimens of the three arms of the study are presented in the table below.
[See table 8 on next page]
Patients entered into the study for evaluation of response must have had at least one unidimensional lesion measuring ≥20mm using conventional CT or MRI scans, or ≥10mm using a spiral CT scan. Tumor response and progression were assessed every 3 cycles (6 weeks) using the Response Evaluation Criteria in Solid Tumors (RECIST) until radiological documentation of progression or for 13 months following the first dose of study drug(s), whichever came first. Confirmed responses were based on two tumor assessments separated by at least 4 weeks.

The demographics of the patient population entered into this study are shown in the table below.
[See table 9 on next page]
The median number of cycles administered per patient was 6 for the ELOXATIN and 5-FU/LV combination and 3 each for 5-FU/LV alone and ELOXATIN alone.

Patients treated with the combination of ELOXATIN and 5-FU/LV had an increased response rate compared to patients given 5-FU/LV or oxaliplatin alone. The efficacy results are summarized in the tables below.
[See table 10 at top of page 332]
[See table 11 at top of page 332]
At the time of the interim analysis 49% of the radiographic progression events had occurred. In this interim analysis an estimated 2-month increase in median time to radiographic progression was observed compared to 5-FU/LV alone.

Of the 13 patients who had tumor response to the combination of ELOXATIN and 5-FU/LV, 5 were female and 8 were male, and responders included patients <65 years old and ≥65 years old. The small number of non-Caucasian participants made efficacy analyses in these populations uninterpretable.

INDICATIONS AND USAGE

ELOXATIN, used in combination with infusional 5-FU/LV, is indicated for adjuvant treatment of stage III colon cancer patients who have undergone complete resection of the primary tumor. The indication is based on an improvement in disease-free survival, with no demonstrated benefit in overall survival after a median follow up of 4 years.

ELOXATIN, used in combination with infusional 5-FU/LV, is indicated for the treatment of advanced carcinoma of the colon or rectum.

CONTRAINDICATIONS

ELOXATIN should not be administered to patients with a history of known allergy to ELOXATIN or other platinum compounds.

Table 8 – Dosing Regimens in Refractory and Relapsed Colorectal Cancer Clinical Trial

Treatment Arm	Dose	Regimen
ELOXATIN + 5-FU/LV (N=152)	**Day 1: ELOXATIN: 85 mg/m^2 (2-hour infusion) + LV 200 mg/m^2 (2-hour infusion), followed by 5-FU: 400 mg/m^2 (bolus), 600 mg/m^2 (22-hour infusion)** **Day 2: LV 200 mg/m^2 (2-hour infusion), followed by 5-FU: 400 mg/m^2 (bolus), 600 mg/m^2 (22-hour infusion)**	**q2w**
5-FU/LV (N=151)	Day 1: LV 200 mg/m^2 (2-hour infusion), followed by 5-FU: 400 mg/m^2 (bolus), 600 mg/m^2 (22-hour infusion) Day 2: LV 200 mg/m^2 (2-hour infusion), followed by 5-FU: 400 mg/m^2 (bolus), 600 mg/m^2 (22-hour infusion)	q2w
ELOXATIN (N=156)	Day 1: ELOXATIN 85 mg/m^2 (2-hour infusion)	q2w

Table 9 – Patient Demographics in Refractory and Relapsed Colorectal Cancer Clinical Trial

	5-FU/LV (N=151)	ELOXATIN (N=156)	ELOXATIN + 5-FU/LV (N=152)
Sex: Male (%)	54.3	60.9	57.2
Female (%)	45.7	39.1	42.8
Median age (years)	60.0	61.0	59.0
Range	21-80	27-79	22-88
Race (%)			
Caucasian	87.4	84.6	88.8
Black	7.9	7.1	5.9
Asian	1.3	2.6	2.6
Other	3.3	5.8	2.6
KPS (%)			
70-100	94.7	92.3	95.4
50-60	2.6	4.5	2.0
Not reported	2.6	3.2	2.6
Prior radiotherapy (%)	25.2	19.2	25.0
Prior pelvic radiation (%)	18.5	13.5	21.1
Number of metastatic sites (%)			
1	27.2	31.4	25.7
≥2	72.2	67.9	74.3
Liver involvement (%)			
Liver only	22.5	25.6	18.4
Liver + other	60.3	59.0	53.3

Table 10 – Response Rates (ITT Analysis)

Best Response	5-FU/LV (N=151)	ELOXATIN (N=156)	ELOXATIN + 5-FU/LV (N=152)
CR	0	0	0
PR	0	2 (1%)	13 (9%)
p-value	0.0002 for **5-FU/LV** vs. **ELOXATIN + 5-FU/LV**		
95% CI	0-2.4%	0.2-4.6%	4.6-14.2%

Table 11 – Summary of Radiographic Time to Progression*

Arm	5-FU/LV (N=151)	ELOXATIN (N=156)	ELOXATIN + 5-FU/LV (N=152)
No. of Progressors	74	101	50
No. of patients with no radiological evaluation beyond baseline	22 (15%)	16 (10%)	17 (11%)
Median TTP (months)	2.7	1.6	4.6
95% CI	1.8-3.0	1.4-2.7	4.2-6.1

*This is not an ITT analysis. Events were limited to radiographic disease progression documented by independent review of radiographs. Clinical progression was not included in this analysis, and 18% of patients were excluded from the analysis based on unavailability of the radiographs for independent review.

WARNINGS

As in the case for other platinum compounds, hypersensitivity and anaphylactic/anaphylactoid reactions to ELOXATIN have been reported (see ADVERSE REACTIONS). These allergic reactions were similar in nature and severity to those reported with other platinum-containing compounds, i.e., rash, urticaria, erythema, pruritus, and, rarely, bronchospasm and hypotension. These reactions occur within minutes of administration and should be managed with appropriate supportive therapy. Drug-related deaths associated with platinum compounds from this reaction have been reported.

Pregnancy Category D

ELOXATIN may cause fetal harm when administered to a pregnant woman. Pregnant rats were administered 1 mg/kg/day oxaliplatin (less than one-tenth the recommended human dose based on body surface area) during gestation days 1-5 (pre-implantation), 6-10, or 11-16 (during organogenesis). Oxaliplatin caused developmental mortality (increased early resorptions) when administered on days 6-10 and 11-16 and adversely affected fetal growth (decreased fetal weight, delayed ossification) when administered on days 6-10. If this drug is used during pregnancy or if the patient becomes pregnant while taking this drug, the patient should be apprised of the potential hazard to the fetus. Women of childbearing potential should be advised to avoid becoming pregnant while receiving treatment with ELOXATIN.

PRECAUTIONS

General

ELOXATIN should be administered under the supervision of a qualified physician experienced in the use of cancer chemotherapeutic agents. Appropriate management of therapy and complications is possible only when adequate diagnostic and treatment facilities are readily available.

Neuropathy

Patients with Stage II or III Colon Cancer

Neuropathy was graded using a prelisted module derived from the Neuro-Sensory section of the NCI CTC scale version 1, as follows:

Table 12 – NCI CTC Grading for Neuropathy in Adjuvant Patients

NCI Grade	Definition
Grade 0	No change or none
Grade 1	Mild paresthesias, loss of deep tendon reflexes
Grade 2	Mild or moderate objective sensory loss, moderate paresthesias
Grade 3	Severe objective sensory loss or paresthesias that interfere with function
Grade 4	Not applicable

Peripheral sensory neuropathy was reported in adjuvant patients treated with the ELOXATIN combination with a frequency of 92% (all grades) and 13% (grade 3). At the 28-day follow-up after the last treatment cycle, 60% of all patients had any grade (Grade 1=39.6%, Grade 2=15.7%, Grade 3=5.0%) peripheral sensory neuropathy decreasing to 39% at 6 months of follow-up (Grade 1=30.5%, Grade 2=7.4%, Grade 3=1.3%) and 21% at 18 months of follow-up (Grade 1=17.2%, Grade 2=3.0%, Grade 3=0.5%).

Previously Untreated and Previously Treated Patients with Advanced Colorectal Cancer

Neuropathy was graded using a study-specific neurotoxicity scale, which was different than the National Cancer Institute Common Toxicity Criteria, version 2.0 (NCI CTC) (see below).

In the previously treated study, neuropathy information was collected to establish that ELOXATIN is associated with two types of neuropathy:

- **An acute, reversible, primarily peripheral, sensory neuropathy that is of early onset, occurring within hours or one to two days of dosing, that resolves within 14 days, and that frequently recurs with further dosing.** The symptoms may be precipitated or exacerbated by exposure to cold temperature or cold objects and they usually present as transient paresthesia, dysesthesia, and hypoesthesia

Table 13 – Adverse Experiences Reported in Patients with Stage II or III Colon Cancer Receiving Adjuvant Treatment (≥5% of all patients and with ≥1% NCI grade 3/4 events)

Adverse Event (WHO/Pref)	ELOXATIN + 5-FU/LV (N=1108)		5-FU/LV (N=1111)	
	All Grades (%)	Grade 3/4 (%)	All Grades (%)	Grade 3/4 (%)
Any Event	100	70	99	31
Allergy/Immunology				
Allergic Reaction	10	3	2	<1
Constitutional Symptoms/Pain				
Fatigue	44	4	38	1
Abdominal Pain	18	1	17	2
Dermatology/Skin				
Skin Disorder	32	2	36	2
Injection Site Reaction[1]	11	3	10	3
Gastrointestinal				
Nausea	74	5	61	2
Diarrhea	56	11	48	7
Vomiting	47	6	24	1
Stomatitis	42	3	40	2
Anorexia	13	1	8	<1
Fever/Infection				
Fever	27	1	12	1
Infection	25	4	25	3
Neurology				
Overall Periphreal Sensory Neuropathy	92	12	16	<1

[1] Includes thrombosis related to the catheter

in the hands, feet, perioral area, or throat. Jaw spasm, abnormal tongue sensation, dysarthria, eye pain, and a feeling of chest pressure have also been observed. The acute, reversible pattern of sensory neuropathy was observed in about 56% of study patients who received ELOXATIN with 5-FU/LV. In any individual cycle acute neurotoxicity was observed in approximately 30% of patients. Ice (mucositis prophylaxis) should be avoided during the infusion of ELOXATIN because cold temperature can exacerbate acute neurological symptoms (see DOSAGE AND ADMINISTRATION: Dose Modifications). An acute syndrome of pharyngolaryngeal dysesthesia seen in 1-2% (grade 3/4) of patients previously untreated for advanced colorectal cancer, and the previously treated patients, is characterized by subjective sensations of dysphagia or dyspnea, without any laryngospasm or bronchospasm (no stridor or wheezing).

• A persistent (>14 days), primarily peripheral, sensory neuropathy that is usually characterized by paresthesias, dysesthesias, hypoesthesias, but may also include deficits in proprioception that can interfere with daily activities (e.g., writing, buttoning, swallowing, and difficulty walking from impaired proprioception). These forms of neuropathy occurred in 48% of the study patients receiving ELOXATIN with 5-FU/LV. Persistent neuropathy can

occur without any prior acute neuropathy event. The majority of the patients (80%) who developed grade 3 persistent neuropathy progressed from prior grade 1 or 2 events. These symptoms may improve in some patients upon discontinuation of ELOXATIN.

Overall, neuropathy was reported in patients previously untreated for advanced colorectal cancer in 82% (all grades) and 19% (grade 3/4), and in the previously treated patients in 74% (all grades) and 7% (grade 3/4) events. Information regarding reversibility of neuropathy was not available from the trial for patients who had not been previously treated for colorectal cancer.

Neurotoxicity scale:
The grading scale for paresthesias/dysesthesias was: grade 1, resolved and did not interfere with functioning; grade 2, interfered with function but not daily activities; grade 3, pain or functional impairment that interfered with daily activities; grade 4, persistent impairment that is disabling or life-threatening.

Pulmonary Toxicity
ELOXATIN has been associated with pulmonary fibrosis (<1% of study patients), which may be fatal. The combined incidence of cough and dyspnea was 7.4% (any grade) and <1% (grade 3) with no grade 4 events in the ELOXATIN plus infusional 5-FU/LV arm compared to 4.5% (any grade)

Table 14 – Adverse Experiences Reported in Patients with Stage II or III Colon Cancer Receiving Adjuvant Treatment (≥5% of all patients, but with <1% NCI grade 3/4 events)

Adverse Event (WHO/Pref)	ELOXATIN + 5-FU/LV N=1108 All Grades (%)	5-FU/LV N=1111 All Grades (%)
Allergy/Immunology		
Rhinitis	6	8
Constitutional Symptoms/Pain/Ocular/Visual		
Epistaxis	16	12
Weight Increase	10	10
Conjunctivitis	9	15
Headache	7	5
Dyspnea	5	3
Pain	5	5
Lacrimation Abnormal	4	12
Dermatology/Skin		
Alopecia	30	28
Gastrointestinal		
Constipation	22	19
Taste Perversion	12	8
Dyspepsia	8	5
Metabolic		
Phosphate Alkaline Increased	42	20
Neurology		
Sensory Disturbance	8	1

and no grade 3 and 0.1% grade 4 events in the infusional 5-FU/LV alone arm in adjuvant colon cancer patients. In this study, one patient died from eosinophilic pneumonia in the ELOXATIN combination arm. The combined incidence of cough, dyspnea, and hypoxia was 43% (any grade) and 7% (grade 3 and 4) in the ELOXATIN plus 5-FU/LV arm compared to 32% (any grade) and 5% (grade 3 and 4) in the irinotecan plus 5-FU/LV arm of unknown duration for patients with previously untreated colorectal cancer. In case of unexplained respiratory symptoms such as non-productive cough, dyspnea, crackles, or radiological pulmonary infiltrates, ELOXATIN should be discontinued until further pulmonary investigation excludes interstitial lung disease or pulmonary fibrosis.

Hepatotoxicity
Hepatotoxicity as evidenced in the adjuvant study, by increase in transaminases (57% vs. 34%) and alkaline phosphatase (42% vs. 20%) was observed more commonly in the ELOXATIN combination arm. The incidence of increased bilirubin was similar on both arms. Changes noted on liver biopsies include: peliosis, nodular regenerative hyperplasia or sinusoidal alterations, perisinusoidal fibrosis, and veno-occlusive lesions. Hepatic vascular disorders should be considered and if appropriate, should be investigated in case of abnormal liver function test results or portal hypertension, which cannot be explained by liver metastases.

Information for Patients
Patients and patients' caregivers should be informed of the expected side effects of ELOXATIN, particularly its neuro-

logic effects, both the acute, reversible effects and the persistent neurosensory toxicity. Patients should be informed that the acute neurosensory toxicity may be precipitated or exacerbated by exposure to cold or cold objects. Patients should be instructed to avoid cold drinks, use of ice, and should cover exposed skin prior to exposure to cold temperature or cold objects.

Patients must be adequately informed of the risk of low blood cell counts and instructed to contact their physician immediately should fever, particularly if associated with persistent diarrhea, or evidence of infection develop.

Patients should be instructed to contact their physician if persistent vomiting, diarrhea, signs of dehydration, cough, or breathing difficulties occur, or signs of allergic reaction appear.

Laboratory Tests
Standard monitoring of the white blood cell count with differential, hemoglobin, platelet count, and blood chemistries (including ALT, AST, bilirubin and creatinine) is recommended before each ELOXATIN cycle (see DOSAGE AND ADMINISTRATION).

Laboratory Test Interactions
None known.

Carcinogenesis, Mutagenesis, Impairment of Fertility
Long-term animal studies have not been performed to evaluate the carcinogenic potential of oxaliplatin. Oxaliplatin was not mutagenic to bacteria (Ames test) but was mutagenic to mammalian cells in vitro (L5178Y mouse lym-

Table 15 – Adverse Experiences Reported in Patients Previously Untreated for Advanced Colorectal Cancer Clinical Trial (≥5% of all patients and with ≥1% NCI grade 3/4 events)

Adverse Event (WHO/Pref)	ELOXATIN + 5-FU/LV (N=259)		Irinotecan + 5-FU/LV (N=256)		ELOXATIN + irinotecan (N=258)	
	All Grades (%)	Grade 3/4 (%)	All Grades (%)	Grade 3/4 (%)	All Grades (%)	Grade 3/4 (%)
Any Event	99	82	98	70	99	76
Allergy/Immunology						
Hypersensitivity	12	2	5	0	6	1
Cardiovascular						
Thrombosis	6	5	6	6	3	3
Hypotension	5	3	6	3	4	3
Constitutional Symptoms/Pain/Ocular/Visual						
Fatigue	70	7	58	11	66	16
Abdominal Pain	29	8	31	7	39	10
Myalgia	14	2	6	0	9	2
Pain	7	1	5	1	6	1
Vision Abnormal	5	0	2	1	6	1
Neuralgia	5	0	0	0	2	1
Dermatology/Skin						
Skin Reaction - hand/foot	7	1	2	1	1	0
Injection Site Reaction	6	0	1	0	4	1
Gastrointestinal						
Nausea	71	6	67	15	83	19
Diarrhea	56	12	65	29	76	25
Vomiting	41	4	43	13	64	23
Stomatitis	38	0	25	1	19	1
Anorexia	35	2	25	4	27	5
Constipation	32	4	27	2	21	2
Diarrhea - colostomy	13	2	16	7	16	3
Gastrointestinal NOS	5	2	4	2	3	2

(Table continued on next page)

phoma assay). Oxaliplatin was clastogenic both *in vitro* (chromosome aberration in human lymphocytes) and *in vivo* (mouse bone marrow micronucleus assay).

In a fertility study, male rats were given oxaliplatin at 0, 0.5, 1, or 2 mg/kg/day for five days every 21 days for a total of three cycles prior to mating with females that received two cycles of oxaliplatin on the same schedule. A dose of 2 mg/kg/day (less than one seventh the recommended human dose on a body surface area basis) did not affect pregnancy rate, but caused developmental mortality (increased early resorptions, decreased live fetuses, decreased live births) and delayed growth (decreased fetal weight).

Testicular damage, characterized by degeneration, hypoplasia, and atrophy, was observed in dogs administered oxaliplatin at 0.75 mg/kg/day × 5 days every 28 days for three cycles. A no effect level was not identified. This daily dose is approximately one sixth of the recommended human dose on a body surface area basis.

Pregnancy Category D - See WARNINGS

Nursing Mothers - It is not known whether ELOXATIN or its derivatives are excreted in human milk. Because many drugs are excreted in human milk and because of the potential for serious adverse reactions in nursing infants from ELOXATIN, a decision should be made whether to discontinue nursing or delay the use of the drug, taking into account the importance of the drug to the mother.

Pediatric Use - The safety and effectiveness of ELOXATIN in pediatric patients have not been established.

Patients with Renal Impairment - The safety and effectiveness of the combination of ELOXATIN and 5-FU/LV in patients with renal impairment have not been evaluated. The

Table 15 *(cont.)* – Adverse Experiences Reported in Patients Previously Untreated for Advanced Colorectal Cancer Clinical Trial (≥5% of all patients and with ≥1% NCI grade 3/4 events)

Adverse Event (WHO/Pref)	ELOXATIN + 5-FU/LV (N=259)		Irinotecan + 5-FU/LV (N=256)		ELOXATIN + irinotecan (N=258)	
	All Grades (%)	Grade 3/4 (%)	All Grades (%)	Grade 3/4 (%)	All Grades (%)	Grade 3/4 (%)
Any Event	99	82	98	70	99	76
Hematology/Infection						
Infection no ANC	10	4	5	1	7	2
Infection – ANC	8	8	12	11	9	8
Lymphopenia	6	2	4	1	5	2
Febrile Neutropenia	4	4	15	14	12	11
Hepatic/Metabolic/Laboratory/Renal						
Hyperglycemia	14	2	11	3	12	3
Hypokalemia	11	3	7	4	6	2
Dehydration	9	5	16	11	14	7
Hypoalbuminemia	8	0	5	2	9	1
Hyponatremia	8	2	7	4	4	1
Urinary Frequency	5	1	2	1	3	1
Neurology						
Overall Neuropathy	82	19	18	2	69	7
Paresthesias	77	18	16	2	62	6
Pharyngo-laryngeal Dysesthesias	38	2	1	0	28	1
Neuro-sensory	12	1	2	0	9	1
Neuro NOS	1	0	1	0	1	0
Pulmonary						
Cough	35	1	25	2	17	1
Dyspnea	18	7	14	3	11	2
Hiccups	5	1	2	0	3	2

combination of ELOXATIN and 5-FU/LV should be used with caution in patients with preexisting renal impairment since the primary route of platinum elimination is renal. Clearance of ultrafilterable platinum is decreased in patients with mild, moderate, and severe renal impairment. A pharmacodynamic relationship between platinum ultrafiltrate levels and clinical safety and effectiveness has not been established (see CLINICAL PHARMACOLOGY and ADVERSE REACTIONS).

Geriatric Use - No significant effect of age on the clearance of ultrafilterable platinum has been observed. In the adjuvant therapy colon cancer randomized clinical trial (see CLINICAL STUDIES), 723 patients treated with ELOXATIN and infusional 5-FU/LV were <65 years and 400 patients were ≥65 years. In the previously untreated for advanced colorectal cancer randomized clinical trial (see CLINICAL STUDIES) of ELOXATIN, 160 patients treated with ELOXATIN and 5-FU/LV were <65 years and 99 patients were ≥65 years. The same efficacy improvements in response rate, time to tumor progression, and overall survival were observed in the ≥65-year-old patients as in the overall study population. In the previously treated randomized clinical trial (see CLINICAL STUDIES) of ELOXATIN, 95 patients treated with ELOXATIN and 5-FU/LV were <65

years and 55 patients were ≥65 years. The rates of overall adverse events, including grade 3 and 4 events, were similar across and within arms in the different age groups in all studies. The incidence of diarrhea, dehydration, hypokalemia, leukopenia, fatigue and syncope were higher in patients ≥65 years old. No adjustment to starting dose was required in patients ≥65 years old.

Drug Interactions - No specific cytochrome P450-based drug interaction studies have been conducted. No pharmacokinetic interaction between 85 mg/m^2 ELOXATIN and 5-FU/LV has been observed in patients treated every 2 weeks. Increases of 5-FU plasma concentrations by approximately 20% have been observed with doses of 130 mg/m^2 ELOXATIN dosed every 3 weeks. Since platinum-containing species are eliminated primarily through the kidney, clearance of these products may be decreased by coadministration of potentially nephrotoxic compounds; although, this has not been specifically studied (see CLINICAL PHARMACOLOGY).

ADVERSE REACTIONS

More than 1100 patients with stage II or III colon cancer and more than 4000 patients with advanced colorectal cancer have been treated in clinical studies with ELOXATIN either as a single agent or in combination with other medications. The most common adverse reactions in patients with stage II or III colon cancer receiving adjuvant therapy were peripheral sensory neuropathy, neutropenia, thrombocytopenia, anemia, nausea, increase in transaminases and alkaline phosphatase, diarrhea, emesis, fatigue, and stomatitis. The most common adverse reactions in previously untreated and treated patients were peripheral sensory neuropathies, fatigue, neutropenia, nausea, emesis, and diarrhea (see PRECAUTIONS).

Combination Adjuvant Therapy with ELOXATIN and Infusional 5-FU/LV in Patients with Stage II or III Colon Cancer
One thousand one hundred eight patients with stage II or III colon cancer, who had undergone complete resection of the primary tumor, have been treated in a clinical study with ELOXATIN in combination with infusional 5-FU/LV (see CLINICAL STUDIES). The incidence of grade 3 or 4 adverse events was 70% on the ELOXATIN combination arm, and 31% on the infusional 5-FU/LV arm. The adverse reactions in this trial are shown in the tables below. Discontinuation of treatment due to adverse events occurred in 15% of the patients receiving ELOXATIN and infusional 5-FU/LV. Both 5-FU/LV and ELOXATIN are associated with gastrointestinal or hematologic adverse events. When ELOXATIN is administered in combination with infusional 5-FU/LV, the incidence of these events is increased.
The incidence of death within 28 days of last treatment, regardless of causality, was 0.5% (n=6) in both the ELOXATIN combination and infusional 5-FU/LV arms, respectively. Deaths within 60 days from initiation of therapy were 0.3% (n=3) in both the ELOXATIN combination and infusional 5-FU/LV arms, respectively. On the ELOXATIN combination arm, 3 deaths were due to sepsis/neutropenic sepsis, 2 from intracerebral bleeding, and one from eosinophilic pneumonia. On the 5-FU/LV arm, one death was due to suicide, 2 from Stevens-Johnson syndrome (1 patient also had sepsis), 1 unknown cause, 1 anoxic cerebral infarction, and 1 probable abdominal aorta rupture.
The following table provides adverse events reported in the adjuvant therapy colon cancer clinical trial (see CLINICAL STUDIES) by body system and decreasing order of frequency in the ELOXATIN and infusional 5-FU/LV arm for events with overall incidences ≥5% and for NCI grade 3/4 events with incidences ≥1%. This table does not include hematologic and blood chemistry abnormalities; these are shown separately below.
[See table 13 at top of page 333]
The following table provides adverse events reported in the adjuvant therapy colon cancer clinical trial (see CLINICAL STUDIES) by body system and decreasing order of frequency in the ELOXATIN and infusional 5-FU/LV arm for events with overall incidences ≥5% but with incidences <1% NCI grade 3/4 events.
[See table 14 at top of page 334]
Although specific events can vary, the overall frequency of adverse events was similar in men and women and in patients <65 and ≥65 years. However, the following grade 3/4 events were more common in females: diarrhea, fatigue, granulocytopenia, nausea; and vomiting. In patients ≥65 years old, the incidence of grade 3/4 diarrhea and granulocytopenia was higher than in younger patients. Insufficient subgroup sizes prevented analysis of safety by race. The following additional adverse events were reported in ≥2% and <5% of the patients in the ELOXATIN and infusional 5-FU/LV combination arm (listed in decreasing order of frequency): pain, leukopenia, weight decrease, coughing.

Patients Previously Untreated for Advanced Colorectal Cancer
Two hundred fifty-nine patients were treated in the ELOXATIN and 5-FU/LV combination arm of the randomized trial in patients previously untreated for advanced colorectal cancer (see CLINICAL STUDIES). The adverse event profile in this study was similar to that seen in other studies, and the adverse reactions in this trial are shown in the tables below.
Both 5-FU and ELOXATIN are associated with gastrointestinal and hematologic adverse events. When ELOXATIN is administered in combination with 5-FU, the incidence of these events is increased.

The incidence of death within 30 days of treatment in the previously untreated for advanced colorectal cancer study, regardless of causality, was 3% with the ELOXATIN and 5-FU/LV combination, 5% with irinotecan plus 5-FU/LV, and 3% with ELOXATIN plus irinotecan. Deaths within 60 days from initiation of therapy were 2.3% with the ELOXATIN and 5-FU/LV combination, 5.1% with irinotecan plus 5-FU/LV, and 3.1% with ELOXATIN plus irinotecan.
The following table provides adverse events reported in the previously untreated for advanced colorectal cancer study (see CLINICAL STUDIES) by body system and decreasing order of frequency in the ELOXATIN and 5-FU/LV combination arm for events with overall incidences ≥5% and for grade 3/4 events with incidences ≥1%. This table does not include hematologic and blood chemistry abnormalities; these are shown separately below.
[See table 15 on pages 335 and 336]
The following table provides adverse events reported in the previously untreated for advanced colorectal cancer study (see CLINICAL STUDIES) by body system and decreasing order of frequency in the ELOXATIN and 5-FU/LV combination arm for events with overall incidences ≥5% but with incidences <1% NCI grade 3/4 events.

Table 16 – Adverse Experiences Reported in Patients Previously Untreated for Advanced Colorectal Cancer Clinical Trial
(≥5% of all patients but with <1% NCI Grade 3/4 events)

Adverse Event (WHO/Pref)	ELOXATIN + 5-FU/LV (N = 259) All Grades (%)	Irinotecan + 5 FU/LV (N = 256) All Grades (%)	ELOXATIN + ironotecan (N = 258) All Grades (%)
Allergy/Immunology			
Rash	11	4	7
Rhinitis Allergic	10	6	6
Cardiovascular			
Edema	15	13	10
Constitutional Symptoms/Pain/Ocular/Visual			
Headache	13	6	9
Weight Loss	11	9	11
Epistaxis	10	2	2
Tearing	9	1	2
Rigors	8	2	7
Dysphasia	5	3	3
Sweating	5	6	12
Arthralgia	5	5	8
Dermatology/Skin			
Alopecia	38	44	67
Flushing	7	2	5
Pruritus	6	4	2
Dry Skin	6	2	5
Gastrointestinal			
Taste Perversion	14	6	8

Dyspepsia	12	7	5
Flatulence	9	6	5
Mouth Dryness	5	2	3
Hematology/Infection			
Fever no ANC	16	9	9
Hepatic/Metabolic/Laboratory/Renal			
Hypocalcemia	7	5	4
Elevated Creatinine	4	4	5
Neurology			
Insomnia	13	9	11
Depression	9	5	7
Dizziness	8	6	10
Anxiety	5	2	6

Adverse events were similar in men and women and in patients <65 and ≥65 years, but older patients may have been more susceptible to diarrhea, dehydration, hypokalemia, leukopenia, fatigue, and syncope. The following additional adverse events, at least possibly related to treatment and potentially important, were reported in ≥2% and <5% of the patients in the ELOXATIN and 5-FU/LV combination arm (listed in decreasing order of frequency): metabolic, pneumonitis, catheter infection, vertigo, prothrombin time, pulmonary, rectal bleeding, dysuria, nail changes, chest pain, rectal pain, syncope, hypertension, hypoxia, unknown infection, bone pain, pigmentation changes, and urticaria.

Previously Treated Patients with Advanced Colorectal Cancer

Four hundred fifty patients (about 150 receiving the combination of ELOXATIN and 5-FU/LV) were studied in a randomized trial in patients with refractory and relapsed colorectal cancer (see CLINICAL STUDIES). The adverse event profile in this study was similar to that seen in other studies, and the adverse reactions in this trial are shown in the tables below.

Thirteen percent of patients in the ELOXATIN and 5-FU/LV combination arm and 18% in the 5-FU/LV arm of the previously treated study had to discontinue treatment because of adverse effects related to gastrointestinal, or hematologic adverse events, or neuropathies. Both 5-FU and ELOXATIN are associated with gastrointestinal and hematologic adverse events. When ELOXATIN is administered in combination with 5-FU, the incidence of these events is increased. The incidence of death within 30 days of treatment in the previously treated study, regardless of causality, was 5% with the ELOXATIN and 5-FU/LV combination, 8% with ELOXATIN alone, and 7% with 5-FU/LV. Of the 7 deaths that occurred on the ELOXATIN and 5-FU/LV combination arm within 30 days of stopping treatment, 3 may have been treatment related, associated with gastrointestinal bleeding or dehydration.

The following table provides adverse events reported in the previously treated study (see CLINICAL STUDIES) by body system and in decreasing order of frequency in the ELOXATIN and 5-FU/LV combination arm for events with overall incidences ≥5% and for grade 3/4 events with incidences ≥1%. This table does not include hematologic and blood chemistry abnormalities; these are shown separately below.

[See table 17 at top of next page]

The following table provides adverse events reported in the previously treated study (see CLINICAL STUDIES) by body system and in decreasing order of frequency in the ELOXATIN and 5-FU/LV combination arm for events with overall incidences ≥5% but with incidences <1% NCI grade 3/4 events.

Table 18 – Adverse Experiences Reported in Previously Treated Colorectal Cancer Clinical Trial
(≥5% of all patients but with <1% NCI grade 3/4 events)

Adverse Event (WHO/Pref)	5-FU/LV (N = 142) All Grades (%)	ELOXATIN (N = 153) All Grades (%)	ELOXATIN + 5-FU/LV (N = 150) All Grades (%)
Allergy/Immunology			
Rhinitis	4	6	15
Allergic Reaction	1	3	10
Rash	5	5	9
Cardiovascular			
Peripheral Edema	11	5	10
Constitutional Symptoms/Pain/Ocular/Visual			
Headache	8	13	17
Arthralgia	10	7	10
Epistaxis	1	2	9
Abnormal Lacrimation	6	1	7
Rigors	6	9	7
Dermatology/Skin			
Hand-Foot Syndrome	13	1	11
Flushing	2	3	10
Alopecia	3	3	7
Gastrointestinal			
Constipation	23	31	32
Dyspepsia	10	7	14
Taste Perversion	1	5	13
Mucositis	10	2	7
Flatulence	6	3	5
Hepatic/Metabolic/Laboratory/Renal			
Hematuria	4	0	6
Dysuria	1	1	6
Neurology			
Dizziness	8	7	13
Insomnia	4	11	9
Pulmonary			
Upper Resp Tract Infection	4	7	10
Pharyngitis	10	2	9
Hiccup	0	2	5

Table 17 – Adverse Experiences Reported in Previously Treated Colorectal Cancer Clinical Trial
(≥5% of all patients and with ≥1% NCI grade 3/4 events)

Adverse Event (WHO/Pref)	5-FU/LV (N=142) All Grades (%)	5-FU/LV (N=142) Grade 3/4 (%)	ELOXATIN (N=153) All Grades (%)	ELOXATIN (N=153) Grade 3/4 (%)	ELOXATIN + 5-FU/LV (N=150) All Grades (%)	ELOXATIN + 5-FU/LV (N=150) Grade 3/4 (%)
Any Event	98	41	100	46	99	73
Cardiovascular						
Dyspnea	11	2	13	7	20	4
Coughing	9	0	11	0	19	1
Edema	13	1	10	1	15	1
Thromboembolism	4	2	2	1	9	8
Chest Pain	4	1	5	1	8	1
Constitutional Symptoms/Pain						
Fatigue	52	6	61	9	68	7
Back Pain	16	4	11	0	19	3
Pain	9	3	14	3	15	2
Dermatology/Skin						
Injection Site Reaction	5	1	9	0	10	3
Gastrointestinal						
Diarrhea	44	3	46	4	67	11
Nausea	59	4	64	4	65	11
Vomiting	27	4	37	4	40	9
Stomatitis	32	3	14	0	37	3
Abdominal Pain	31	5	31	7	33	4
Anorexia	20	1	20	2	29	3
Gastroesophageal Reflux	3	0	1	0	5	2
Hematology/Infection						
Fever	23	1	25	1	29	1
Febrile Neutropenia	1	1	0	0	6	6
Hepatic/Metabolic/Laboratory/Renal						
Hypokalemia	3	1	3	2	9	4
Dehydration	6	4	5	3	8	3
Neurology						
Neuropathy	17	0	76	7	74	7
Acute	10	0	65	5	56	2
Persistent	9	0	43	3	48	6

Adverse events were similar in men and women and in patients <65 and ≥65 years, but older patients may have been more susceptible to dehydration, diarrhea, hypokalemia and fatigue. The following additional adverse events, at least possibly related to treatment and potentially important, were reported in ≥2% and <5% of the patients in the ELOXATIN and 5-FU/LV combination arm (listed in decreasing order of frequency): anxiety, myalgia, erythematous rash, increased sweating, conjunctivitis, weight decrease, dry mouth, rectal hemorrhage, depression, ataxia, ascites, hemorrhoids, muscle weakness, nervousness, tachycardia, abnormal micturition frequency, dry skin, pruritus, hemoptysis, purpura, vaginal hemorrhage, melena, somnolence, pneumonia, proctitis, involuntary muscle contractions, intestinal obstruction, gingivitis, tenesmus, hot flashes, enlarged abdomen, urinary incontinence.

Table 19 – Adverse Hematologic Experiences in Patients with Stage II or III Colon Cancer Receiving Adjuvant Therapy (≥5% of patients)

Hematology Parameter	ELOXATIN + 5-FU/LV (N=1108)		5-FU/LV (N=1111)	
	All Grades (%)	Grade 3/4 (%)	All Grades (%)	Grade 3/4 (%)
Anemia	76	1	67	<1
Neutropenia	79	41	40	5
Thrombocytopenia	77	2	19	<1

Table 20 – Adverse Hematologic Experiences in Patients Previously Untreated for Advanced Colorectal Cancer (≥5% of patients)

Hematology Parameter	ELOXATIN + 5-FU/LV (N=259)		Irinotecan + 5-FU/LV (N=256)		ELOXATIN + irinotecan (N=258)	
	All Grades (%)	Grade 3/4 (%)	All Grades (%)	Grade 3/4 (%)	All Grades (%)	Grade 3/4 (%)
Anemia	27	3	28	4	25	3
Leukopenia	85	20	84	23	76	24
Neutropenia	81	53	77	44	71	36
Thrombocytopenia	71	5	26	2	44	4

Hematologic
The following tables list the hematologic changes occurring in ≥5% of patients, based on laboratory values and NCI grade, with the exception of those events occurring in adjuvant patients and anemia in the patients previously untreated for advanced colorectal cancer, respectively, which are based on AE reporting and NCI grade alone.
[See table 19 above]
[See table 20 above]
[See table 21 below]
Thrombocytopenia
Thrombocytopenia was frequently reported with the combination of ELOXATIN and infusional 5-FU/LV. The incidence of all hemorrhagic events in the adjuvant and previously treated patients was higher on the ELOXATIN combination arm compared to the infusional 5-FU/LV arm. These events included gastrointestinal bleeding, hematuria, and epistaxis. In the adjuvant trial, two patients died from intracerebral hemorrhages.
The incidence of grade 3/4 thrombocytopenia was 2% in adjuvant patients with colon cancer. In patients treated for advanced colorectal cancer the incidence of grade 3/4 thrombocytopenia was 3-5%, and the incidence of these events was greater for the combination of ELOXATIN and 5-FU/LV over the irinotecan plus 5-FU/LV or 5-FU/LV control groups. Grade 3/4 gastrointestinal bleeding was reported in 0.2% of adjuvant patients receiving ELOXATIN and 5-FU/LV. In the previously untreated patients, the incidence of epistaxis

was 10% in the ELOXATIN and 5-FU/LV arm, and 2% and 1%, respectively, in the irinotecan plus 5-FU/LV or irinotecan plus ELOXATIN arms.
Neutropenia
Neutropenia was frequently observed with the combination of ELOXATIN and 5-FU/LV, with grade 3 and 4 events reported in 29% and 12% of adjuvant patients with colon cancer, respectively. In the adjuvant trial, 3 patients died from sepsis/neutropenic sepsis. Grade 3 and 4 events were reported in 35% and 18% of the patients previously untreated for advanced colorectal cancer, respectively. Grade 3 and 4 events were reported in 27% and 17% of previously treated patients, respectively. In adjuvant patients the incidence of either febrile neutropenia (0.7%) or documented infection with concomitant grade 3/4 neutropenia (1.1%) was 1.8% in the ELOXATIN and 5-FU/LV arm. The incidence of febrile neutropenia in the patients previously untreated for advanced colorectal cancer was 15% (3% of cycles) in the irinotecan plus 5-FU/LV arm and 4% (less than 1% of cycles) in the ELOXATIN and 5-FU/LV combination arm. Additionally, in this same population, infection with grade 3 or 4 neutropenia was 12% in the irinotecan plus 5-FU/LV and 8% in the ELOXATIN and 5-FU/LV combination. The incidence of febrile neutropenia in the previously treated patients was 1% in the 5-FU/LV arm and 6% (less than 1% of cycles) in the ELOXATIN and 5-FU/LV combination arm.
Gastrointestinal
In patients receiving the combination of ELOXATIN plus infusional 5-FU/LV for adjuvant treatment for colon cancer

Table 21 – Adverse Hematologic Experiences in Previously Treated Patients (≥5% of patients)

Hematology Parameter	5-FU/LV (N=142)		ELOXATIN (N=153)		ELOXATIN + 5-FU/LV (N=150)	
	All Grades (%)	Grade 3/4 (%)	All Grades (%)	Grade 3/4 (%)	All Grades (%)	Grade 3/4 (%)
Anemia	68	2	64	1	81	2
Leukopenia	34	1	13	0	76	19
Neutropenia	25	5	7	0	73	44
Thrombocytopenia	20	0	30	3	64	4

Table 22 – Adverse Hepatic Experiences in Patients with Stage II or III Colon Cancer Receiving Adjuvant Therapy (≥5% of patients)

Hepatic Parameter	ELOXATIN + 5-FU/LV (N=1108)		5-FU/LV (N=1111)	
	All Grades (%)	Grade 3/4 (%)	All Grades (%)	Grade 3/4 (%)
Increase in transaminases	57	2	34	1
ALP Increased	42	<1	20	<1
Bilirubinaemia	20	4	20	5

Table 23 – Adverse Hepatic – Clinical Chemistry Experience in Patients Previously Untreated for Advanced Colorectal Cancer (≥5% of patients)

Clinical Chemistry	ELOXATIN + 5-FU/LV (N=259)		Irinotecan + 5-FU/LV (N=256)		ELOXATIN + ironicetan (N=258)	
	All Grades (%)	Grade 3/4 (%)	All Grades (%)	Grade 3/4 (%)	All Grades (%)	Grade 3/4 (%)
ALT (SGPT-ALAT)	6	1	2	0	5	2
AST (SGOT-ASAT)	17	1	2	1	11	1
Alkaline Phosphatase	16	0	8	0	14	2
Total Bilirubin	6	1	3	1	3	2

the incidence of grade 3/4 nausea and vomiting was greater than in those receiving infusional 5-FU/LV alone (see table). In patients previously untreated for advanced colorectal cancer receiving the combination of ELOXATIN and 5-FU/LV, the incidence of grade 3 and 4 vomiting and diarrhea was less compared to irinotecan plus 5-FU/LV controls (see table). In previously treated patients receiving the combination of ELOXATIN and 5-FU/LV, the incidence of grade 3 and 4 nausea, vomiting, diarrhea, and mucositis/stomatitis increased compared to 5-FU/LV controls (see table).

The incidence of gastrointestinal adverse events in the previously untreated and previously treated patients appears to be similar across cycles. Premedication with antiemetics, including 5-HT$_3$ blockers, is recommended. Diarrhea and mucositis may be exacerbated by the addition of ELOXATIN to 5-FU/LV, and should be managed with appropriate supportive care. Since cold temperature can exacerbate acute neurological symptoms, ice (mucositis prophylaxis) should be avoided during the infusion of ELOXATIN.

Dermatologic
ELOXATIN did not increase the incidence of alopecia compared to 5-FU/LV alone. No complete alopecia was reported. The incidence of grade 3/4 skin disorders was 2% in both the ELOXATIN plus infusional 5-FU/LV and the infusional 5-FU/LV alone arms in the adjuvant colon cancer patients. The incidence of hand-foot syndrome in patients previously untreated for advanced colorectal cancer was 2% in the irinotecan plus 5-FU/LV arm and 7% in the ELOXATIN and 5-FU/LV combination arm. The incidence of hand-foot syndrome in previously treated patients was 13% in the 5-FU/LV arm and 11% in the ELOXATIN and 5-FU/LV combination arm.

Care of Intravenous Site:
Extravasation may result in local pain and inflammation that may be severe and lead to complications, including necrosis. Injection site reaction, including redness, swelling, and pain, has been reported.

Neurologic
Peripheral sensory neuropathy was reported in adjuvant patients treated with the ELOXATIN combination with a frequency of 92% (all grades) and 13% (grade 3), and by 18 months of follow-up, 21% had persistent peripheral sensory neuropathy (all grades). In these patients the median cycle of onset for grade 3 peripheral sensory neuropathy was 9. In patients previously untreated for advanced colorectal cancer neuropathy was reported in 82% (all grades) and 19% (grade 3/4), and in the previously treated patients in 74% (all grades) and 7% (grade 3/4) events. ELOXATIN is consistently associated with two types of peripheral neuropathy (see PRECAUTIONS, Neuropathy). In the previously treated patients, the incidence of overall and grade 3/4 persistent peripheral neuropathy was 48% and 6%, respectively. The majority of the patients (80%) that developed grade 3 persistent neuropathy progressed from prior grade 1 or 2 events. The median number of cycles administered on the ELOXATIN with 5-FU/LV combination arm in the previously treated patients was 6.

Pulmonary
ELOXATIN has been associated with pulmonary fibrosis (see PRECAUTIONS, Pulmonary Toxicity). One patient treated with the ELOXATIN combination regimen in the adjuvant trial died from eosinophilic pneumonia.

Allergic Reactions
Grade 3/4 hypersensitivity to ELOXATIN has been observed in 2-3% of colon cancer patients. These allergic reactions, which can be fatal, can occur at any cycle, and were similar in nature and severity to those reported with other platinum-containing compounds, such as rash, urticaria, erythema, pruritus, and, rarely, bronchospasm and hypotension. The symptoms associated with hypersensitivity reactions reported in the previously untreated patients were urticaria, pruritus, flushing of the face, diarrhea associated with oxaliplatin infusion, shortness of breath, bronchospasm, diaphoresis, chest pains, hypotension, disorientation, and syncope. These reactions are usually managed with standard epinephrine, corticosteroid, antihistamine therapy, and may require discontinuation of therapy (see WARNINGS for anaphylactic/ anaphylactoid reactions).

Anticoagulation and Hemorrhage
There have been reports while on study and from postmarketing surveillance of prolonged prothrombin time and INR occasionally associated with hemorrhage in patients who received ELOXATIN plus 5-FU/LV while on anticoagulants. Patients receiving ELOXATIN plus 5-FU/LV and requiring oral anticoagulants may require closer monitoring.

Renal
About 5-10% of patients in all groups had some degree of elevation of serum creatinine. The incidence of grade 3/4 el-

Table 24 – Adverse Hepatic – Clinical Chemistry Experience in Previously Treated Patients (≥5% of patients)

Clinical Chemistry	5-FU/LV (N=142)		ELOXATIN (N=153)		ELOXATIN + 5-FU/LV (N=150)	
	All Grades (%)	Grade 3/4 (%)	All Grades (%)	Grade 3/4 (%)	All Grades (%)	Grade 3/4 (%)
ALT (SGPT-ALAT)	28	3	36	1	31	0
AST (SGOT-ASAT)	39	2	54	4	47	0
Total Bilirubin	22	6	13	5	13	1

Figure 4

evations in serum creatinine in the ELOXATIN and 5-FU/LV combination arm was 1% in the previously treated patients. Serum creatinine measurements were not reported in the adjuvant trial.

Hepatic

Hepatotoxicity (defined as elevation of liver enzymes) appears to be related to ELOXATIN combination therapy (see PRECAUTIONS). The following tables list the clinical chemistry changes associated with hepatic toxicity occurring in ≥5% of patients, based on adverse events reported and NCI CTC grade for adjuvant patients and patients previously untreated for advanced colorectal cancer, laboratory values, and NCI CTC grade for previously treated patients.
[See table 22 at top of previous page]
[See table 23 at top of previous page]
[See table 24 above]

Thromboembolism

The incidence of thromboembolic events in adjuvant patients with colon cancer was 6% (1.8% grade 3/4) in the infusional 5-FU/LV arm and 6% (1.2% grade 3/4) in the ELOXATIN and infusional 5-FU/LV combined arm, respectively. The incidence was 6 and 9% of the patients previously untreated for advanced colorectal cancer and previously treated patients in the ELOXATIN and 5-FU/LV combination arm, respectively.

Postmarketing Experience

The following events have been reported from worldwide postmarketing experience.
Body as a whole:
-angioedema, anaphylactic shock
Central and peripheral nervous system disorders:
-loss of deep tendon reflexes, dysarthria, Lhermitte's sign, cranial nerve palsies, fasciculations
Liver and gastrointestinal system disorders:
-severe diarrhea/vomiting resulting in hypokalemia, colitis (including *Clostridium difficile* diarrhea), metabolic acidosis; ileus; intestinal obstruction, pancreatitis; veno-occlusive disease of liver also known as sinusoidal obstruction syndrome, and perisinusoidal fibrosis, which rarely may progress
Hearing and vestibular system disorders:
-deafness
Platelet, bleeding, and clotting disorders:
-immuno-allergic thrombocytopenia
-prolongation of prothrombin time and of INR in patients receiving anticoagulants
Red blood cell disorders:
-hemolytic uremic syndrome, immuno-allergic hemolytic anemia

Respiratory system disorders:
-pulmonary fibrosis and other interstitial lung diseases
Vision disorders:
-decrease of visual acuity, visual field disturbance, optic neuritis

OVERDOSAGE

There have been five ELOXATIN overdoses reported. One patient received two 130 mg/m² doses of ELOXATIN (cumulative dose of 260 mg/m²) within a 24-hour period. The patient experienced grade 4 thrombocytopenia (<25,000/mm³) without any bleeding, which resolved. Two other patients were mistakenly administered ELOXATIN instead of carboplatin. One patient received a total ELOXATIN dose of 500 mg and the other received 650 mg. The first patient experienced dyspnea, wheezing, paresthesia, profuse vomiting, and chest pain on the day of administration. She developed respiratory failure and severe bradycardia, and subsequently did not respond to resuscitation efforts. The other patient also experienced dyspnea, wheezing, paresthesia, and vomiting. Her symptoms resolved with supportive care. Another patient who was mistakenly administered a 700 mg dose experienced rapid onset of dysesthesia. Inpatient supportive care was given, including hydration, electrolyte support, and platelet transfusion. Recovery occurred 15 days after the overdose. The last patient received an overdose of oxaliplatin at 360 mg instead of 120 mg over a 1-hour infusion by mistake. At the end of the infusion, the patient experienced 2 episodes of vomiting, laryngospasm, and paresthesia. The patient fully recovered from the laryngospasm within half an hour. At the time of reporting, 1 hour after onset of the event, the patient was recovering from paresthesia. There is no known antidote for ELOXATIN overdose. In addition to thrombocytopenia, the anticipated complications of an ELOXATIN overdose include myelosuppression, nausea and vomiting, diarrhea, and neurotoxicity. Patients suspected of receiving an overdose should be monitored, and supportive treatment should be administered.

DOSAGE AND ADMINISTRATION

Adjuvant Therapy in Patients with Stage III Colon Cancer

Adjuvant treatment in patients with stage III colon cancer is recommended for a total of 6 months, i.e., 12 cycles, every 2 weeks, according to the dose schedule described below for previously treated patients with advanced colorectal cancer.

Therapy in Previously Untreated and Previously Treated Patients with Advanced Colorectal Cancer

The recommended dose schedule given every two weeks is as follows:

ay 1: ELOXATIN 85 mg/m^2 IV infusion in 250-500 mL 5W and leucovorin 200 mg/m^2 IV infusion in D5W both ven over 120 minutes at the same time in separate bags ing a Y-line, followed by 5-FU 400 mg/m^2 IV bolus given er 2-4 minutes, followed by 5-FU 600 mg/m^2 IV infusion 500 mL D5W (recommended) as a 22-hour continuous fusion.

ay 2: Leucovorin 200 mg/m^2 IV infusion over 120 minutes, llowed by 5-FU 400 mg/m^2 IV bolus given over 2-4 min-es, followed by 5-FU 600 mg/m^2 IV infusion in 500 mL 5W (recommended) as a 22-hour continuous infusion.

ee figure 4 at top of previous page]

epeat cycle every 2 weeks.

ne administration of ELOXATIN does not require ehydration.

emedication with antiemetics, including 5-HT$_3$ blockers ith or without dexamethasone, is recommended.

or information on 5-fluorouracil and leucovorin, see the re-ective package inserts.

ose Modification Recommendations
rior to subsequent therapy cycles, patients should be eval-ated for clinical toxicities and laboratory tests (see Labo-atory Tests). Prolongation of infusion time for ELOXATIN om 2 hours to 6 hours decreases the C_{max} by an estimated ?% and may mitigate acute toxicities. The infusion times r 5-FU and leucovorin do not need to be changed.

djuvant Therapy in Patients with Stage III Colon Cancer
europathy and other toxicities were graded using the NCI TC scale, version 1 (see PRECAUTIONS, Neuropathy). or patients who experience persistent grade 2 neuro-ensory events that do not resolve, a dose reduction of LOXATIN to 75 mg/m^2 should be considered. For patients ith persistent Grade 3 neurosensory events, discontinuing herapy should be considered. The infusional 5-FU/LV regi-en need not be altered.

dose reduction of ELOXATIN to 75 mg/m^2 and infusional FU to 300 mg/m^2 bolus and 500 mg/m^2 22 hour infusion is ecommended for patients after recovery from grade 3/4 astrointestinal (despite prophylactic treatment) or grade 4 eutropenia or grade 3/4 thrombocytopenia. The next dose hould be delayed until: neutrophils $\geq$1.5 $\times$ 10^9/L and atelets $\geq$75 $\times$ 10^9/L.

ose Modifications in Therapy in Previously Untreated and reviously Treated Patients with Advanced Colorectal ancer
europathy was graded using a study-specific neurotoxicity cale (see PRECAUTIONS, Neuropathy). Other toxicities ere graded by the NCI CTC, version 2.0.

or patients who experience persistent Grade 2 neuro-ensory events that do not resolve, a dose reduction of LOXATIN to 65 mg/m^2 should be considered. For patients ith persistent grade 3 neurosensory events, discontinuing herapy should be considered. The 5-FU/LV regimen need ot be altered.

dose reduction of ELOXATIN to 65 mg/m^2 and 5-FU by 0% (300 mg/m^2 bolus and 500 mg/m^2 22-hour infusion) is ecommended for patients after recovery from grade 3/4 astrointestinal (despite prophylactic treatment) or grade 4 eutropenia or grade 3/4 thrombocytopenia. The next dose hould be delayed until: neutrophils $\geq$1.5 $\times$ 10^9/L and plate-ets $\geq$75 $\times$10^9/L.

reparation of Infusion Solution
)o not freeze and protect from light the concentrated olution.

FINAL DILUTION MUST NEVER BE PERFORMED WITH A ODIUM CHLORIDE SOLUTION OR OTHER CHLORIDE-:ONTAINING SOLUTIONS.

he solution must be further diluted in an infusion solution f 250-500 mL of 5% Dextrose Injection, USP.

After dilution with 250-500 mL of 5% Dextrose Injection, JSP, the shelf life is 6 hours at room temperature [20-25°C 68-77°F)] or up to 24 hours under refrigeration [2-8°C (36-16°F)]. After final dilution, protection from light is not re-uired. ELOXATIN is incompatible in solution with alka-ine medications or media (such as basic solutions of 5-FU) nd must not be mixed with these or administered simulta-

neously through the same infusion line. **The infusion line should be flushed with D5W prior to administration of any concomitant medication.**
Parenteral drug products should be inspected visually for particulate matter and discoloration prior to administration and discarded if present.
Needles or intravenous administration sets containing alu-minum parts that may come in contact with ELOXATIN should not be used for the preparation or mixing of the drug. Aluminum has been reported to cause degradation of plati-num compounds.

HOW SUPPLIED
ELOXATIN is supplied in clear, glass, single-use vials with gray elastomeric stoppers and aluminum flip-off seals con-taining 50 mg or 100 mg of oxaliplatin as a sterile, preservative-free, aqueous solution at a concentration of 5 mg/mL. Water for Injection, USP is present as an inactive ingredient.
NDC 0024-0590-10: 50 mg single-use vial with green flip-off seal individually packaged in a carton.
NDC 0024-0591-20: 100 mg single-use vial with dark blue flip-off seal individually packaged in a carton.
Storage
Store at 25°C (77°F); excursions permitted to 15-30°C (59-86°F). Do not freeze and protect from light (keep in original outer carton).
Handling and Disposal
As with other potentially toxic anticancer agents, care should be exercised in the handling and preparation of in-fusion solutions prepared from ELOXATIN. The use of gloves is recommended. If a solution of ELOXATIN contacts the skin, wash the skin immediately and thoroughly with soap and water. If ELOXATIN contacts the mucous mem-branes, flush thoroughly with water.
Procedures for the handling and disposal of anticancer drugs should be considered. Several guidelines on the sub-ject have been published [1–8]. There is no general agree-ment that all of the procedures recommended in the guide-lines are necessary or appropriate.

REFERENCES
1. ONS Clinical Practice Committee. Cancer Chemotherapy Guidelines and Recommendations for Practice. Pitts-burgh, Pa: Oncology Nursing Society; 1999:32-41.
2. Recommendations for the safe handling of parenteral an-tineoplastic drugs. NIH Publication No. 83-2621. For sale by the Superintendent of Documents, U.S. Government Printing Office, Washington, D.C. 20402.
3. AMA Council Report. Guidelines for handling parenteral antineoplastics. *JAMA* 1985;253(11):1590-1592.
4. National Study Commission on Cytotoxic Exposure. Rec-ommendations for handling cytotoxic agents. Available from Louis P. Jeffrey, Sc.D., Chairman, National Study Commission on Cytotoxic Exposure, Massachusetts Col-lege of Pharmacy and Allied Health Sciences, 179 Long-wood Avenue, Boston, MA 02115.
5. Clinical Oncological Society of Australia. Guidelines and recommendations for safe handling of antineoplastic agents. *Med J Australia* 1983;1:426-428.
6. Jones RB, et al. Safe handling of chemotherapeutic agents: a report from the Mount Sinai Medical Center. *Ca - A Cancer Journal for Clinicians*. Sept./Oct. 1983:258-263.
7. American Society of Hospital Pharmacists. ASHP Techni-cal Assistance Bulletin on handling cytotoxic and hazard-ous drugs. *Am J Hosp Pharm* 1990;47:1033-1049.
8. Controlling Occupational Exposure to Hazardous Drugs. (OSHA Work-Practice Guidelines). *Am J Hosp Pharm* 1996;53:1669-1685.

sanofi-synthelabo
Distributed by Sanofi-Synthelabo Inc.
New York, NY 10016
Manufactured for Sanofi-Synthelabo Inc. by Ben Venue Laboratories
Bedford, OH 44146-0568
ESS-5C   Printed in USA
Copyright, Sanofi-Synthelabo Inc. 2002, 2004
Rev. April 2005

ERBITUX™   ℞
[ər-bĭ-tŭks]
(Cetuximab)
℞ ONLY

For intravenous use only.

WARNING

Infusion Reactions: Severe infusion reactions occurred with the administration of ERBITUX in approximately 3% of patients, rarely with fatal outcome (<1 in 1000). Approximately 90% of severe infusion reactions were associated with the first infusion of ERBITUX. Severe infusion reactions are characterized by rapid onset of airway obstruction (bronchospasm, stridor, hoarseness), urticaria, and hypotension (see **WARNINGS** and **ADVERSE REACTIONS**). Severe infusion reactions require immediate interruption of the ERBITUX infusion and permanent discontinuation from further treatment. (See **WARNINGS: Infusion Reactions** and **DOSAGE AND ADMINISTRATION: Dose Modifications**.)

DESCRIPTION

ERBITUX™ (Cetuximab) is a recombinant, human/mouse chimeric monoclonal antibody that binds specifically to the extracellular domain of the human epidermal growth factor receptor (EGFR). ERBITUX is composed of the Fv regions of a murine anti-EGFR antibody with human IgG1 heavy and kappa light chain constant regions and has an approximate molecular weight of 152 kDa. ERBITUX is produced in mammalian (murine myeloma) cell culture.

ERBITUX is a sterile, clear, colorless liquid of pH 7.0 to 7.4, which may contain a small amount of easily visible, white, amorphous, Cetuximab particulates. Each single-use, 50-mL vial contains 100 mg of Cetuximab at a concentration of 2 mg/mL and is formulated in a preservative-free solution containing 8.48 mg/mL sodium chloride, 1.88 mg/mL sodium phosphate dibasic heptahydrate, 0.42 mg/mL sodium phosphate monobasic monohydrate, and Water for Injection, USP.

CLINICAL PHARMACOLOGY
General

ERBITUX binds specifically to the epidermal growth factor receptor (EGFR, HER1, c-ErbB-1) on both normal and tumor cells, and competitively inhibits the binding of epidermal growth factor (EGF) and other ligands, such as transforming growth factor–alpha. Binding of ERBITUX to the EGFR blocks phosphorylation and activation of receptor-associated kinases, resulting in inhibition of cell growth, induction of apoptosis, and decreased matrix metalloproteinase and vascular endothelial growth factor production. The EGFR is a transmembrane glycoprotein that is a member of a subfamily of type I receptor tyrosine kinases including EGFR (HER1), HER2, HER3, and HER4. The EGFR is constitutively expressed in many normal epithelial tissues, including the skin and hair follicle. Over-expression of EGFR is also detected in many human cancers including those of the colon and rectum.

In vitro assays and *in vivo* animal studies have shown that ERBITUX inhibits the growth and survival of tumor cells that over-express the EGFR. No anti-tumor effects of ERBITUX were observed in human tumor xenografts lacking EGFR expression. The addition of ERBITUX to irinotecan or irinotecan plus 5-fluorouracil in animal studies resulted in an increase in anti-tumor effects compared to chemotherapy alone.

Human Pharmacokinetics

ERBITUX administered as monotherapy or in combination with concomitant chemotherapy or radiotherapy exhibits nonlinear pharmacokinetics. The area under the concentration time curve (AUC) increased in a greater than dose proportional manner as the dose increased from 20 to 400 mg/m^2. ERBITUX clearance (CL) decreased from 0.08 to 0.02 L/h/m^2 as the dose increased from 20 to 200 mg/m^2, and

at doses >200 mg/m^2, it appeared to plateau. The volume the distribution (Vd) for ERBITUX appeared to be independent of dose and approximated the vascular space 2-3 L/m^2.

Following a 2-hour infusion of 400 mg/m^2 of ERBITUX, th maximum mean serum concentration (C$_{max}$) was 184 µg/m (range: 92-327 µg/mL) and the mean elimination half-li was 97 hours (range 41-213 hours). A 1-hour infusion 250 mg/m^2 produced a mean C$_{max}$ of 140 µg/mL (range 12(170 µg/mL). Following the recommended dose regime (400 mg/m^2 initial dose/250 mg/m^2 weekly dose), ERBITU concentrations reached steady-state levels by the thir weekly dose with mean peak and trough concentration across studies ranging from 168 to 235 and 41 to 85 µg/m respectively. The mean half-life was 114 hours (range 7 188 hours).

Special Populations

A population pharmacokinetic analysis was performed explore the potential effects of selected covariates includin race, gender, age, and hepatic and renal function o ERBITUX pharmacokinetics.

Female patients had a 25% lower intrinsic ERBITUX clea ance than male patients. The toxicity profile was similar i males and females. Definitive conclusions regarding compa rability in efficacy cannot be made given the small numbe of patients with objective tumor responses. None of th other covariates explored appeared to have an impact o ERBITUX pharmacokinetics.

ERBITUX has not been studied in pediatric populations.

CLINICAL STUDIES

The efficacy and safety of ERBITUX alone or in combinatio with irinotecan were studied in a randomized, controlle trial (329 patients) and in combination with irinotecan in a open-label, single-arm trial (138 patients). ERBITUX wa further evaluated as a single agent in a third clinical tria (57 patients). Safety data from 111 patients treated wit single-agent ERBITUX was also evaluated. All trials stud ied patients with EGFR-expressing, metastatic colorecta cancer, whose disease had progressed after receiving a irinotecan-containing regimen.

Randomized, Controlled Trial

A multicenter, randomized, controlled clinical trial was con ducted in 329 patients randomized to receive eithe ERBITUX plus irinotecan (218 patients) or ERBITU monotherapy (111 patients). In both arms of the study ERBITUX was administered as a 400 mg/m^2 initial dose followed by 250 mg/m^2 weekly until disease progression o unacceptable toxicity. All patients received a 20-mg tes dose on Day 1. In the ERBITUX plus irinotecan arm, irino tecan was added to ERBITUX using the same dose an schedule for irinotecan as the patient had previously failed Acceptable irinotecan schedules were 350 mg/m^2 every weeks, 180 mg/m^2 every 2 weeks, or 125 mg/m^2 weekl times four doses every 6 weeks. An Independent Radio graphic Review Committee (IRC), blinded to the treatmen arms, assessed both the progression on prior irinotecan an the response to protocol treatment for all patients.

Of the 329 randomized patients, 206 (63%) were male. The median age was 59 years (range 26-84), and the majority was Caucasian (323, 98%). Eighty-eight percent of patients had baseline Karnofsky Performance Status ≥80. Fifty eight percent of patients had colon cancer and 40% recta cancer. Approximately two-thirds (63%) of patients had previously failed oxaliplatin treatment.

The efficacy of ERBITUX plus irinotecan or ERBITUX monotherapy was evaluated in all randomized patients.

Analyses were also conducted in two pre-specified subpopu lations: irinotecan refractory and irinotecan and oxaliplatin failures. The irinotecan refractory population was defined as randomized patients who had received at least two cycles of irinotecan-based chemotherapy prior to treatment with ERBITUX, and had independent confirmation of disease progression within 30 days of completion of the last cycle o irinotecan-based chemotherapy.

The irinotecan and oxaliplatin failure population was de fined as irinotecan refractory patients who had previously been treated with and failed an oxaliplatin-containing regimen.

Table 1: Objective Response Rates per Independent Review

Populations	ERBITUX + Irinotecan		ERBITUX Monotherapy		Difference (95% CI[a])	
	n	ORR (%)	n	ORR (%)	%	p-value CMH[b]
All Patients	218	22.9	111	10.8	12.1 (4.1 - 20.2)	0.007
Irinotecan-Oxaliplatin Failure	80	23.8	44	11.4	12.4 (-0.8 - 25.6)	0.09
Irinotecan Refractory	132	25.8	69	14.5	11.3 (0.1 - 22.4)	0.07

95% confidence interval for the difference in objective response rates.
Cochran-Mantel-Haenszel test.

Table 2: Time to Progression per Independent Review

Populations	ERBITUX + Irinotecan (median)	ERBITUX Monotherapy (median)	Hazard Ratio (95% CI[a])	Log-rank p-value
All Patients	4.1 mo	1.5 mo	0.54 (0.42 - 0.71)	<0.001
Irinotecan-Oxaliplatin Failure	2.9 mo	1.5 mo	0.48 (0.31 - 0.72)	<0.001
Irinotecan Refractory	4.0 mo	1.5 mo	0.52 (0.37 - 0.73)	<0.001

Hazard ratio of ERBITUX + irinotecan: ERBITUX monotherapy with 95% confidence interval.

The objective response rates (ORR) in these populations are presented in Table 1.
See table 1 above
The median duration of response in the overall population was 5.7 months in the combination arm and 4.2 months in the monotherapy arm. Compared with patients randomized to ERBITUX alone, patients randomized to ERBITUX and irinotecan experienced a significantly longer median time to disease progression (see Table 2).
[See table 2 above]

Single-Arm Trials
ERBITUX, in combination with irinotecan, was studied in a single-arm, multicenter, open-label clinical trial in 138 patients with EGFR-expressing metastatic colorectal cancer who had progressed following an irinotecan-containing regimen. Patients received a 20-mg test dose of ERBITUX on Day 1, followed by a 400-mg/m^2 initial dose, and 250 mg/m^2 weekly until disease progression or unacceptable toxicity. Patients received the same dose and schedule for irinotecan as the patient had previously failed. Acceptable irinotecan schedules were 350 mg/m^2 every 3 weeks or 125 mg/m^2 weekly times four doses every 6 weeks. Of 138 patients enrolled, 74 patients had documented progression to irinotecan as determined by an IRC. The overall response rate was 15% for the overall population and 12% for the irinotecan-failure population. The median durations of response were 6.5 and 6.7 months, respectively.
ERBITUX was studied as a single agent in a multicenter, open-label, single-arm clinical trial in patients with EGFR-expressing, metastatic colorectal cancer who progressed following an irinotecan-containing regimen. Of 57 patients enrolled, 28 patients had documented progression to irinotecan. The overall response rate was 9% for the all-treated group and 14% for the irinotecan-failure group. The median times to progression were 1.4 and 1.3 months, respectively. The median duration of response was 4.2 months for both groups.

EGFR Expression and Response
Patients enrolled in the clinical studies were required to have immunohistochemical evidence of positive EGFR expression. Primary tumor or tumor from a metastatic site was tested with the DakoCytomation EGFR pharmDx™ test kit. Specimens were scored based on the percentage of cells expressing EGFR and intensity (barely/faint, weak to moderate, and strong). Response rate did not correlate with either the percentage of positive cells or the intensity of EGFR expression.

INDICATIONS AND USAGE
ERBITUX, used in combination with irinotecan, is indicated for the treatment of EGFR-expressing, metastatic colorectal carcinoma in patients who are refractory to irinotecan-based chemotherapy.

ERBITUX (Cetuximab) administered as a single agent is indicated for the treatment of EGFR-expressing, metastatic colorectal carcinoma in patients who are intolerant to irinotecan-based chemotherapy.
The effectiveness of ERBITUX is based on objective response rates (see **CLINICAL STUDIES**). Currently, no data are available that demonstrate an improvement in disease-related symptoms or increased survival with ERBITUX.

CONTRAINDICATIONS
None.

WARNINGS
Infusion Reactions (See BOXED WARNING: Infusion Reactions, ADVERSE REACTIONS: Infusion Reactions, and DOSAGE AND ADMINISTRATION: Dose Modifications.)
Severe infusion reactions occurred with the administration of ERBITUX in approximately 3% (20/774) of patients, rarely with fatal outcome (<1 in 1000). Approximately 90% of severe infusion reactions were associated with the first infusion of ERBITUX despite the use of prophylactic antihistamines. These reactions were characterized by the rapid onset of airway obstruction (bronchospasm, stridor, hoarseness), urticaria, and/or hypotension. Caution must be exercised with every ERBITUX infusion, as there were patients who experienced their first severe infusion reaction during later infusions.
Severe infusion reactions require the immediate interruption of ERBITUX therapy and permanent discontinuation from further treatment. Appropriate medical therapy including epinephrine, corticosteroids, intravenous antihistamines, bronchodilators, and oxygen should be available for use in the treatment of such reactions. Patients should be carefully observed until the complete resolution of all signs and symptoms.
In clinical trials, mild to moderate infusion reactions were managed by slowing the infusion rate of ERBITUX and by continued use of antihistamine medications (eg, diphenhydramine) in subsequent doses (see **DOSAGE AND ADMINISTRATION: Dose Modifications**).

Pulmonary Toxicity
Interstitial lung disease (ILD) was reported in 3 of 774 (<0.5%) patients with advanced colorectal cancer receiving ERBITUX. Interstitial pneumonitis with non-cardiogenic pulmonary edema resulting in death was reported in one case. Two patients had pre-existing fibrotic lung disease and experienced an acute exacerbation of their disease while receiving ERBITUX in combination with irinotecan. In the clinical investigational program, an additional case of interstitial pneumonitis was reported in a patient with head and

neck cancer treated with ERBITUX and cisplatin. The onset of symptoms occurred between the fourth and eleventh doses of treatment in all reported cases.

In the event of acute onset or worsening pulmonary symptoms, ERBITUX therapy should be interrupted and a prompt investigation of these symptoms should occur. If ILD is confirmed, ERBITUX should be discontinued and the patient should be treated appropriately.

Dermatologic Toxicity (See ADVERSE REACTIONS: Dermatologic Toxicity and DOSAGE AND ADMINISTRATION: Dose Modifications.)

In cynomolgus monkeys, ERBITUX, when administered at doses of approximately 0.4 to 4 times the weekly human exposure (based on total body surface area), resulted in dermatologic findings, including inflammation at the injection site and desquamation of the external integument. At the highest dose level, the epithelial mucosa of the nasal passage, esophagus, and tongue were similarly affected, and degenerative changes in the renal tubular epithelium occurred. Deaths due to sepsis were observed in 50% (5/10) of the animals at the highest dose level beginning after approximately 13 weeks of treatment.

In clinical studies of ERBITUX, dermatologic toxicities, including acneform rash, skin drying and fissuring, and inflammatory and infectious sequelae (eg, blepharitis, cheilitis, cellulitis, cyst) were reported. In patients with advanced colorectal cancer, acneform rash was reported in 89% (686/774) of all treated patients, and was severe (Grade 3 or 4) in 11% (84/774) of these patients. Subsequent to the development of severe dermatologic toxicities, complications including S. aureus sepsis and abscesses requiring incision and drainage were reported.

Patients developing dermatologic toxicities while receiving ERBITUX should be monitored for the development of inflammatory or infectious sequelae, and appropriate treatment of these symptoms initiated. Dose modifications of any future ERBITUX infusions should be instituted in case of severe acneform rash (see **DOSAGE AND ADMINISTRATION**, Table 4). Treatment with topical and/or oral antibiotics should be considered; topical corticosteroids are not recommended.

PRECAUTIONS

General

ERBITUX therapy should be used with caution in patients with known hypersensitivity to Cetuximab, murine proteins, or any component of this product.

It is recommended that patients wear sunscreen and hats and limit sun exposure while receiving ERBITUX as sunlight can exacerbate any skin reactions that may occur.

EGF Receptor Testing

Patients enrolled in the clinical studies were required to have immunohistochemical evidence of positive EGFR expression using the DakoCytomation EGFR pharmDx™ test kit. Assessment for EGFR expression should be performed by laboratories with demonstrated proficiency in the specific technology being utilized. Improper assay performance, including use of suboptimally fixed tissue, failure to utilize specified reagents, deviation from specific assay instructions, and failure to include appropriate controls for assay validation, can lead to unreliable results. Refer to the DakoCytomation test kit package insert for full instructions on assay performance. (See **CLINICAL STUDIES: EGFR Expression and Response.**)

Drug Interactions

A drug interaction study was performed in which ERBITUX was administered in combination with irinotecan. There was no evidence of any pharmacokinetic interactions between ERBITUX and irinotecan.

Immunogenicity

As with all therapeutic proteins, there is potential for immunogenicity. Potential immunogenic responses to ERBITUX were assessed using either a double antigen radiometric assay or an enzyme-linked immunosorbant assay. Due to limitations in assay performance and sampling timing, the incidence of antibody development in patients receiving ERBITUX has not been adequately determined. The incidence of antibodies to ERBITUX was measured by collecting and analyzing serum pre-study, prior to selected infusions and during treatment follow-up. Patients were considered evaluable if they had a negative pre-treatment sample and a post-treatment sample. Non-neutralizing anti-ERBITUX antibodies were detected in 5% (28 of 530) of evaluable patients. In patients positive for anti-ERBITUX antibody, the median time to onset was 44 days (range 8-28 days). Although the number of sero-positive patients is limited, there does not appear to be any relationship between the appearance of antibodies to ERBITUX and the safety or antitumor activity of the molecule.

The observed incidence of anti-ERBITUX antibody responses may be influenced by the low sensitivity of available assays, inadequate to reliably detect lower antibody titers. Other factors which might influence the incidence of anti-ERBITUX antibody response include sample handling, timing of sample collection, concomitant medications, and underlying disease. For these reasons, comparison of the incidence of antibodies to ERBITUX with the incidence of antibodies to other products may be misleading.

Carcinogenesis, Mutagenesis, Impairment of Fertility

Long-term animal studies have not been performed to test ERBITUX for carcinogenic potential. No mutagenic or clastogenic potential of ERBITUX was observed in the Salmonella-Escherichia coli (Ames) assay or in the in vivo rat micronucleus test. A 39-week toxicity study in cynomolgus monkeys receiving 0.4 to 4 times the human dose of ERBITUX (based on total body surface area) revealed a tendency for impairment of menstrual cycling in treated female monkeys, including increased incidences of irregularity or absence of cycles, when compared to control animals, and beginning from week 25 of treatment and continuing through the 6-week recovery period. Serum testosterone levels and analysis of sperm counts, viability, and motility were not remarkably different between ERBITUX-treated and control male monkeys. It is not known if ERBITUX can impair fertility in humans.

Pregnancy Category C

Animal reproduction studies have not been conducted with ERBITUX. However, the EGFR has been implicated in the control of prenatal development and may be essential for normal organogenesis, proliferation, and differentiation in the developing embryo. In addition, human IgG1 is known to cross the placental barrier; therefore, ERBITUX has the potential to be transmitted from the mother to the developing fetus. It is not known whether ERBITUX can cause fetal harm when administered to a pregnant woman or whether ERBITUX can affect reproductive capacity. There are no adequate and well-controlled studies of ERBITUX in pregnant women. ERBITUX should only be given to a pregnant woman, or any woman not employing adequate contraception if the potential benefit justifies the potential risk to the fetus. All patients should be counseled regarding the potential risk of ERBITUX treatment to the developing fetus prior to initiation of therapy. If the patient becomes pregnant while receiving this drug, she should be apprised of the potential hazard to the fetus and/or the potential risk for loss of the pregnancy.

Nursing Mothers

It is not known whether ERBITUX (Cetuximab) is secreted in human milk. Because human IgG1 is secreted in human milk, the potential for absorption and harm to the infant after ingestion is unknown. Based on the mean half-life of ERBITUX after multiple dosing of 114 hours [range 75-188 hours] (see **CLINICAL PHARMACOLOGY: Human Pharmacokinetics**), women should be advised to discontinue nursing during treatment with ERBITUX and for 60 days following the last dose of ERBITUX.

Pediatric Use

The safety and effectiveness of ERBITUX in pediatric patients have not been established.

Geriatric Use

Of the 774 patients who received ERBITUX with irinotecan or ERBITUX monotherapy in four advanced colorectal cancer studies, 253 patients (33%) were 65 years of age or older. No overall differences in safety or efficacy were observed between these patients and younger patients.

Table 3: Incidence of Adverse Events (≥10%) in Patients with Advanced Colorectal Carcinoma

Body System	ERBITUX plus Irinotecan (n=354)		ERBITUX Monotherapy (n=420)	
	Grades 1 - 4	Grades 3 and 4	Grades 1 - 4	Grades 3 and 4
Preferred Term[1]	% of Patients			
Body as a Whole				
Asthenia/Malaise[2]	73	16	48	10
Abdominal Pain	45	8	26	9
Fever[3]	34	4	27	<1
Pain	23	6	17	5
Infusion Reaction[4]	19	3	21	2
Infection	16	1	14	1
Back Pain	16	3	10	2
Headache	14	2	26	2
Digestive				
Diarrhea	72	22	25	2
Nausea	55	6	29	2
Vomiting	41	7	25	3
Anorexia	36	4	23	2
Constipation	30	2	26	2
Stomatitis	26	2	10	<1
Dyspepsia	14	0	6	0
Hematic/Lymphatic				
Leukopenia	25	17	<1	0
Anemia	16	5	9	3
Metabolic/Nutritional				
Weight Loss	21	0	7	1
Peripheral Edema	16	1	10	1
Dehydration	15	6	10	3
Nervous				
Insomnia	12	0	10	<1
Depression	10	0	7	0
Respiratory				
Dyspnea[3]	23	2	17	7
Cough Increased	20	0	11	1
Skin/Appendages				
Acneform Rash[5]	88	14	90	8
Alopecia	21	0	4	0
Skin Disorder	15	1	4	0
Nail Disorder	12	<1	16	<1
Pruritus	10	1	11	<1
Conjunctivitis	14	1	7	<1

[1] Adverse events that occurred (toxicity Grades 1 through 4) in ≥10% of patients with refractory colorectal carcinoma treated with ERBITUX plus irinotecan or in ≥10% of patients with refractory colorectal carcinoma treated with ERBITUX monotherapy.
[2] Asthenia/malaise is defined as any event described as "asthenia", "malaise", or "somnolence".
[3] Includes cases reported as infusion reaction.
[4] Infusion reaction is defined as any event described at any time during the clinical study as "allergic reaction" or "anaphylactoid reaction", or any event occurring on the first day of dosing described as "allergic reaction", "anaphylactoid reaction", "fever", "chills", "chills and fever", or "dyspnea".
[5] Acneform rash is defined as any event described as "acne", "rash", "maculopapular rash", "pustular rash", "dry skin", or "exfoliative dermatitis".

ADVERSE REACTIONS

Except where indicated, the data described below reflect exposure to ERBITUX in 774 patients with advanced metastatic colorectal cancer. ERBITUX was studied in combination with irinotecan (n=354) or as monotherapy (n=420). Patients receiving ERBITUX plus irinotecan received a median of 12 doses (with 88/354 [25%] treated for over 6 months), and patients receiving ERBITUX monotherapy received a median of 7 doses (with 36/420 [9%] treated for over 6 months). The population had a median age of 59 and was 59% male and 91% Caucasian. The range of dosing for patients receiving ERBITUX plus irinotecan was 1-84 infusions, and the range of dosing for patients receiving ERBITUX monotherapy was 1-63 infusions.

The most **serious adverse reactions** associated with ERBITUX were:

- Infusion reaction (3%) (see **BOXED WARNING, WARNINGS**, and **DOSAGE AND ADMINISTRATION: Dose Modifications**);
- Dermatologic toxicity (1%) (see **WARNINGS** and **DOSAGE AND ADMINISTRATION: Dose Modifications**);
- Interstitial lung disease (0.4%) (see **WARNINGS**);
- Fever (5%);
- Sepsis (3%);
- Kidney failure (2%);
- Pulmonary embolus (1%);
- Dehydration (5%) in patients receiving ERBITUX plus irinotecan, 2% in patients receiving ERBITUX monotherapy;
- Diarrhea (6%) in patients receiving ERBITUX plus irinotecan, 0.2% in patients receiving ERBITUX monotherapy.

Thirty-seven (10%) patients receiving ERBITUX plus irinotecan and 17 (4%) patients receiving ERBITUX monotherapy discontinued treatment primarily because of adverse events.

The most common adverse events seen in 354 patients receiving ERBITUX plus irinotecan were acneform rash

Table 4: ERBITUX Dose Modification Guidelines

Severe Acneform Rash	ERBITUX	Outcome	ERBITUX Dose Modification
1st occurrence	Delay infusion 1 to 2 weeks	Improvement No Improvement	Continue at 250 mg/m^2 Discontinue ERBITUX
2nd occurrence	Delay infusion 1 to 2 weeks	Improvement No Improvement	Reduce dose to 200 mg/m^2 Discontinue ERBITUX
3rd occurrence	Delay infusion 1 to 2 weeks	Improvement No Improvement	Reduce dose to 150 mg/m^2 Discontinue ERBITUX
4th occurrence	Discontinue ERBITUX		

(88%), asthenia/malaise (73%), diarrhea (72%), nausea (55%), abdominal pain (45%), and vomiting (41%).
The most common adverse events seen in 420 patients receiving ERBITUX monotherapy were acneform rash (90%), asthenia/malaise (48%), nausea (29%), fever (27%), constipation (26%), abdominal pain (26%), headache (26%), and diarrhea (25%).

Because clinical trials are conducted under widely varying conditions, adverse reaction rates observed in the clinical trials of a drug cannot be directly compared to rates in the clinical trials of another drug and may not reflect the rates observed in practice. The adverse reaction information from clinical trials does, however, provide a basis for identifying the adverse events that appear to be related to drug use and for approximating rates.

Data in patients with advanced colorectal carcinoma in Table 3 are based on the experience of 354 patients treated with ERBITUX plus irinotecan and 420 patients treated with ERBITUX monotherapy.
[See table 3 at top of previous page]

Infusion Reactions (see BOXED WARNING: Infusion Reactions.)

In clinical trials, severe, potentially fatal infusion reactions were reported. These events include the rapid onset of airway obstruction (bronchospasm, stridor, hoarseness), urticaria, and/or hypotension. In studies in advanced colorectal cancer, severe infusion reactions were observed in 3% of patients receiving ERBITUX plus irinotecan and 2% of patients receiving ERBITUX monotherapy. Grade 1 and 2 infusion reactions, including chills, fever, and dyspnea usually occurring on the first day of initial dosing, were observed in 16% of patients receiving ERBITUX plus irinotecan and 19% of patients receiving ERBITUX monotherapy. (See **WARNINGS: Infusion Reactions** and **DOSAGE AND ADMINISTRATION: Dose Modifications.**)

In the clinical studies described above, a 20-mg test dose was administered intravenously over 10 minutes prior to the loading dose to all patients. The test dose did not reliably identify patients at risk for severe allergic reactions.

Dermatologic Toxicity and Related Disorders

Non-suppurative acneform rash described as "acne", "rash", "maculopapular rash", "pustular rash", "dry skin", or "exfoliative dermatitis" was observed in patients receiving ERBITUX (Cetuximab) plus irinotecan or ERBITUX monotherapy. One or more of the dermatological adverse events were reported in 88% (14% Grade 3) of patients receiving ERBITUX plus irinotecan and in 90% (8% Grade 3) of patients receiving ERBITUX monotherapy. Acneform rash most commonly occurred on the face, upper chest, and back, but could extend to the extremities and was characterized by multiple follicular- or pustular-appearing lesions. Skin drying and fissuring were common in some instances, and were associated with inflammatory and infectious sequelae (eg, blepharitis, cellulitis, cyst). Two cases of *S. aureus* sepsis were reported. The onset of acneform rash was generally within the first two weeks of therapy. Although in a majority of the patients the event resolved following cessation of treatment, in nearly half of the cases, the event continued beyond 28 days. (See **WARNINGS: Dermatologic Tox-**

icity and **DOSAGE AND ADMINISTRATION: Dose Modifications.**)

A related nail disorder, occurring in 14% of patients (0.4% Grade 3), was characterized as a paronychial inflammation with associated swelling of the lateral nail folds of the toe and fingers, with the great toes and thumbs as the most commonly affected digits.

Use with Radiation Therapy

In a study of 21 patients with locally advanced squamous cell cancer of the head and neck, patients treated with ERBITUX, cisplatin, and radiation had a 95% incidence of rash (19% Grade 3). The incidence and severity of cutaneous reactions with combined modality therapy appears to be additive, particularly within the radiation port. The addition of radiation to ERBITUX therapy in patients with colorectal cancer should be done with appropriate caution.

OVERDOSAGE

Single doses of ERBITUX higher than 500 mg/m^2 have not been tested. There is no experience with overdosage in human clinical trials.

DOSAGE AND ADMINISTRATION

The recommended dose of ERBITUX, in combination with irinotecan or as monotherapy, is 400 mg/m^2 as an initial loading dose (first infusion) administered as a 120-minute IV infusion (maximum infusion rate 5 mL/min). The recommended weekly maintenance dose (all other infusions) is 250 mg/m^2 infused over 60 minutes (maximum infusion rate 5 mL/min). Premedication with an H$_1$ antagonist (eg, 50 mg of diphenhydramine IV) is recommended. Appropriate medical resources for the treatment of severe infusion reactions should be available during ERBITUX infusions. (See **WARNINGS: Infusion Reactions.**)

Dose Modifications

Infusion Reactions

If the patient experiences a mild or moderate (Grade 1 or 2) infusion reaction, the infusion rate should be permanently reduced by 50%.

ERBITUX should be immediately and permanently discontinued in patients who experience severe (Grade 3 or 4) infusion reactions. (See **WARNINGS** and **ADVERSE REACTIONS.**)

Dermatologic Toxicity and Related Disorders

If a patient experiences severe acneform rash, ERBITUX treatment adjustments should be made according to Table 4. In patients with mild and moderate skin toxicity, treatment should continue without dose modification. (See **WARNINGS** and **ADVERSE REACTIONS.**)
[See table 4 above]

Preparation for Administration

DO NOT ADMINISTER ERBITUX AS AN IV PUSH OR BOLUS.

ERBITUX must be administered with the use of a low protein binding 0.22-micrometer in-line filter.

ERBITUX is supplied as a 50-mL, single-use vial containing 100 mg of Cetuximab at a concentration of 2 mg/mL in phosphate buffered saline. The solution should be clear and colorless and may contain a small amount of easily visible, white, amorphous, Cetuximab particulates. **DO NOT SHAKE OR DILUTE.**

ERBITUX CAN BE ADMINISTERED VIA INFUSION PUMP OR SYRINGE PUMP.

Infusion Pump:
- Draw up the volume of a vial using a sterile syringe attached to an appropriate needle (a vented spike or other appropriate transfer device may be used).
- Fill ERBITUX into a sterile evacuated container or bag such as glass containers, polyolefin bags (eg, Baxter Intravia), ethylene vinyl acetate bags (eg, Baxter Clintec), DEHP plasticized PVC bags (eg, Abbott Lifecare), or PVC bags.
- Repeat procedure until the calculated volume has been put into the container. Use a new needle for each vial.
- Administer through a low protein binding 0.22-micrometer in-line filter (placed as proximal to the patient as practical).
- Affix the infusion line and prime it with ERBITUX before starting the infusion.
- Maximum infusion rate should not exceed 5 mL/min.
- Use 0.9% saline solution to flush line at the end of infusion.

Syringe Pump:
- Draw up the volume of a vial using a sterile syringe attached to an appropriate needle (a vented spike may be used).
- Place the syringe into the syringe driver of a syringe pump and set the rate.
- Administer through a low protein binding 0.22-micrometer in-line filter rated for syringe pump use (placed as proximal to the patient as practical).
- Connect up the infusion line and start the infusion after priming the line with ERBITUX.
- Repeat procedure until the calculated volume has been infused.
- Use a new needle and filter for each vial.
- Maximum infusion rate should not exceed 5 mL/min.
- Use 0.9% saline solution to flush line at the end of infusion.

ERBITUX should be piggybacked to the patient's infusion line.
Following the ERBITUX infusion, a 1-hour observation period is recommended.

HOW SUPPLIED

ERBITUX™ (Cetuximab) is supplied as a single-use, 50-mL vial containing 100 mg of Cetuximab as a sterile, preservative-free, injectable liquid. Each carton contains one ERBITUX vial (NDC 66733-948-23).

Stability and Storage

Store vials under refrigeration at 2° C to 8° C (36° F to 46° F). **DO NOT FREEZE.** Increased particulate formation may occur at temperatures at or below 0° C. This product contains no preservatives. Preparations of ERBITUX in infusion containers are chemically and physically stable for up to 12 hours at 2° C to 8° C (36° F to 46° F) and up to 8 hours at controlled room temperature (20° C to 25° C; 68° F to 77° F). Discard any remaining solution in the infusion container after 8 hours at controlled room temperature or after 12 hours at 2° to 8° C. Discard any unused portion of the vial.

US Patent No. 6,217,866
ERBITUX™ is a trademark of ImClone Systems Incorporated.
Manufactured by ImClone Systems Incorporated, Branchburg, NJ 08876
Distributed and Marketed by Bristol-Myers Squibb Company, Princeton, NJ 08543

ImClone Systems Incorporated
Bristol-Myers Squibb Company

ER-B0001-06-04   Revised June 2004
Based on 51-022606-01, 1169848A1

GLEEVEC® ℞
[glē-věk]
(imatinib mesylate)
Tablets
Rx only

Prescribing Information
The following prescribing information is based on official labeling in effect July 2005.

DESCRIPTION
Gleevec® (imatinib mesylate) film-coated tablets contain imatinib mesylate equivalent to 100 mg or 400 mg of imatinib free base. Imatinib mesylate is designated chemically as 4-[(4-Methyl-1-piperazinyl)methyl]-N-[4-methyl-3-[[4-(3-pyridinyl)-2-pyrimidinyl]amino]-phenyl]benzamide methanesulfonate and its structural formula is

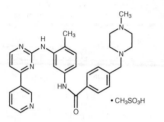

Imatinib mesylate is a white to off-white to brownish or yellowish tinged crystalline powder. Its molecular formula is $C_{29}H_{31}N_7O \cdot CH_4SO_3$ and its molecular weight is 589.7. Imatinib mesylate is soluble in aqueous buffers ≤pH 5.5 but is very slightly soluble to insoluble in neutral/alkaline aqueous buffers. In non-aqueous solvents, the drug substance is freely soluble to very slightly soluble in dimethyl sulfoxide, methanol and ethanol, but is insoluble in n-octanol, acetone and acetonitrile.

Inactive Ingredients: colloidal silicon dioxide (NF); crospovidone (NF); hydroxypropyl methylcellulose (USP); magnesium stearate (NF); and microcrystalline cellulose (NF). *Tablet coating:* ferric oxide, red (NF); ferric oxide, yellow (NF); hydroxypropyl methylcellulose (USP); polyethylene glycol (NF) and talc (USP).

CLINICAL PHARMACOLOGY
Mechanism of Action
Imatinib mesylate is a protein-tyrosine kinase inhibitor that inhibits the bcr-abl tyrosine kinase, the constitutive abnormal tyrosine kinase created by the Philadelphia chromosome abnormality in chronic myeloid leukemia (CML). It inhibits proliferation and induces apoptosis in bcr-abl positive cell lines as well as fresh leukemic cells from Philadelphia chromosome positive chronic myeloid leukemia. In colony formation assays using *ex vivo* peripheral blood and bone marrow samples, imatinib shows inhibition of bcr-abl positive colonies from CML patients.

In vivo, it inhibits tumor growth of bcr-abl transfected murine myeloid cells as well as bcr-abl positive leukemia lines derived from CML patients in blast crisis.

Imatinib is also an inhibitor of the receptor tyrosine kinases for platelet-derived growth factor (PDGF) and stem cell factor (SCF), c-kit, and inhibits PDGF- and SCF-mediated cellular events. *In vitro*, imatinib inhibits proliferation and induces apoptosis in gastrointestinal stromal tumor (GIST) cells, which express an activating c-kit mutation.

Pharmacokinetics
The pharmacokinetics of Gleevec® (imatinib mesylate) have been evaluated in studies in healthy subjects and in population pharmacokinetic studies in over 900 patients. Imatinib is well absorbed after oral administration with C_{max} achieved within 2-4 hours post-dose. Mean absolute bioavailability is 98%. Following oral administration in healthy volunteers, the elimination half-lives of imatinib and its major active metabolite, the N-desmethyl derivative, are approximately 18 and 40 hours, respectively. Mean

imatinib AUC increases proportionally with increasing doses ranging from 25 mg-1,000 mg. There is no significant change in the pharmacokinetics of imatinib on repeated dosing, and accumulation is 1.5- to 2.5-fold at steady state when Gleevec is dosed once daily. At clinically relevant concentrations of imatinib, binding to plasma proteins in *in vitro* experiments is approximately 95%, mostly to albumin and α_1-acid glycoprotein.

The pharmacokinetics of Gleevec are similar in CML and GIST patients.

Metabolism and Elimination
CYP3A4 is the major enzyme responsible for metabolism of imatinib. Other cytochrome P450 enzymes, such as CYP1A2, CYP2D6, CYP2C9, and CYP2C19, play a minor role in its metabolism. The main circulating active metabolite in humans is the N-demethylated piperazine derivative, formed predominantly by CYP3A4. It shows *in vitro* potency similar to the parent imatinib. The plasma AUC for this metabolite is about 15% of the AUC for imatinib. The plasma protein binding of the N-demethylated metabolite CGP71588 is similar to that of the parent compound.

Elimination is predominately in the feces, mostly as metabolites. Based on the recovery of compound(s) after an oral ^{14}C-labeled dose of imatinib, approximately 81% of the dose was eliminated within 7 days, in feces (68% of dose) and urine (13% of dose). Unchanged imatinib accounted for 25% of the dose (5% urine, 20% feces), the remainder being metabolites.

Typically, clearance of imatinib in a 50-year-old patient weighing 50 kg is expected to be 8 L/h, while for a 50-year-old patient weighing 100 kg the clearance will increase to 14 L/h. However, the inter-patient variability of 40% in clearance does not warrant initial dose adjustment based on body weight and/or age but indicates the need for close monitoring for treatment-related toxicity.

Special Populations
Pediatric: As in adult patients, imatinib was rapidly absorbed after oral administration in pediatric patients, with a C_{max} of 2-4 hours. Apparent oral clearance was similar to adult values (11.0 L/hr/m^2 in children vs. 10.0 L/hr/m^2 in adults), as was the half-life (14.8 hours in children vs. 17.1 hours in adults). Dosing in children at both 260 mg/m^2 and 340 mg/m^2 achieved an AUC similar to the 400-mg dose in adults. The comparison of AUC$_{(0-24)}$ on Day 8 vs. Day 1 at 260 mg/m^2 and 340 mg/m^2 dose levels revealed a 1.5- and 2.2-fold drug accumulation, respectively, after repeated once-daily dosing. Mean imatinib AUC did not increase proportionally with increasing dose.

Hepatic Insufficiency: No clinical studies were conducted with Gleevec in patients with impaired hepatic function.

Renal Insufficiency: No clinical studies were conducted with Gleevec in patients with decreased renal function (studies excluded patients with serum creatinine concentration more than 2 times the upper limit of the normal range). Imatinib and its metabolites are not significantly excreted via the kidney.

Drug-Drug Interactions
CYP3A4 Inhibitors: There was a significant increase in exposure to imatinib (mean C_{max} and AUC increased by 26% and 40%, respectively) in healthy subjects when Gleevec was coadministered with a single dose of ketoconazole (a CYP3A4 inhibitor). *(See PRECAUTIONS.)*

CYP3A4 Substrates: Gleevec increased the mean C_{max} and AUC of simvastatin (CYP3A4 substrate) by 2- and 3.5-fold, respectively, indicating an inhibition of CYP3A4 by Gleevec. *(See PRECAUTIONS.)*

CYP3A4 Inducers: Pretreatment of 14 healthy volunteers with multiple doses of rifampin, 600 mg daily for 8 days, followed by a single 400-mg dose of Gleevec, increased Gleevec oral-dose clearance by 3.8-fold (90% confidence interval = 3.5- to 4.3-fold), which represents mean decreases in C_{max}, AUC$_{(0-24)}$ and AUC$_{(0-∞)}$ by 54%, 68% and 74%, of the respective values without rifampin treatment. *(See PRECAUTIONS and DOSAGE AND ADMINISTRATION.)*

In Vitro Studies of CYP Enzyme Inhibition: Human liver microsome studies demonstrated that Gleevec is a potent competitive inhibitor of CYP2C9, CYP2D6, and CYP3A4/5

Table 1
Response in Newly Diagnosed CML Study (30-Month Data)

(Best Response Rates)	Gleevec® n=553	IFN+Ara-C n=553
Hematologic Response[1]		
CHR Rate n (%)	527 (95.3%)*	308 (55.7%)*
[95% CI]	[93.2%, 96.9%]	[51.4%, 59.9%]
Cytogenetic Response[2]		
Major Cytogenetic Response n (%)	461 (83.4%)*	90 (16.3%)*
[95% CI]	[80.0%, 86.4%]	[13.3%, 19.6%]
Unconfirmed[3]	87.2%*	23.0%*
Complete Cytogenetic Response n (%)	378 (68.4%)*	30 (5.4%)*
Unconfirmed[3]	78.8%*	10.7%*
Molecular Response[4]		
Major Response at 12 Months (%)	40%*	2%*
Major Response at 24 Months (%)	54%*	N/A[5]

*p<0.001, Fischer's exact test
[1] **Hematologic response criteria (all responses to be confirmed after ≥4 weeks):** WBC $<10 \times 10^9$/L, platelet $<450 \times 10^9$/L, myelocyte + metamyelocyte <5% in blood, no blasts and promyelocytes in blood, basophils <20%, no extramedullary involvement.
[2] **Cytogenetic response criteria (confirmed after ≥4 weeks):** complete (0% Ph+ metaphases) or partial (1%-35%). A major response (0%-35%) combines both complete and partial responses.
[3] Unconfirmed cytogenetic response is based on a single bone marrow cytogenetic evaluation, therefore unconfirmed complete or partial cytogenetic responses might have had a lesser cytogenetic response on a subsequent bone marrow evaluation.
[4] **Major molecular response criteria:** In the peripheral blood, after 12 months of therapy, reduction of ≥3 logarithms in the amount of bcr-abl transcripts (measured by real-time quantitative reverse transcriptase PCR assay) over a standardized baseline.
[5] Not Applicable: Insufficient data, only two patients available with samples.

with K_i values of 27, 7.5 and 8 µM, respectively. Gleevec is likely to increase the blood level of drugs that are substrates of CYP2C9, CYP2D6 and CYP3A4/5. (*See PRECAUTIONS.*)

CLINICAL STUDIES
Chronic Myeloid Leukemia
Chronic Phase, Newly Diagnosed: An open-label, multi-center, international randomized Phase 3 study has been conducted in patients with newly diagnosed Philadelphia chromosome positive (Ph+) chronic myeloid leukemia (CML) in chronic phase. This study compared treatment with either single-agent Gleevec® (imatinib mesylate) or a combination of interferon-alfa (IFN) plus cytarabine (Ara-C). Patients were allowed to cross over to the alternative treatment arm if they failed to show a complete hematologic response (CHR) at 6 months, a major cytogenetic response (MCyR) at 12 months, or if they lost a CHR or MCyR. Patients with increasing WBC or severe intolerance to treatment were also allowed to cross over to the alternative treatment arm with the permission of the study monitoring committee (SMC). In the Gleevec arm, patients were treated initially with 400 mg daily. In the IFN arm, patients were treated with a target dose of IFN of 5 MIU/m^2/day subcutaneously in combination with subcutaneous Ara-C 20 mg/m^2/day for 10 days/month.
A total of 1,106 patients were randomized from 177 centers in 16 countries, 553 to each arm. Baseline characteristics were well balanced between the two arms. Median age was 51 years (range 18-70 years), with 21.9% of patients ≥60 years of age. There were 59% males and 41% females; 89.9% Caucasian and 4.7% Black patients. With a median follow-up of 31 and 30 months for Gleevec and IFN, respectively, 79% of patients randomized to Gleevec were still receiving first-line treatment. Due to discontinuations and cross-overs, only 7% of patients randomized to IFN were still on first-line treatment. In the IFN arm, withdrawal of consent (13.6%) was the most frequent reason for discontinuation of first-line therapy, and the most frequent reason for cross-over to the Gleevec arm was severe intolerance to treatment (25.1%).
The primary efficacy endpoint of the study was progression-free survival (PFS). Progression was defined as any of the following events: progression to accelerated phase or blast crisis, death, loss of CHR or MCyR, or in patients not

achieving a CHR an increasing WBC despite appropriate therapeutic management. The protocol specified that the progression analysis would compare the intent to treat (ITT) population: patients randomized to receive Gleevec were compared with patients randomized to receive interferon. Patients that crossed over prior to progression were not censored at the time of cross-over, and events that occurred in these patients following cross-over were attributed to the original randomized treatment. The estimated rate of progression-free survival at 30 months in the ITT population was 87.8% in the Gleevec arm and 68.3% in the IFN arm (p<0.001), (Figure 1). The estimated rate of patients free of progression to accelerated phase (AP) or blast crisis (BC) at 30 months was 94.8% in the Gleevec arm compared to 89.6%, (p=0.0016) in the IFN arm, (Figure 2). There were 33 and 46 deaths reported in the Gleevec and IFN arm, respectively, with an estimated 30-month survival rate of 94.6% and 91.6%, respectively (differences not significant). The probability of remaining progression-free at 30 months was 100% for patients who were in complete cytogenetic response with major molecular response (≥3-log reduction in bcr-abl transcripts as measured by quantitative reverse transcriptase polymerase chain reaction) at 12 months, compared to 93% for patients in complete cytogenetic response but without a major molecular response, and 82% in patients who were not in complete cytogenetic response at this time point (p<0.001).

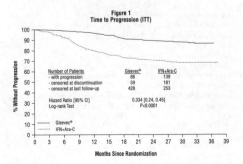

Figure 1
Time to Progression (ITT)

Number of Patients	Gleevec®	IFN+Ara-C
- with progression	66	139
- censored at discontinuation	59	161
- censored at last follow-up	428	253
Hazard Ratio [95% CI]	0.334 [0.24, 0.45]	
Log-rank Test	P<0.0001	

Months Since Randomization

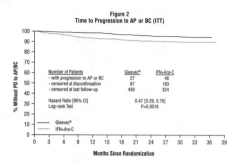

Figure 2
Time to Progression to AP or BC (ITT)

Number of Patients	Gleevec®	IFN+Ara-C
- with progression to AP or BC	27	46
- censored at discontinuation	87	183
- censored at last follow-up	439	324
Hazard Ratio [95% CI]	0.47 [0.29, 0.76]	
Log-rank Test	P=0.0016	

Gleevec®
IFN+Ara-C

Months Since Randomization

Major cytogenetic response, hematologic response, evaluation of minimal residual disease (molecular response), time to accelerated phase or blast crisis and survival were main secondary endpoints. Response data are shown in Table 1. Complete hematologic response, major cytogenetic response and complete cytogenetic response were also statistically significantly higher in the Gleevec arm compared to the IFN + Ara-C arm.

[See table 1 at top of previous page]

Physical, functional, and treatment-specific biologic response modifier scales from the FACT-BRM (Functional Assessment of Cancer Therapy - Biologic Response Modifier) instrument were used to assess patient-reported general effects of interferon toxicity in 1,067 patients with CML in chronic phase. After one month of therapy to six months of therapy, there was a 13%-21% decrease in median index from baseline in patients treated with interferon, consistent with increased symptoms of interferon toxicity. There was no apparent change from baseline in median index for patients treated with Gleevec.

Late Chronic Phase CML and Advanced Stage CML: Three international, open-label, single-arm Phase 2 studies were conducted to determine the safety and efficacy of Gleevec in patients with Ph+ CML: 1) in the chronic phase after failure of IFN therapy, 2) in accelerated phase disease, or 3) in myeloid blast crisis. About 45% of patients were women and 6% were Black. In clinical studies 38%-40% of patients were ≥60 years of age and 10%-12% of patients were ≥70 years of age.

Chronic Phase, Prior Interferon-Alpha Treatment: 532 patients were treated at a starting dose of 400 mg; dose escalation to 600 mg was allowed. The patients were distributed in three main categories according to their response to prior interferon: failure to achieve (within 6 months), or loss of a complete hematologic response (29%), failure to achieve (within 1 year) or loss of a major cytogenetic response (35%), or intolerance to interferon (36%). Patients had received a median of 14 months of prior IFN therapy at doses ≥25 × 10^6 IU/week and were all in late chronic phase, with a median time from diagnosis of 32 months. Effectiveness was evaluated on the basis of the rate of hematologic response and by bone marrow exams to assess the rate of major cytogenetic response (up to 35% Ph+ metaphases) or complete cytogenetic response (0% Ph+ metaphases). Median duration of treatment was 29 months with 81% of patients treated for ≥24 months (maximum=31.5 months). Efficacy results are reported in Table 2. Confirmed major cytogenetic response rates were higher in patients with IFN intolerance (66%) and cytogenetic failure (64%), than in patients with hematologic failure (47%). Hematologic response was achieved in 98% of patients with cytogenetic failure, 94% of patients with hematologic failure, and 92% of IFN-intolerant patients.

Accelerated Phase: 235 patients with accelerated phase disease were enrolled. These patients met one or more of the following criteria: ≥15%-<30% blasts in PB or BM; ≥30% blasts + promyelocytes in PB or BM; ≥20% basophils in PB; and <100 × 10^9/L platelets. The first 77 patients were started at 400 mg, with the remaining 158 patients starting at 600 mg.

Effectiveness was evaluated primarily on the basis of the rate of hematologic response, reported as either complete hematologic response, no evidence of leukemia (i.e., clearance of blasts from the marrow and the blood, but without a full peripheral blood recovery as for complete responses), or return to chronic phase CML. Cytogenetic responses were also evaluated. Median duration of treatment was 18 months with 45% of patients treated for ≥24 months (maximum= 35 months). Efficacy results are reported in Table 2. Response rates in accelerated phase CML were higher for the 600-mg dose group than for the 400-mg group: hematologic response (75% vs. 64%), confirmed and unconfirmed major cytogenetic response (31% vs. 19%).

Myeloid Blast Crisis: 260 patients with myeloid blast crisis were enrolled. These patients had ≥30% blasts in PB or BM and/or extramedullary involvement other than spleen or liver; 95 (37%) had received prior chemotherapy for treatment of either accelerated phase or blast crisis ("pretreated patients") whereas 165 (63%) had not ("untreated patients"). The first 37 patients were started at 400 mg; the remaining 223 patients were started at 600 mg.

Effectiveness was evaluated primarily on the basis of rate of hematologic response, reported as either complete hematologic response, no evidence of leukemia, or return to chronic phase CML using the same criteria as for the study in accelerated phase. Cytogenetic responses were also assessed. Median duration of treatment was 4 months with 21% of patients treated for ≥12 months and 10% for ≥24 months (maximum=35 months). Efficacy results are reported in Table 2. The hematologic response rate was higher in untreated patients than in treated patients (36% vs. 22%, respectively) and in the group receiving an initial dose of 600 mg rather than 400 mg (33% vs. 16%). The confirmed and unconfirmed major cytogenetic response rate was also higher for the 600-mg dose group than for the 400-mg dose group (17% vs. 8%).

[See table 2 at top of next page]

The median time to hematologic response was 1 month. In late chronic phase CML, with a median time from diagnosis of 32 months, an estimated 87.8% of patients who achieved MCyR maintained their response 2 years after achieving their initial response. After 2 years of treatment, an estimated 85.4% of patients were free of progression to AP or BC, and estimated overall survival 90.8% [88.3, 93.2]. In accelerated phase, median duration of hematologic response was 28.8 months for patients with an initial dose of 600 mg (16.5 months for 400 mg, p=0.0035). An estimated 63.8% of patients who achieved MCyR were still in response 2 years after achieving initial response. The median survival was 20.9 [13.1, 34.4] months for the 400-mg group and was not yet reached for the 600-mg group (p=0.0097). An estimated 46.2% [34.7, 57.7] vs. 65.8% [58.4, 73.3] of patients were still alive after 2 years of treatment in the 400-mg vs. 600-mg dose groups, respectively (p=0.0088). In blast crisis, the estimated median duration of hematologic response is 10 months. An estimated 27.2% [16.8, 37.7] of hematologic responders maintained their response 2 years after achieving their initial response. Median survival was 6.9 [5.8, 8.6] months, and an estimated 18.3% [13.4, 23.3] of all patients with blast crisis were alive 2 years after start of study.

Efficacy results were similar in men and women and in patients younger and older than age 65. Responses were seen in Black patients, but there were too few Black patients to allow a quantitative comparison.

Pediatric CML: One open-label, single-arm study enrolled 14 pediatric patients with Ph+ chronic phase CML recurrent after stem cell transplant or resistant to interferon-alpha therapy. Patients ranged in age from 3-20 years old; 3 were 3-11 years old, 9 were 12-18 years old, and 2 were >18 years old. Patients were treated at doses of 260 mg/m²/day (n=3), 340 mg/m²/day (n=4), 440 mg/m²/day (n=5) and 570 mg/m²/day (n=2). In the 13 patients for whom cytogenetic data are available, 4 achieved a major cytogenetic response, 7 achieved a complete cytogenetic response, and 2 had a minimal cytogenetic response. At the recommended dose of 260 mg/m²/day, 2 of 3 patients achieved a complete

Table 2
Response in CML Studies

	Chronic Phase IFN Failure (n=532) 400 mg	Accelerated Phase (n=235) 600 mg n=158 400 mg n=77	Myeloid Blast Crisis (n=260) 600 mg n=223 400 mg n=37
	% of patients [$CI_{95\%}$]		
Hematologic Response[1]	95% [92.3-96.3]	71% [64.8-76.8]	31% [25.2-36.8]
Complete Hematologic Response (CHR)	95%	38%	7%
No evidence of Leukemia (NEL)	Not applicable	13%	5%
Return to Chronic Phase (RTC)	Not applicable	20%	18%
Major Cytogenetic Response[2]	60% [55.3-63.8]	21% [16.2-27.1]	7% [4.5-11.2]
(Unconfirmed[3])	(65%)	(27%)	(15%)
Complete[4] (Unconfirmed[3])	39% (47%)	16% (20%)	2% (7%)

Hematologic response criteria (all responses to be confirmed after ≥4 weeks):
CHR: Chronic phase study [WBC <10 ×10^9/L, platelet <450 ×10^9/L, myelocytes + metamyelocytes <5% in blood, no blasts and promyelocytes in blood, basophils <20%, no extramedullary involvement] and in the accelerated and blast crisis studies [ANC ≥1.5 ×10^9/L, platelets ≥100 ×10^9/L, no blood blasts, BM blasts <5% and no extramedullary disease]
NEL: Same criteria as for CHR but ANC ≥1 ×10^9/L and platelets ≥20 ×10^9/L (accelerated and blast crisis studies).
RTC: <15% blasts BM and PB, <30% blasts + promyelocytes in BM and PB, <20% basophils in PB, no extramedullary disease other than spleen and liver (accelerated and blast crisis studies).
M=bone marrow, PB=peripheral blood
Cytogenetic response criteria (confirmed after ≥4 weeks): complete (0% Ph+ metaphases) or partial (1%-35%). A major response (0%-35%) combines both complete and partial responses.
Unconfirmed cytogenetic response is based on a single bone marrow cytogenetic evaluation, therefore unconfirmed complete or partial cytogenetic responses might have had a lesser cytogenetic response on a subsequent bone marrow evaluation.
Complete cytogenetic response confirmed by a second bone marrow cytogenetic evaluation performed at least 1 month after the initial bone marrow study.

cytogenetic response. Cytogenetic response rate was similar at all dose levels.

In a second study, 2 of 3 patients with Ph+ chronic phase CML resistant to interferon-alpha therapy achieved a complete cytogenetic response at doses of 242 and 257 mg/m^2/day.

Gastrointestinal Stromal Tumors

One open-label, multinational study was conducted in patients with unresectable and/or metastatic malignant gastrointestinal stromal tumors (GIST). In this study, 147 patients were enrolled and randomized to receive either 400 mg or 600 mg orally q.d. for up to 24 months. The study was not powered to show a statistically significant difference in response rates between the two dose groups. Patients ranged in age from 18-83 years old and had a pathologic diagnosis of Kit (CD117) positive unresectable and/or metastatic malignant GIST. Immunohistochemistry was routinely performed with Kit antibody (A-4502, rabbit polyclonal antiserum, 1:100; DAKO Corporation, Carpinteria, CA) according to analysis by an avidin-biotin-peroxidase complex method after antigen retrieval.

The primary outcome of the study was objective response rate. Tumors were required to be measurable at entry in at least one site of disease, and response characterization was based on Southwestern Oncology Group (SWOG) criteria. Results are shown in Table 3.

Table 3
Tumor Response in GIST Study

Total Patients	N	Confirmed Partial Response N (%)	95% Confidence Interval
400 mg Daily	73	24 (33%)	22%, 45%
600 mg Daily	74	32 (43%)	32%, 55%
Total	147	56 (38%)	30%, 46%

statistically significant difference in response rates between the two dose groups was not demonstrated. At the time of interim analysis, when the median follow-up was less than 7 months, 55 of 56 patients with a confirmed partial response (PR) had a maintained PR. The data were too immature to determine a meaningful response duration. No responses were observed in 12 patients with progressive disease on 400 mg daily whose doses were increased to 600 mg daily.

INDICATIONS AND USAGE

Gleevec® (imatinib mesylate) is indicated for the treatment of newly diagnosed adult patients with Philadelphia chromosome positive chronic myeloid leukemia (CML) in chronic phase. Follow-up is limited.

Gleevec is also indicated for the treatment of patients with Philadelphia chromosome positive chronic myeloid leukemia (CML) in blast crisis, accelerated phase, or in chronic phase after failure of interferon-alpha therapy. Gleevec is also indicated for the treatment of pediatric patients with Ph+ chronic phase CML whose disease has recurred after stem cell transplant or who are resistant to interferon-alpha therapy. There are no controlled trials in pediatric patients demonstrating a clinical benefit, such as improvement in disease-related symptoms or increased survival.

Gleevec is also indicated for the treatment of patients with Kit (CD117) positive unresectable and/or metastatic malignant gastrointestinal stromal tumors (GIST). (See CLINICAL STUDIES, Gastrointestinal Stromal Tumors.) The effectiveness of Gleevec in GIST is based on objective response rate (see CLINICAL STUDIES). There are no controlled trials demonstrating a clinical benefit, such as improvement in disease-related symptoms or increased survival.

CONTRAINDICATIONS

Use of Gleevec® (imatinib mesylate) is contraindicated in patients with hypersensitivity to imatinib or to any other component of Gleevec.

WARNINGS

Pregnancy

Women of childbearing potential should be advised to avoid becoming pregnant.

Imatinib mesylate was teratogenic in rats when administered during organogenesis at doses ≥100 mg/kg, approximately equal to the maximum clinical dose of 800 mg/day based on body surface area. Teratogenic effects included exencephaly or encephalocele, absent/reduced frontal and absent parietal bones. Female rats administered doses

≥45 mg/kg (approximately one-half the maximum human dose of 800 mg/day based on body surface area) also experienced significant post-implantation loss as evidenced by either early fetal resorption or stillbirths, nonviable pups and early pup mortality between postpartum Days 0 and 4. At doses higher than 100 mg/kg, total fetal loss was noted in all animals. Fetal loss was not seen at doses ≤30 mg/kg (one-third the maximum human dose of 800 mg).

Male and female rats were exposed *in utero* to a maternal imatinib mesylate dose of 45 mg/kg (approximately one-half the maximum human dose of 800 mg) from Day 6 of gestation and through milk during the lactation period. These animals then received no imatinib exposure for nearly 2 months. Body weights were reduced from birth until terminal sacrifice in these rats. Although fertility was not affected, fetal loss was seen when these male and female animals were then mated.

There are no adequate and well-controlled studies in pregnant women. If Gleevec® (imatinib mesylate) is used during pregnancy, or if the patient becomes pregnant while taking (receiving) Gleevec, the patient should be apprised of the potential hazard to the fetus.

PRECAUTIONS
General
Dermatologic Toxicities: Bullous dermatologic reactions, including erythema multiforme and Stevens-Johnson syndrome, have been reported with use of Gleevec® (imatinib mesylate). In some cases reported during post-marketing surveillance, a recurrent dermatologic reaction was observed upon rechallenge. Several foreign post-marketing reports have described cases in which patients tolerated the reintroduction of Gleevec therapy after resolution or improvement of the bullous reaction. In these instances, Gleevec was resumed at a dose lower than that at which the reaction occurred and some patients also received concomitant treatment with corticosteroids or antihistamines.

Fluid Retention and Edema: Gleevec is often associated with edema and occasionally serious fluid retention *(see ADVERSE REACTIONS)*. Patients should be weighed and monitored regularly for signs and symptoms of fluid retention. An unexpected rapid weight gain should be carefully investigated and appropriate treatment provided. The probability of edema was increased with higher Gleevec dose and age >65 years in the CML studies. Severe superficial edema was reported in 1.1% of newly diagnosed CML patients taking Gleevec, and in 2%-6% of other adult CML patients taking Gleevec. In addition, other severe fluid retention (e.g., pleural effusion, pericardial effusion, pulmonary edema, and ascites) events were reported in 0.7% of newly diagnosed CML patients taking Gleevec, and in 2%-6% of other adult CML patients taking Gleevec. Severe superficial edema and severe fluid retention (pleural effusion, pulmonary edema and severe fluid retention) were reported in 1%-6% of patients taking Gleevec for GIST.

There have been post-marketing reports, including fatalities, of cardiac tamponade, cerebral edema, increased intracranial pressure, and papilledema in patients treated with Gleevec.

GI Irritation: Gleevec is sometimes associated with GI irritation. Gleevec should be taken with food and a large glass of water to minimize this problem.

Hemorrhage: In the newly diagnosed CML trial, 1.1% of patients had Grade 3/4 hemorrhage. In the GIST clinical trial, seven patients (5%), four in the 600-mg dose group and three in the 400-mg dose group, had a total of eight events of CTC Grade 3/4 - gastrointestinal (GI) bleeds (3 patients), intra-tumoral bleeds (3 patients) or both (1 patient). Gastrointestinal tumor sites may have been the source of GI bleeds.

Hematologic Toxicity: Treatment with Gleevec is associated with anemia, neutropenia, and thrombocytopenia. Complete blood counts should be performed weekly for the first month, biweekly for the second month, and periodically thereafter as clinically indicated (for example, every 2-3 months). In CML, the occurrence of these cytopenias is dependent on the stage of disease and is more frequent in patients with accelerated phase CML or blast crisis than in patients with chronic phase CML. (See *DOSAGE AND ADMINISTRATION*.)

Hepatotoxicity: Hepatotoxicity, occasionally severe, may occur with Gleevec *(see ADVERSE REACTIONS)*. Liver function (transaminases, bilirubin, and alkaline phosphatase) should be monitored before initiation of treatment and monthly, or as clinically indicated. Laboratory abnormalities should be managed with interruption and/or dose reduction of the treatment with Gleevec. (See *DOSAGE AND ADMINISTRATION*.) Patients with hepatic impairment should be closely monitored because exposure to Gleevec may be increased. As there are no clinical studies of Gleevec in patients with impaired liver function, no specific advice concerning initial dosing adjustment can be given.

Toxicities From Long-Term Use: It is important to consider potential toxicities suggested by animal studies, specifically, *liver and kidney toxicity and immunosuppression*. Severe liver toxicity was observed in dogs treated for 2 weeks, with elevated liver enzymes, hepatocellular necrosis, bile duct necrosis, and bile duct hyperplasia. Renal toxicity was observed in monkeys treated for 2 weeks, with focal mineralization and dilation of the renal tubules and tubular nephrosis. Increased BUN and creatinine were observed in several of these animals. An increased rate of opportunistic infections was observed with chronic imatinib treatment in laboratory animal studies. In a 39-week monkey study, treatment with imatinib resulted in worsening of normally suppressed malarial infections in these animals. Lymphopenia was observed in animals (as in humans).

Drug Interactions
Drugs that may alter imatinib plasma concentrations
Drugs that may **increase** imatinib plasma concentrations: Caution is recommended when administering Gleevec with inhibitors of the CYP3A4 family (e.g., ketoconazole, itraconazole, erythromycin, clarithromycin). Substances that inhibit the cytochrome P450 isoenzyme (CYP3A4) activity may decrease metabolism and increase imatinib concentrations. There is a significant increase in exposure to imatinib when Gleevec is coadministered with ketoconazole (CYP3A4 inhibitor).

Drugs that may **decrease** imatinib plasma concentrations: Substances that are inducers of CYP3A4 activity may increase metabolism and decrease imatinib plasma concentrations. Co-medications that induce CYP3A4 (e.g. dexamethasone, phenytoin, carbamazepine, rifampin phenobarbital or St. John's Wort) may significantly reduce exposure to Gleevec. Pretreatment of healthy volunteers with multiple doses of rifampin followed by a single dose of Gleevec, increased Gleevec oral-dose clearance by 3.8-fold which significantly (p<0.05) decreased mean C_{max} and $AUC_{(0-\infty)}$. In patients where rifampin or other CYP3A4 inducers are indicated, alternative therapeutic agents with less enzyme induction potential should be considered *(See CLINICAL PHARMACOLOGY and DOSAGE AND ADMINISTRATION.)*

Drugs that may have their plasma concentration altered by Gleevec
Gleevec increases the mean C_{max} and AUC of simvastatin (CYP3A4 substrate) 2- and 3.5-fold, respectively, suggesting an inhibition of the CYP3A4 by Gleevec. Particular caution is recommended when administering Gleevec with CYP3A4 substrates that have a narrow therapeutic window (e.g., cyclosporine or pimozide). Gleevec will increase plasma concentration of other CYP3A4 metabolized drugs (e.g., triazolo-benzodiazepines, dihydropyridine calcium channel blockers, certain HMG-CoA reductase inhibitors).

Because *warfarin* is metabolized by CYP2C9 and CYP3A4, patients who require anticoagulation should receive low-molecular weight or standard heparin.

In vitro, Gleevec inhibits the cytochrome P450 isoenzyme CYP2D6 activity at similar concentrations that affect CYP3A4 activity. Systemic exposure to substrates of CYP2D6 is expected to be increased when coadministered with Gleevec. No specific studies have been performed and caution is recommended.

Table 4
Adverse Experiences Reported in Newly Diagnosed CML Clinical Trial (≥10% of all patients)[1]

Preferred Term	All Grades		CTC Grades 3/4	
	Gleevec® N=551 (%)	IFN+Ara-C N=533 (%)	Gleevec® N=551 (%)	IFN+Ara-C N=533 (%)
Fluid Retention	59.2	10.7	1.8	0.9
– Superficial Edema	57.5	9.2	1.1	0.4
– Other Fluid Retention Events	6.9	1.9	0.7	0.6
Nausea	47.0	61.5	0.9	5.1
Muscle Cramps	43.2	11.4	1.6	0.2
Musculoskeletal Pain	39.9	44.1	3.4	8.1
Diarrhea	38.5	42.0	2.0	3.2
Rash and Related Terms	37.2	25.7	2.4	2.4
Fatigue	37.0	66.8	1.6	25.0
Headache	33.6	43.3	0.5	3.6
Joint Pain	30.3	39.4	2.5	7.3
Abdominal Pain	29.9	25.0	2.5	3.9
Nasopharyngitis	26.9	8.4	0	0.2
Hemorrhage	24.1	20.8	1.1	1.5
–GI Hemorrhage	1.3	1.1	0.5	0.2
–CNS Hemorrhage	0.2	0.2	0	0.2
Myalgia	22.5	38.8	1.5	8.1
Vomiting	20.5	27.4	1.5	3.4
Dyspepsia	17.8	9.2	0	0.8
Cough	17.4	23.1	0.2	0.6
Pharyngolaryngeal Pain	16.9	11.3	0.2	0
Upper Respiratory Tract Infection	16.5	8.4	0.2	0.4
Dizziness	15.8	24.2	0.9	3.6
Pyrexia	15.4	42.4	0.9	3.0
Weight Increased	15.2	2.1	1.6	0.4
Insomnia	13.2	18.8	0	2.3
Depression	12.7	35.8	0.5	13.1
Influenza	11.1	6.0	0.2	0.2

[1] All adverse events occurring in ≥10% of patients are listed regardless of suspected relationship to treatment.

In vitro, Gleevec inhibits acetaminophen O-glucuronidation (K_i value of 58.5 µM) at therapeutic levels. Systemic exposure to acetaminophen is expected to be increased when co-administered with Gleevec. No specific studies in humans have been performed and caution is recommended.

Carcinogenesis, Mutagenesis, Impairment of Fertility
The urogenital tract from a 2-year carcinogenicity study in rats receiving doses of 15, 30 and 60 mg/kg/day of imatinib mesylate showed renal adenomas/carcinomas, urinary bladder papillomas and papillomas/carcinomas of the preputial and clitoral gland. Evaluation of other organs in the rats is ongoing.

The papilloma/carcinoma of the preputial/clitoral gland were noted at 30 and 60 mg/kg/day (approximately 0.5 to 4 times the human daily exposure at 400 mg/day). The kidney adenoma/carcinoma and the urinary bladder papilloma were noted at 60 mg/kg/day. No tumors in the urogenital tract were observed at 15 mg/kg/day.

Positive genotoxic effects were obtained for imatinib in an *in vitro* mammalian cell assay (Chinese hamster ovary) for clastogenicity (chromosome aberrations) in the presence of metabolic activation. Two intermediates of the manufacturing process, which are also present in the final product, are positive for mutagenesis in the Ames assay. One of these intermediates was also positive in the mouse lymphoma assay. Imatinib was not genotoxic when tested in an *in vitro* bacterial cell assay (Ames test), an *in vitro* mammalian cell assay (mouse lymphoma) and an *in vivo* rat micronucleus assay.

In a study of fertility, in male rats dosed for 70 days prior to mating, testicular and epididymal weights and percent motile sperm were decreased at 60 mg/kg, approximately three-fourths the maximum clinical dose of 800 mg/day based on body surface area. This was not seen at doses ≤20 mg/kg (one-fourth the maximum human dose of 800 mg). When female rats were dosed 14 days prior to mating and through to gestational Day 6, there was no effect on mating or on number of pregnant females.

In female rats dosed with imatinib mesylate at 45 mg/kg (approximately one-half the maximum human dose of 800 mg/day based on body surface area) from gestational Day 6 until the end of lactation, red vaginal discharge was noted on either gestational Day 14 or 15.

Pregnancy
Pregnancy Category D. (See WARNINGS).

Nursing Mothers
It is not known whether imatinib mesylate or its metabolites are excreted in human milk. However, in lactating female rats administered 100 mg/kg, a dose approximately equal to the maximum clinical dose of 800 mg/day based on body surface area, imatinib and its metabolites were extensively excreted in milk. Concentration in milk was approximately three-fold higher than in plasma. It is estimated that approximately 1.5% of a maternal dose is excreted into milk, which is equivalent to a dose to the infant of 30% of the maternal dose per unit body weight. Because many drugs are excreted in human milk and because of the potential for serious adverse reactions in nursing infants, women should be advised against breast-feeding while taking Gleevec.

Pediatric Use
Gleevec safety and efficacy have been demonstrated only in children with Ph+ chronic phase CML with recurrence after stem cell transplantation or resistance to interferon-alpha therapy. There are no data in children under 3 years of age.

Geriatric Use
In the CML clinical studies, approximately 40% of patients were older than 60 years and 10% were older than 70 years. In the study of patients with newly diagnosed CML, 22% of patients were 60 years of age or older. No difference was observed in the safety profile in patients older than 65 years as compared to younger patients, with the exception of a higher frequency of edema. *(See PRECAUTIONS.)* The efficacy of Gleevec was similar in older and younger patients. In the GIST study, 29% of patients were older than 60 years and 10% of patients were older than 70 years. No obvious differences in the safety or efficacy profile were noted in pa-

tients older than 65 years as compared to younger patients, but the small number of patients does not allow a formal analysis.

ADVERSE REACTIONS
Chronic Myeloid Leukemia
The majority of Gleevec-treated patients experienced adverse events at some time. Most events were of mild-to-moderate grade, but drug was discontinued for drug-related adverse events in 3.1% of newly diagnosed patients, 4% of patients in chronic phase after failure of interferon-alpha therapy, 4% in accelerated phase and 5% in blast crisis.
The most frequently reported drug-related adverse events were edema, nausea and vomiting, muscle cramps, musculoskeletal pain, diarrhea and rash (Table 4 for newly diagnosed CML, Table 5 for other CML patients). Edema was most frequently periorbital or in lower limbs and was managed with diuretics, other supportive measures, or by reducing the dose of Gleevec® (imatinib mesylate). (See DOSAGE AND ADMINISTRATION.) The frequency of severe superficial edema was 0.9%-6%.

A variety of adverse events represent local or general fluid retention including pleural effusion, ascites, pulmonary edema and rapid weight gain with or without superficial edema. These events appear to be dose related, were more common in the blast crisis and accelerated phase studies (where the dose was 600 mg/day), and are more common in the elderly. These events were usually managed by interrupting Gleevec treatment and with diuretics or other appropriate supportive care measures. However, a few of these events may be serious or life threatening, and one patient with blast crisis died with pleural effusion, congestive heart failure, and renal failure.
Adverse events, regardless of relationship to study drug, that were reported in at least 10% of the patients treated in the Gleevec studies are shown in Tables 4 and 5.
[See table 4 at top of previous page]
[See table 5 below]
Hematologic Toxicity
Cytopenias, and particularly neutropenia and thrombocytopenia, were a consistent finding in all studies, with a higher

Table 5
Adverse Experiences Reported in Other CML Clinical Trials (≥10% of all patients in any trial)[1]

Preferred Term	Myeloid Blast Crisis (n=260) % All Grades	Grade 3/4	Accelerated Phase (n=235) % All Grades	Grade 3/4	Chronic Phase, IFN Failure (n=532) % All Grades	Grade 3/4
Fluid Retention	72	11	76	6	69	4
– Superficial Edema	66	6	74	3	67	2
– Other Fluid Retention Events[2]	22	6	15	4	7	2
Nausea	71	5	73	5	63	3
Muscle Cramps	28	1	47	0.4	62	2
Vomiting	54	4	58	3	36	2
Diarrhea	43	4	57	5	48	3
Hemorrhage	53	19	49	11	30	2
– CNS Hemorrhage	9	7	3	3	2	1
– GI Hemorrhage	8	4	6	5	2	0.4
Musculoskeletal Pain	42	9	49	9	38	2
Fatigue	30	4	46	4	48	1
Skin Rash	36	5	47	5	47	3
Pyrexia	41	7	41	8	21	2
Arthralgia	25	5	34	6	40	1
Headache	27	5	32	2	36	0.6
Abdominal Pain	30	6	33	4	32	1
Weight Increased	5	1	17	5	32	7
Cough	14	0.8	27	0.9	20	0
Dyspepsia	12	0	22	0	27	0
Myalgia	9	0	24	2	27	0.2
Nasopharyngitis	10	0	17	0	22	0.2
Asthenia	18	5	21	5	15	0.2
Dyspnea	15	4	21	7	12	0.9
Upper Respiratory Tract Infection	3	0	12	0.4	19	0
Anorexia	14	2	17	2	7	0
Night Sweats	13	0.8	17	1	14	0.2
Constipation	16	2	16	0.9	9	0.4
Dizziness	12	0.4	13	0	16	0.2
Pharyngitis	10	0	12	0	15	0
Insomnia	10	0	14	0	14	0.2
Pruritus	8	1	14	0.9	14	0.8
Hypokalemia	13	4	9	2	6	0.8
Pneumonia	13	7	10	7	4	1
Anxiety	8	0.8	12	0	8	0.4
Liver Toxicity	10	5	12	6	6	3
Rigors	10	0	12	0.4	10	0
Chest Pain	7	2	10	0.4	11	0.8
Influenza	0.8	0.4	6	0	11	0.2
Sinusitis	4	0.4	11	0.4	9	0.4

[1] All adverse events occurring in ≥10% of patients are listed regardless of suspected relationship to treatment.
[2] Other fluid retention events include pleural effusion, ascites, pulmonary edema, pericardial effusion, anasarca, edema aggravated, and fluid retention not otherwise specified.

Table 6
Lab Abnormalities in Newly Diagnosed CML Trial

CTC Grades	Gleevec® N=551 %		IFN+Ara-C N=533 %	
	Grade 3	Grade 4	Grade 3	Grade 4
Hematology Parameters				
- Neutropenia*	12.3	3.1	20.8	4.3
- Thrombocytopenia*	8.3	0.2	15.9	0.6
- Anemia	3.1	0.9	4.1	0.2
Biochemistry Parameters				
- Elevated Creatinine	0	0	0.4	0
- Elevated Bilirubin	0.7	0.2	0.2	0
- Elevated Alkaline Phosphatase	0.2	0	0.8	0
- Elevated SGOT (AST)	2.9	0.2	3.8	0.4
- Elevated SGPT (ALT)	3.1	0.4	5.6	0

*$p<0.001$ (difference in Grade 3 plus 4 abnormalities between the two treatment groups)

Table 7
Lab Abnormalities in Other CML Clinical Trials

CTC Grades	Myeloid Blast Crisis (n=260) 600 mg n=223 400 mg n=37 %		Accelerated Phase (n=235) 600 mg n=158 400 mg n=77 %		Chronic Phase, IFN Failure (n=532) 400 mg %	
	Grade 3	Grade 4	Grade 3	Grade 4	Grade 3	Grade 4
Hematology Parameters						
- Neutropenia	16	48	23	36	27	9
- Thrombocytopenia	30	33	31	13	21	<1
- Anemia	42	11	34	7	6	1
Biochemistry Parameters						
- Elevated Creatinine	1.5	0	1.3	0	0.2	0
- Elevated Bilirubin	3.8	0	2.1	0	0.6	0
- Elevated Alkaline Phosphatase	4.6	0	5.5	0.4	0.2	0
- Elevated SGOT (AST)	1.9	0	3.0	0	2.3	0
- Elevated SGPT (ALT)	2.3	0.4	4.3	0	2.1	0

CTC Grades: neutropenia (Grade 3 $\geq 0.5\text{-}1.0 \times 10^9$/L, Grade 4 $<0.5 \times 10^9$/L), thrombocytopenia (Grade 3 $\geq 10\text{-}50 \times 10^9$/L, Grade 4 $<10 \times 10^9$/L), anemia (hemoglobin $\geq 65\text{-}80$ g/L, Grade 4 <65 g/L), elevated creatinine (Grade 3 $>3\text{-}6 \times$ upper limit normal range [ULN], Grade 4 $>6 \times$ ULN), elevated bilirubin (Grade 3 $>3\text{-}10 \times$ ULN, Grade 4 $>10 \times$ ULN), elevated alkaline phosphatase (Grade 3 $>5\text{-}20 \times$ ULN, Grade 4 $>20 \times$ ULN), elevated SGOT or SGPT (Grade 3 $>5\text{-}20 \times$ ULN, Grade 4 $>20 \times$ ULN)

frequency at doses ≥ 750 mg (Phase 1 study). However, the occurrence of cytopenias in CML patients was also dependent on the stage of the disease.

In patients with newly diagnosed CML, cytopenias were less frequent than in the other CML patients (see Tables 6 and 7). The frequency of Grade 3 or 4 neutropenia and thrombocytopenia was between 2- and 3-fold higher in blast crisis and accelerated phase compared to chronic phase (see Tables 6 and 7). The median duration of the neutropenic and thrombocytopenic episodes varied from 2 to 3 weeks, and from 2 to 4 weeks, respectively.

These events can usually be managed with either a reduction of the dose or an interruption of treatment with Gleevec, but in rare cases require permanent discontinuation of treatment.

Hepatotoxicity

Severe elevation of transaminases or bilirubin occurred in 3%-6% (see Table 5) and were usually managed with dose reduction or interruption (the median duration of these episodes was approximately 1 week). Treatment was discontinued permanently because of liver laboratory abnormalities in less than 1% of patients. However, one patient, who was taking acetaminophen regularly for fever, died of acute liver failure.

Adverse Reactions in Pediatric Population

The overall safety profile of pediatric patients treated with Gleevec in 39 children studied was similar to that found in studies with adult patients, except that musculoskeletal pain was less frequent (20.5%) and peripheral edema was not reported.

Adverse Effects in Other Subpopulations

In older patients (≥ 65 years old), with the exception of edema, where it was more frequent, there was no evidence of an increase in the incidence or severity of adverse events. In women there was an increase in the frequency of neutropenia, as well as Grade 1/2 superficial edema, headache, nausea, rigors, vomiting, rash, and fatigue. No differences were seen related to race but the subsets were too small for proper evaluation.

[See table 6 above]
[See table 7 above]

Gastrointestinal Stromal Tumors

The majority of Gleevec-treated patients experienced adverse events at some time. The most frequently reported adverse events were edema, nausea, diarrhea, abdominal pain, muscle cramps, fatigue, and rash. Most events were of mild-to-moderate severity. Drug was discontinued for adverse events in 6 patients (8%) in both dose levels studied. Superficial edema, most frequently periorbital or lower extremity edema, was managed with diuretics, other supportive measures, or by reducing the dose of Gleevec® (imatinib mesylate). (See DOSAGE AND ADMINISTRATION.) Severe (CTC grade 3/4) superficial edema was observed in 3

Table 8
Adverse Experiences Reported in GIST Trial (≥10% of all patients at either dose)[1]

	All CTC Grades Initial Dose (mg/day)		CTC Grade 3/4 Initial Dose (mg/day)	
	400 mg (n=73)	600 mg (n=74)	400 mg (n=73)	600 mg (n=74)
Preferred Term	%	%	%	%
Fluid Retention	71	76	6	3
- Superficial Edema	71	76	4	0
- Pleural Effusion or Ascites	6	4	1	3
Diarrhea	56	60	1	4
Nausea	53	56	3	3
Fatigue	33	38	1	0
Muscle Cramps	30	41	0	0
Abdominal Pain	37	37	7	3
Skin Rash	26	38	3	3
Headache	25	35	0	0
Vomiting	22	23	1	3
Musculoskeletal Pain	19	11	3	0
Flatulence	16	23	0	0
Any Hemorrhage	18	19	5	8
- Tumor Hemorrhage	1	4	1	4
- Cerebral Hemorrhage	1	0	1	0
- GI Tract Hemorrhage	6	4	4	1
Nasopharyngitis	12	14	0	0
Pyrexia	12	5	0	0
Insomnia	11	11	0	0
Back Pain	11	10	1	0
Lacrimation Increased	6	11	0	0
Upper Respiratory Tract Infection	6	11	0	0
Taste Disturbance	1	14	0	0

[1] All adverse events occurring in ≥10% of patients are listed regardless of suspected relationship to treatment.

patients (2%), including face edema in one patient. Grade 3/4 pleural effusion or ascites was observed in 3 patients (2%).

Adverse events, regardless of relationship to study drug, that were reported in at least 10% of the patients treated with Gleevec are shown in Table 8. No major differences were seen in the severity of adverse events between the 400-mg or 600-mg treatment groups, although overall incidence of diarrhea, muscle cramps, headache, dermatitis, and edema was somewhat higher in the 600-mg treatment group.

[See table 8 above]

Clinically relevant or severe abnormalities of routine hematologic or biochemistry laboratory values are presented in Table 9.

[See table 9 below]

Additional Data from Multiple Clinical Trials

The following less common (estimated 1%-10%), infrequent (estimated 0.1%-1%), and rare (estimated less than 0.1%) adverse events have been reported during clinical trials of Gleevec. These events are included based on clinical relevance.

Cardiovascular: Infrequent: cardiac failure, tachycardia, hypertension, hypotension, flushing, peripheral coldness *Rare:* pericarditis

Clinical Laboratory Tests: Infrequent: blood CPK increased, blood LDH increased

Dermatologic: Less common: dry skin, alopecia *Infrequent:* exfoliative dermatitis, bullous eruption, nail disorder, skin pigmentation changes, photosensitivity reaction, purpura, psoriasis

Rare: vesicular rash, Stevens-Johnson syndrome, acute generalized exanthematous pustulosis

Table 9
Laboratory Abnormalities in GIST Trial

	400 mg (n=73) %		600 mg (n=74) %	
CTC Grades	Grade 3	Grade 4	Grade 3	Grade 4
Hematology Parameters				
- Anemia	3	0	4	1
- Thrombocytopenia	0	0	1	0
- Neutropenia	3	3	5	4
Biochemistry Parameters				
- Elevated Creatinine	0	1	3	0
- Reduced Albumin	3	0	4	0
- Elevated Bilirubin	1	0	1	3
- Elevated Alkaline Phosphatase	0	0	· 1	0
- Elevated SGOT (AST)	3	0	1	1
- Elevated SGPT (ALT)	3	0	4	0

CTC Grades: neutropenia (Grade 3 ≥0.5-1.0 × 10^9/L, Grade 4 <0.5 × 10^9/L), thrombocytopenia (Grade 3 ≥10-50 × 10^9/L, Grade 4 <10 × 10^9/L), anemia (Grade 3 ≥65-80 g/L, Grade 4 <65 g/L), elevated creatinine (Grade 3 >3-6 × upper limit normal range [ULN], Grade 4 >6 × ULN), elevated bilirubin (Grade 3 >3-10 × ULN, Grade 4 >10 × ULN), elevated alkaline phosphatase SGOT or SGPT (Grade 3 >5-20 × ULN, Grade 4 >20 × ULN), albumin (Grade 3 <20 g/L)

Digestive: *Less common:* abdominal distention, gastro-esophageal reflux, mouth ulceration
Infrequent: gastric ulcer, gastroenteritis, gastritis
Rare: colitis, ileus/intestinal obstruction, pancreatitis
General Disorders and Administration Site Conditions:
Rare: tumor necrosis
Hematologic: *Infrequent:* pancytopenia
Rare: aplastic anemia
Hypersensitivity: *Rare:* angioedema
Infections: *Infrequent:* sepsis, herpes simplex, herpes zoster
Metabolic and Nutritional: *Infrequent:* hypophosphatemia, dehydration, gout, appetite disturbances, weight decreased
Rare: hyperkalemia, hyponatremia
Musculoskeletal: *Less common:* joint swelling
Infrequent: sciatica, joint and muscle stiffness
Nervous System/Psychiatric: *Less common:* paresthesia
Infrequent: depression, anxiety, syncope, peripheral neuropathy, somnolence, migraine, memory impairment
Rare: increased intracranial pressure, cerebral edema (including fatalities), confusion, convulsions
Renal: *Infrequent:* renal failure, urinary frequency, hematuria
Reproductive: *Infrequent:* breast enlargement, menorrhagia, sexual dysfunction
Respiratory: *Rare:* interstitial pneumonitis, pulmonary fibrosis
Special Senses: *Less common:* conjunctivitis, vision blurred
Infrequent: conjunctival hemorrhage, dry eye, vertigo, tinnitus
Rare: macular edema, papilledema, retinal hemorrhage, glaucoma, vitreous hemorrhage
Vascular Disorders: *Rare:* thrombosis/embolism

OVERDOSAGE

Experience with doses greater than 800 mg is limited. Isolated cases of Gleevec® (imatinib mesylate) overdose have been reported. In the event of overdosage, the patient should be observed and appropriate supportive treatment given.

A patient with myeloid blast crisis experienced Grade 1 elevations of serum creatinine, Grade 2 ascites and elevated liver transaminase levels, and Grade 3 elevations of bilirubin after inadvertently taking 1,200 mg of Gleevec daily for 6 days. Therapy was temporarily interrupted and complete reversal of all abnormalities occurred within 1 week. Treatment was resumed at a dose of 400 mg daily without recurrence of adverse events. Another patient developed severe muscle cramps after taking 1,600 mg of Gleevec daily for 6 days. Complete resolution of muscle cramps occurred following interruption of therapy and treatment was subsequently resumed. Another patient that was prescribed 400 mg daily, took 800 mg of Gleevec on Day 1 and 1,200 mg on Day 2. Therapy was interrupted, no adverse events occurred and the patient resumed therapy.

DOSAGE AND ADMINISTRATION

Therapy should be initiated by a physician experienced in the treatment of patients with chronic myeloid leukemia or gastrointestinal stromal tumors.

The recommended dosage of Gleevec® (imatinib mesylate) is 400 mg/day for adult patients in chronic phase CML and 600 mg/day for adult patients in accelerated phase or blast crisis. The recommended Gleevec dosage is 260 mg/m²/day for children with Ph+ chronic phase CML recurrent after stem cell transplant or who are resistant to interferon-alpha therapy. The recommended dosage of Gleevec is 400 mg/day or 600 mg/day for adult patients with unresectable and/or metastatic, malignant GIST.

The prescribed dose should be administered orally, with a meal and a large glass of water. Doses of 400 mg or 600 mg should be administered once daily, whereas a dose of 800 mg should be administered as 400 mg twice a day.

In children, Gleevec treatment can be given as a once-daily dose or alternatively the daily dose may be split into two -

once in the morning and once in the evening. There is no experience with Gleevec treatment in children under 3 years of age.

For patients unable to swallow the film-coated tablets, the tablets may be dispersed in a glass of water or apple juice. The required number of tablets should be placed in the appropriate volume of beverage (approximately 50 mL for a 100-mg tablet, and 200 mL for a 400-mg tablet) and stirred with a spoon. The suspension should be administered immediately after complete disintegration of the tablet(s).

Treatment may be continued as long as there is no evidence of progressive disease or unacceptable toxicity.

In CML, a dose increase from 400 mg to 600 mg in adult patients with chronic phase disease, or from 600 mg to 800 mg (given as 400 mg twice daily) in adult patients in accelerated phase or blast crisis may be considered in the absence of severe adverse drug reaction and severe non-leukemia related neutropenia or thrombocytopenia in the following circumstances: disease progression (at any time), failure to achieve a satisfactory hematologic response after at least 3 months of treatment, failure to achieve a cytogenetic response after 6-12 months of treatment, or loss of a previously achieved hematologic or cytogenetic response. In children with chronic phase CML, daily doses can be increased under circumstances similar to those leading to an increase in adult chronic phase disease, from 260 mg/m²/day to 340 mg/m²/day, as clinically indicated.

Dosage of Gleevec should be increased by at least 50%, and clinical response should be carefully monitored, in patients receiving Gleevec with a potent CYP3A4 inducer such as rifampin or phenytoin.

For daily dosing of 800 mg and above, dosing should be accomplished using the 400-mg tablet to reduce exposure to iron. Patients at a total dose of 1,200 mg daily may have an increased susceptibility to excess iron. If routine blood sampling indicates sustained increases in iron levels, attempts to lower other sources of iron exposure should be undertaken.

Dose Adjustment for Hepatotoxicity and Other Non-Hematologic Adverse Reactions

If a severe non-hematologic adverse reaction develops (such as severe hepatotoxicity or severe fluid retention), Gleevec should be withheld until the event has resolved. Thereafter, treatment can be resumed as appropriate depending on the initial severity of the event.

If elevations in bilirubin >3 × institutional upper limit of normal (IULN) or in liver transaminases >5 × IULN occur, Gleevec should be withheld until bilirubin levels have returned to a <1.5 × IULN and transaminase levels to <2.5 × IULN. In adults, treatment with Gleevec may then be continued at a reduced daily dose (i.e., 400 mg to 300 mg or 600 mg to 400 mg). In children, daily doses can be reduced under the same circumstances from 260 mg/m²/day to 200 mg/m²/day or from 340 mg/m²/day to 260 mg/m²/day, respectively.

Dose Adjustment for Hematologic Adverse Reactions

Dose reduction or treatment interruptions for severe neutropenia and thrombocytopenia are recommended as indicated in Table 10.

[See table 10 at top of next page]

HOW SUPPLIED

Each film-coated tablet contains 100 mg or 400 mg of imatinib free base.

100-mg Tablets

Very dark yellow to brownish orange, film-coated tablets, round, biconvex with bevelled edges, debossed with "NVR" on one side, and "SA" with score on the other side.
Bottles of 100 tablets .... NDC 0078-0401-05

400-mg Tablets

Very dark yellow to brownish orange, film-coated tablets, ovaloid, biconvex with bevelled edges, debossed with "400" on one side with score on the other side, and "SL" on each side of the score.
Bottles of 30 tablets .... NDC 0078-0438-15

Table 10
Dose Adjustments for Neutropenia and Thrombocytopenia

Chronic Phase CML (starting dose 400 mg[1]) or GIST (starting dose either 400 mg or 600 mg)	$ANC <1.0 \times 10^9/L$ and/or Platelets $<50 \times 10^9/L$	1. Stop Gleevec until $ANC \geq1.5 \times 10^9/L$ and platelets $\geq75 \times10^9/L$ 2. Resume treatment with Gleevec at the original starting dose of 400 mg[1] or 600 mg 3. If recurrence of $ANC <1.0 \times 10^9/L$ and/or platelets $<50 \times 10^9/L$, repeat step 1 and resume Gleevec at a reduced dose (300 mg[2] if starting dose was 400 mg[1], 400 mg if starting dose was 600 mg)
Accelerated Phase CML and Blast Crisis (starting dose 600 mg)	[3]$ANC <0.5 \times 10^9/L$ and/or Platelets $<10 \times 10^9/L$	1. Check if cytopenia is related to leukemia (marrow aspirate or biopsy) 2. If cytopenia is unrelated to leukemia, reduce dose of Gleevec to 400 mg 3. If cytopenia persists 2 weeks, reduce further to 300 mg 4. If cytopenia persists 4 weeks and is still unrelated to leukemia, stop Gleevec until $ANC \geq1 \times 10^9/L$ and platelets $\geq20 \times 10^9/L$ and then resume treatment at 300 mg

[1]or 260 mg/m^2 in children
[2]or 200 mg/m^2 in children
[3]occurring after at least 1 month of treatment

Storage
Store at 25°C (77°F); excursions permitted to 15-30°C (59-86°F) [see USP Controlled Room Temperature]. Protect from moisture.
Dispense in a tight container, USP.

REV: MARCH 2005   Printed in U.S.A.   T2005-18   5000305

Manufactured by:
Novartis Pharma Stein AG
Stein, Switzerland
Distributed by:
Novartis Pharmaceuticals Corporation
East Hanover, New Jersey 07936
©Novartis

VIRAZOLE® ℞
[*vira 'zahl '*]
(Ribavirin for Inhalation Solution)
℞ only

PRESCRIBING INFORMATION

> **WARNINGS:**
> USE OF AEROSOLIZED VIRAZOLE IN PATIENTS REQUIRING MECHANICAL VENTILATOR ASSISTANCE SHOULD BE UNDERTAKEN ONLY BY PHYSICIANS AND SUPPORT STAFF FAMILIAR WITH THE SPECIFIC VENTILATOR BEING USED AND THIS MODE OF ADMINISTRATION OF THE DRUG. STRICT ATTENTION MUST BE PAID TO PROCEDURES THAT HAVE BEEN SHOWN TO MINIMIZE THE ACCUMULATION OF DRUG PRECIPITATE, WHICH CAN RESULT IN MECHANICAL VENTILATOR DYSFUNCTION AND ASSOCIATED INCREASED PULMONARY PRESSURES (SEE WARNINGS).
> SUDDEN DETERIORATION OF RESPIRATORY FUNCTION HAS BEEN ASSOCIATED WITH INITIATION OF AEROSOLIZED VIRAZOLE USE IN INFANTS. RESPIRATORY FUNCTION SHOULD BE CAREFULLY MONITORED DURING TREATMENT. IF INITIATION OF AEROSOLIZED VIRAZOLE TREATMENT APPEARS TO PRODUCE SUDDEN DETERIORATION OF RESPIRATORY FUNCTION, TREATMENT SHOULD BE STOPPED AND REINSTITUTED ONLY WITH EXTREME CAUTION, CONTINUOUS MONITORING AND CONSIDERATION OF CONCOMITANT ADMINISTRATION OF BRONCHODILATORS (SEE WARNINGS).
> VIRAZOLE IS NOT INDICATED FOR USE IN ADULTS. PHYSICIANS AND PATIENTS SHOULD BE AWARE THAT RIBAVIRIN HAS BEEN SHOWN TO PRODUCE TESTICULAR LESIONS IN RODENTS AND TO BE TERATOGENIC IN ALL ANIMAL SPECIES IN WHICH ADEQUATE STUDIES HAVE BEEN CONDUCTED (RODENTS AND RABBITS); (SEE CONTRAINDICATIONS).

DESCRIPTION

Virazole® is a brand name for ribavirin, a synthetic nucleoside with antiviral activity. VIRAZOLE for inhalation solution is a sterile, lyophilized powder to be reconstituted for aerosol administration. Each 100 mL glass vial contains 6 grams of ribavirin, and when reconstituted to the recommended volume of 300 mL with sterile water for injection or sterile water for inhalation (no preservatives added), will contain 20 mg of ribavirin per mL, pH approximately 5.5. Aerosolization is to be carried out in a Small Particle Aerosol Generator (SPAG-2) nebulizer only.
Ribavirin is 1-beta-D-ribofuranosyl-1H-1,2,4-triazole-3-carboxamide, with the following structural formula:

Ribavirin is a stable, white crystalline compound with a maximum solubility in water of 142 mg/mL at 25°C and with only a slight solubility in ethanol. The empirical formula is $C_8H_{12}N_4O_5$ and the molecular weight is 244.21.

CLINICAL PHARMACOLOGY
Mechanism of Action
In cell cultures the inhibitory activity of ribavirin for respiratory syncytial virus (RSV) is selective. The mechanism of action is unknown. Reversal of the *in vitro* antiviral activity by guanosine or xanthosine suggests ribavirin may act as an analogue of these cellular metabolites.

Microbiology
Ribavirin has demonstrated antiviral activity against RSV *in vitro*[1] and in experimentally infected cotton rats.[2] Several clinical isolates of RSV were evaluated for ribavirin susceptibility by plaque reduction in tissue culture. Plaques were reduced 85–98% by 16 µg/mL; however, results may vary with the test system. The development of resistance has not been evaluated *in vitro* or in clinical trials.
In addition to the above, ribavirin has been shown to have *in vitro* activity against influenza A and B viruses and herpes simplex virus, but the clinical significance of these data is unknown.

Immunologic Effects
Neutralizing antibody responses to RSV were decreased in aerosolized VIRAZOLE treated infants compared to placebo treated infants.[3] One study also showed that RSV-specific IgE antibody in bronchial secretions was decreased in patients treated with aerosolized VIRAZOLE. In rats, ribavirin administration resulted in lymphoid atrophy of the thymus, spleen, and lymph nodes. Humoral immunity was reduced in guinea pigs and ferrets. Cellular immunity was also mildly depressed in animal studies. The clinical significance of these observations is unknown.

Pharmacokinetics
Assay for VIRAZOLE in human materials is by a radioimmunoassay which detects ribavirin and at least one metabolite.
VIRAZOLE brand of ribavirin, when administered by aerosol, is absorbed systemically. Four pediatric patients inhaling VIRAZOLE aerosol administered by face mask for 2.5 hours each day for 3 days had plasma concentrations ranging from 0.44 to 1.55 µM, with a mean concentration of 0.76 µM. The plasma half-life was reported to be 9.5 hours. Three pediatric patients inhaling aerosolized VIRAZOLE administered by face mask or mist tent for 20 hours each day for 5 days had plasma concentrations ranging from 1.5 to 14.3 µM, with a mean concentration of 6.8 µM.
The bioavailability of aerosolized VIRAZOLE is unknown and may depend on the mode of aerosol delivery. After aerosol treatment, peak plasma concentrations of ribavirin are 85% to 98% less than the concentration that reduced RSV plaque formation in tissue culture. After aerosol treatment, respiratory tract secretions are likely to contain ribavirin in concentrations many fold higher than those required to reduce plaque formation. However, RSV is an intracellular virus and it is unknown whether plasma concentrations or respiratory secretion concentrations of the drug better reflect intracellular concentrations in the respiratory tract.
In man, rats, and rhesus monkeys, accumulation of ribavirin and/or metabolites in the red blood cells have been noted, plateauing in red cells in man in about 4 days and gradually declining with an apparent half-life of 40 days (the half-life of erythrocytes). The extent of accumulation of ribavirin following inhalation therapy is not well defined.

Animal Toxicology
Ribavirin, when administered orally or as an aerosol, produced cardiac lesions in mice, rats, and monkeys, when given at doses of 30, 36 and 120 mg/kg or greater for 4 weeks or more (estimated human equivalent doses of 4.8, 12.3 and 111.4 mg/kg for a 5 kg child, or 2.5, 5.1 and 40 mg/kg for a 60 kg adult, based on body surface area adjustment). Aerosolized ribavirin administered to developing ferrets at 60 mg/kg for 10 or 30 days resulted in inflammatory and possibly emphysematous changes in the lungs. Proliferative changes were seen in the lungs following exposure at 131 mg/kg for 30 days. The significance of these findings to human administration is unknown.

INDICATIONS AND USAGE

VIRAZOLE is indicated for the treatment of hospitalized infants and young children with severe lower respiratory tract infections due to respiratory syncytial virus. Treatment early in the course of severe lower respiratory tract infection may be necessary to achieve efficacy.

Only severe RSV lower respiratory tract infection should be treated with VIRAZOLE. The vast majority of infants and children with RSV infection have disease that is mild, self-limited, and does not require hospitalization or antiviral treatment. Many children with mild lower respiratory tract involvement will require shorter hospitalization than would be required for a full course of VIRAZOLE aerosol (3 to 7 days) and should not be treated with the drug. Thus the decision to treat with VIRAZOLE should be based on the severity of the RSV infection.

The presence of an underlying condition such as prematurity, immunosuppression or cardiopulmonary disease may increase the severity of clinical manifestations and complications of RSV infection.

Use of aerosolized VIRAZOLE in patients requiring mechanical ventilator assistance should be undertaken only by physicians and support staff familiar with this mode of administration and the specific ventilator being used (see WARNINGS, and DOSAGE AND ADMINISTRATION).

Diagnosis

RSV infection should be documented by a rapid diagnostic method such as demonstration of viral antigen in respiratory tract secretions by immunofluorescence[3,4] or ELISA[5] before or during the first 24 hours of treatment. Treatment may be initiated while awaiting rapid diagnostic test results. However, treatment should not be continued without documentation of RSV infection.

Non-culture antigen detection techniques may have false positive or false negative results. Assessment of the clinical situation, the time of year and other parameters may warrant reevaluation of the laboratory diagnosis.

Description of Studies

Non-Mechanically-Ventilated Infants: In two placebo controlled trials in infants hospitalized with RSV lower respiratory tract infection, aerosolized VIRAZOLE treatment had a therapeutic effect, as judged by the reduction in severity of clinical manifestations of disease by treatment day 3.[3,4] Treatment was most effective when instituted within the first 3 days of clinical illness. Virus titers in respiratory secretions were also significantly reduced with VIRAZOLE in one of these original studies.[4] Additional controlled studies conducted since these initial trials of aerosolized VIRAZOLE in the treatment of RSV infection have supported these data.

Mechanically-Ventilated Infants: A randomized, double-blind, placebo controlled evaluation of aerosolized VIRAZOLE at the recommended dose was conducted in 28 infants requiring mechanical ventilation for respiratory failure caused by documented RSV infection.[6] Mean age was 1.4 months (SD, 1.7 months). Seven patients had underlying diseases predisposing them to severe infection and 21 were previously normal. Aerosolized VIRAZOLE treatment significantly decreased the duration of mechanical ventilation required (4.9 vs. 9.9 days, p=0.01) and duration of required supplemental oxygen (8.7 vs 13.5 days, p=0.01). Intensive patient management and monitoring techniques were employed in this study. These included endotracheal tube suctioning every 1 to 2 hours; recording of proximal airway pressure, ventilatory rate, and F_1O_2 every hour; and arterial blood gas monitoring every 2 to 6 hours. To reduce the risk of VIRAZOLE precipitation and ventilator malfunction, heated wire tubing, two bacterial filters connected in series in the expiratory limb of the ventilator (with filter changes every 4 hours), and water column pressure release valves to monitor internal ventilator pressures were used in connecting ventilator circuits to the SPAG-2.

Employing these techniques, no technical difficulties with VIRAZOLE administration were encountered during the study. Adverse events consisted of bacterial pneumonia in one case, staphyloccus bacteremia in one case and two cases of post-extubation stridor. None were felt to be related to VIRAZOLE administration.

CONTRAINDICATIONS

VIRAZOLE is contraindicated in individuals who have shown hypersensitivity to the drug or its components, and in women who are or may become pregnant during exposure

to the drug. Ribavirin has demonstrated significant teratogenic and/or embryocidal potential in all animal species in which adequate studies have been conducted (rodents and rabbits). Therefore, although clinical studies have not been performed, it should be assumed that VIRAZOLE may cause fetal harm in humans. Studies in which the drug has been administered systemically demonstrate that ribavirin is concentrated in the red blood cells and persists for the life of the erythrocyte.

WARNINGS

SUDDEN DETERIORATION OF RESPIRATORY FUNCTION HAS BEEN ASSOCIATED WITH INITIATION OF AEROSOLIZED VIRAZOLE USE IN INFANTS. Respiratory function should be carefully monitored during treatment. If initiation of aerosolized VIRAZOLE treatment appears to produce sudden deterioration of respiratory function, treatment should be stopped and reinstituted only with extreme caution, continuous monitoring, and consideration of concomitant administration of bronchodilators.

Use with Mechanical Ventilators

USE OF AEROSOLIZED VIRAZOLE IN PATIENTS REQUIRING MECHANICAL VENTILATOR ASSISTANCE SHOULD BE UNDERTAKEN ONLY BY PHYSICIANS AND SUPPORT STAFF FAMILIAR WITH THIS MODE OF ADMINISTRATION AND THE SPECIFIC VENTILATOR BEING USED. Strict attention must be paid to procedures that have been shown to minimize the accumulation of drug precipitate, which can result in mechanical ventilator dysfunction and associated increased pulmonary pressures. These procedures include the use of bacteria filters in series in the expiratory limb of the ventilator circuit with frequent changes (every 4 hours), water column pressure release valves to indicate elevated ventilator pressures, frequent monitoring of these devices and verification that ribavirin crystals have not accumulated within the ventilator circuitry, and frequent suctioning and monitoring of the patient (see Clinical Studies).

Those administering aerosolized VIRAZOLE in conjunction with mechanical ventilator use should be thoroughly familiar with detailed descriptions of these procedures as outlined in the SPAG-2 manual.

PRECAUTIONS

General: Patients with severe lower respiratory tract infection due to respiratory syncytial virus require optimum monitoring and attention to respiratory and fluid status (see SPAG-2 manual).

Drug Interactions

Clinical studies of interactions of VIRAZOLE with other drugs commonly used to treat infants with RSV infections, such as digoxin, bronchodilators, other antiviral agents, antibiotics, or anti-metabolites have not been conducted. Interference by VIRAZOLE with laboratory tests has not been evaluated.

Carcinogenesis and Mutagenesis

Ribavirin increased the incidence of cell transformations and mutations in mouse Balb/c 3T3 (fibroblasts) and L5178Y (lymphoma) cells at concentrations of 0.015 and 0.03–5.0 mg/mL, respectively (without metabolic activation.) Modest increases in mutation rates (3–4x) were observed at concentrations between 3.75–10.0 mg/mL in L5178Y cells in vitro with the addition of a metabolic activation fraction. In the mouse micronucleus assay, ribavirin was clastogenic at intravenous doses of 20–200 mg/kg, (estimated human equivalent of 1.67–16.7 mg/kg, based on body surface area adjustment for a 60 kg adult). Ribavirin was not mutagenic in a dominant lethal assay in rats at intraperitoneal doses between 50–200 mg/kg when administered for 5 days (estimated human equivalent of 7.14–28.6 mg/kg, based on body surface area adjustment; see Pharmacokinetics).

In vivo carcinogenicity studies with ribavirin are incomplete. However, results of a chronic feeding study with ribavirin in rats, at doses of 16–100 mg/kg/day (estimated human equivalent of 2.3–14.3 mg/kg/day, based on body surface area adjustment for the adult), suggest that ribavirin may induce benign mammary, pancreatic, pituitary and drenal tumors. Preliminary results of 2 oral gavage onco-enicity studies in the mouse and rat (18–24 months; doses f 20–75 and 10–40 mg/kg/day, respectively [estimated human equivalent of 1.67–6.25 and 1.43–5.71 mg/kg/day, respectively, based on body surface area adjustment for the adult]) are inconclusive as to the carcinogenic potential of ribavirin (see Pharmacokinetics). However, these studies have demonstrated a relationship between chronic ribavirin xposure and increased incidences of vascular lesions (microscopic hemorrhages in mice) and retinal degeneration (in ats).

mpairment of Fertility

The fertility of ribavirin-treated animals (male or female) has not been fully investigated. However, in the mouse, administration of ribavirin at doses between 35–150 mg/kg/day (estimated human equivalent of 2.92–12.5 mg/kg/day, based on body surface area adjustment for the adult) resulted in significant seminiferous tubule atrophy, decreased sperm concentrations, and increased numbers of sperm with abnormal morphology. Partial recovery of sperm production was apparent 3–6 months following dose cessation. In several additional toxicology studies, ribavirin has been shown to cause testicular lesions (tubular atrophy), in adult rats at oral dose levels as low as 16 mg/kg/day (estimated human equivalent of 2.29 mg/kg/day, based on body surface area adjustment; see Pharmacokinetics). Lower doses were not tested. The reproductive capacity of treated male animals has not been studied.

Pregnancy: Category X

Ribavirin has demonstrated significant teratogenic and/or embryocidal potential in all animal species in which adequate studies have been conducted. Teratogenic effects were evident after single oral doses of 2.5 mg/kg or greater in the hamster, and after daily oral doses of 0.3 and 1.0 mg/kg in the rabbit and rat, respectively (estimated human equivalent doses of 0.12 and 0.14 mg/kg, based on body surface area adjustment for the adult). Malformations of the skull, palate, eye, jaw, limbs, skeleton, and gastrointestinal tract were noted. The incidence and severity of teratogenic effects increased with escalation of the drug dose. Survival of fetuses and offspring was reduced. Ribavirin caused embryolethality in the rabbit at daily oral dose levels as low as 1 mg/kg. No teratogenic effects were evident in the rabbit and rat administered daily oral doses of 0.1 and 0.3 mg/kg, respectively with estimated human equivalent doses of 0.01 and 0.04 mg/kg, based on body surface area adjustment (see Pharmacokinetics). These doses are considered to define the "No Observable Teratogenic Effects Level" (NOTEL) for ribavirin in the rabbit and rat.

Following oral administration of ribavirin in the pregnant rat (1.0 mg/kg) and rabbit (0.3 mg/kg), mean plasma levels of drug ranged from 0.10–0.20 µM [0.024–0.049 µg/mL] at 1 hour after dosing, to undetectable levels at 24 hours. At 1 hour following the administration of 0.3 or 0.1 mg/kg in the rat and rabbit (NOTEL), respectively, mean plasma levels of drug in both species were near or below the limit of detection (0.05 µM; see Pharmacokinetics).

Although clinical studies have not been performed, VIRAZOLE may cause fetal harm in humans. As noted previously, ribavirin is concentrated in red blood cells and persists for the life of the cell. Thus the terminal half-life for the systemic elimination of ribavirin is essentially that of the half-life of circulating erythrocytes. The minimum interval following exposure to VIRAZOLE before pregnancy may be safely initiated is unknown (see CONTRAINDICATIONS, WARNINGS, and Information for Health Care Personnel).

Nursing Mothers

VIRAZOLE has been shown to be toxic to lactating animals and their offspring. It is not known if VIRAZOLE is excreted in human milk.

Information for Health Care Personnel

Health care workers directly providing care to patients receiving aerosolized VIRAZOLE should be aware that ribavirin has been shown to be teratogenic in all animal species in which adequate studies have been conducted (rodents and rabbits). Although no reports of teratogenesis in offspring of mothers who were exposed to aerosolized VIRAZOLE during pregnancy have been confirmed, no controlled studies have been conducted in pregnant women. Studies of environmental exposure in treatment settings have shown that the drug can disperse into the immediate bedside area during routine patient care activities with highest ambient levels closest to the patient and extremely low levels outside of the immediate bedside area. Adverse reactions resulting from actual occupational exposure in adults are described below (see Adverse Events in Health Care Workers). Some studies have documented ambient drug concentrations at the bedside that could potentially lead to systemic exposures above those considered safe for exposure during pregnancy (1/1000 of the NOTEL dose in the most sensitive animal species).[7,8,9]

A 1992 study conducted by the National Institute of Occupational Safety and Health (NIOSH) demonstrated measurable urine levels of ribavirin in health care workers exposed to aerosol in the course of direct patient care.[7] Levels were lowest in workers caring for infants receiving aerosolized VIRAZOLE with mechanical ventilation and highest in those caring for patients being administered the drug via an oxygen tent or hood. This study employed a more sensitive assay to evaluate ribavirin levels in urine than was available for several previous studies of environmental exposure that failed to detect measurable ribavirin levels in exposed workers. Creatinine adjusted urine levels in the NIOSH study ranged from less than 0.001 to 0.140 µM of ribavirin per gram of creatinine in exposed workers. However, the relationship between urinary ribavirin levels in exposed workers, plasma levels in animal studies, and the specific risk of teratogenesis in exposed pregnant women is unknown.

It is good practice to avoid unnecessary occupational exposure to chemicals wherever possible. Hospitals are encouraged to conduct training programs to minimize potential occupational exposure to VIRAZOLE. Health care workers who are pregnant should consider avoiding direct care of patients receiving aerosolized VIRAZOLE. If close patient contact cannot be avoided, precautions to limit exposure should be taken. These include administration of VIRAZOLE in negative pressure rooms; adequate room ventilation (at least six air exchanges per hour); the use of VIRAZOLE aerosol scavenging devices; turning off the SPAG-2 device for 5 to 10 minutes prior to prolonged patient contact, and wearing appropriately fitted respirator masks. Surgical masks do not provide adequate filtration of VIRAZOLE particles. Further information is available from NIOSH's Hazard Evaluation and Technical Assistance Branch and additional recommendations have been published in an Aerosol Consensus Statement by the American Respiratory Care Foundation and the American Association for Respiratory Care.[10]

ADVERSE REACTIONS

The description of adverse reactions is based on events from clinical studies (approximately 200 patients) conducted prior to 1986, and the controlled trial of aerosolized VIRAZOLE conducted in 1989–1990. Additional data from spontaneous post-marketing reports of adverse events in individual patients have been available since 1986.

Deaths

Deaths during or shortly after treatment with aerosolized VIRAZOLE have been reported in 20 cases of patients treated with VIRAZOLE (12 of these patients were being treated for RSV infections). Several cases have been characterized as "possibly related" to VIRAZOLE by the treating physician; these were in infants who experienced worsening respiratory status related to bronchospasm while being treated with the drug. Several other cases have been attributed to mechanical ventilator malfunction in which VIRAZOLE precipitation within the ventilator apparatus led to excessively high pulmonary pressures and diminished oxygenation. In these cases the monitoring procedures described in the current package insert were not employed (see Description of Studies, WARNINGS, and DOSAGE AND ADMINISTRATION).

Pulmonary and Cardiovascular

Pulmonary function significantly deteriorated during aerosolized VIRAZOLE treatment in six of six adults with chronic obstructive lung disease and in four of six asthmatic adults. Dyspnea and chest soreness were also reported in the latter group. Minor abnormalities in pulmonary function were also seen in healthy adult volunteers.

In the original study population of approximately 200 infants who received aerosolized VIRAZOLE, several serious adverse events occurred in severely ill infants with life-threatening underlying diseases, many of whom required assisted ventilation. The role of VIRAZOLE in these events is indeterminate. Since the drug's approval in 1986, additional reports of similar serious, though non-fatal, events have been filed infrequently. Events associated with aerosolized VIRAZOLE use have included the following:

Pulmonary: Worsening of respiratory status, bronchospasm, pulmonary edema, hypoventilation, cyanosis, dyspnea, bacterial pneumonia, pneumothorax, apnea, atelectasis and ventilator dependence.

Cardiovascular: Cardiac arrest, hypotension, bradycardia and digitalis toxicity. Bigeminy, bradycardia and tachycardia have been described in patients with underlying congenital heart disease.

Some subjects requiring assisted ventilation experienced serious difficulties, due to inadequate ventilation and gas exchange. Precipitation of drug within the ventilatory apparatus, including the endotracheal tube, has resulted in increased positive end expiratory pressure and increased positive inspiratory pressure. Accumulation of fluid in tubing ("rain out") has also been noted. Measures to avoid these complications should be followed carefully (see DOSAGE AND ADMINISTRATION).

Hematologic

Although anemia was not reported with use of aerosolized VIRAZOLE in controlled clinical trials, most infants treated with the aerosol have not been evaluated 1 to 2 weeks post-treatment when anemia is likely to occur. Anemia has been shown to occur frequently with experimental oral and intravenous VIRAZOLE in humans. Also, cases of anemia (type unspecified), reticulocytosis and hemolytic anemia associated with aerosolized VIRAZOLE use have been reported through post-marketing reporting systems. All have been reversible with discontinuation of the drug.

Other

Rash and conjunctivitis have been associated with the use of aerosolized VIRAZOLE. These usually resolve within hours of discontinuing therapy. Seizures and asthenia associated with experimental intravenous VIRAZOLE therapy have also been reported.

Adverse Events in Health Care Workers

Studies of environmental exposure to aerosolized VIRAZOLE in health care workers administering care to patients receiving the drug have not detected adverse signs or symptoms related to exposure. However, 152 health care workers have reported experiencing adverse events through post-marketing surveillance. Nearly all were in individuals providing direct care to infants receiving aerosolized VIRAZOLE. Of 358 events from these 152 individual health care worker reports, the most common signs and symptoms were headache (51% of reports), conjunctivitis (32%), and rhinitis, nausea, rash, dizziness, pharyngitis, or lacrimation (10–20% each). Several cases of bronchospasm and/or chest pain were also reported, usually in individuals with known underlying reactive airway disease. Several case reports of damage to contact lenses after prolonged close exposure to aerosolized VIRAZOLE have also been reported. Most signs and symptoms reported as having occurred in exposed health care workers resolved within minutes to hours of discontinuing close exposure to aerosolized VIRAZOLE (also see Information for Health Care Personnel).

The symptoms of RSV in adults can include headache, conjunctivitis, sore throat and/or cough, fever, hoarseness, nasal congestion and wheezing, although RSV infections in adults are typically mild and transient. Such symptoms represent a potential hazard to uninfected hospital patients. It is unknown whether certain symptoms cited in reports from health care workers were due to exposure to the drug or infection with RSV. Hospitals should implement appropriate infection control procedures.

Overdosage

No overdosage with VIRAZOLE by aerosol administration has been reported in humans. The LD_{50} in mice is 2 g orally and is associated with hypoactivity and gastrointestinal symptoms (estimated human equivalent dose of 0.17 g/kg, based on body surface area conversion). The mean plasma half-life after administration of aerosolized VIRAZOLE for pediatric patients is 9.5 hours. VIRAZOLE is concentrated and persists in red blood cells for the life of the erythrocyte (see Pharmacokinetics).

DOSAGE AND ADMINISTRATION

BEFORE USE, READ THOROUGHLY THE ICN SMALL PARTICLE AEROSOL GENERATOR MODEL SPAG-2 OPERATOR'S MANUAL FOR SMALL PARTICLE AEROSOL GENERATOR OPERATING INSTRUCTIONS. AEROSOLIZED VIRAZOLE SHOULD NOT BE ADMINISTERED WITH ANY OTHER AEROSOL GENERATING DEVICE.

The recommended treatment regimen is 20 mg/mL VIRAZOLE as the starting solution in the drug reservoir of the SPAG-2 unit, with continuous aerosol administration for 12–18 hours per day for 3 to 7 days. Using the recommended drug concentration of 20 mg/mL the average aerosol concentration for a 12 hour delivery period would be 190 micrograms/liter of air. Aerosolized VIRAZOLE should not be administered in a mixture for combined aerosolization or simultaneously with other aerosolized medications.

Non-mechanically ventilated infants

VIRAZOLE should be delivered to an infant oxygen hood from the SPAG-2 aerosol generator. Administration by face mask or oxygen tent may be necessary if a hood cannot be employed (see SPAG-2 manual). However, the volume and condensation area are larger in a tent and this may alter delivery dynamics of the drug.

Mechanically ventilated infants

The recommended dose and administration schedule for infants who require mechanical ventilation is the same as for those who do not. Either a pressure or volume cycle ventilator may be used in conjunction with the SPAG-2. In either case, patients should have their endotracheal tubes suctioned every 1–2 hours, and their pulmonary pressures monitored frequently (every 2–4 hours). For both pressure and volume ventilators, heated wire connective tubing and bacteria filters in series in the expiratory limb of the system (which must be changed frequently, i.e., every 4 hours) must be used to minimize the risk of VIRAZOLE precipitation in the system and the subsequent risk of ventilator dysfunction. Water column pressure release valves should be used in the ventilator circuit for pressure cycled ventilators, and may be utilized with volume cycled ventilators (SEE SPAG-2 MANUAL FOR DETAILED INSTRUCTIONS).

Method of Preparation

VIRAZOLE brand of ribavirin is supplied as 6 grams of lyophilized powder per 100 mL vial for aerosol administration only. By sterile technique, reconstitute drug with a minimum of 75 mL of **sterile USP water for injection or inhalation** in the original 100 mL glass vial. Shake well. Transfer to the clean, sterilized 500 mL SPAG-2 reservoir and dilute to a final volume of 300 mL with Sterile Water for Injection, USP, or Inhalation. The final concentration should be 20 mg/mL. **Important:** This water should NOT have had any antimicrobial agent or other substance added. The solution should be inspected visually for particulate matter and discoloration prior to administration. Solutions that have been placed in the SPAG-2 unit should be discarded at least every 24 hours and when the liquid level is low before adding newly reconstituted solution.

HOW SUPPLIED

VIRAZOLE (Ribavirin for Inhalation Solution, USP) is supplied in four packs containing 100 mL glass vials with 6 grams of Sterile, lyophilized drug (NDC 0187-0007-14) which is to be reconstituted with 300 mL Sterile Water for Injection or Sterile Water for Inhalation (no preservatives added) and administered only by a small particle aerosol generator (SPAG-2). Vials containing the lyophilized drug powder should be stored in a dry place at 25°C (77°F); excursions permitted to 15°C–30°C (59°F–86°F). Reconstituted solutions may be stored, under sterile conditions, at room temperature (20–30°C, 68–86°F) for 24 hours. Solutions which have been placed in the SPAG-2 unit should be discarded at least every 24 hours.

REFERENCES

1. Hruska JF, Bernstein JM, Douglas Jr., RG, and Hall CB. Effects of Virazole on respiratory syncytial virus in vitro. Antimicrob Agents Chemother 17:770–775, 1 1980.
2. Hruska JF, Morrow PE, Suffin SC, and Douglas Jr., RG. In vivo inhibition of respiratory syncytial virus by Virazole. Antimicrob Agents Chemother 21:125–130, 1982.
3. Taber LH, Knight V, Gilbert BE, McClung HW et al. Virazole aerosol treatment of bronchiolitis associated with respiratory tract infection in infants. Pediatrics 72:613–618, 1983.
4. Hall CB, McBride JT, Walsh EE, Bell DM et al. Aerosolized Virazole treatment of infants with respiratory syncytial viral infection. N Engl J Med 308:1443–7, 1983.
5. Hendry RM, McIntosh K, Fahnestock ML, and Pierik LT. Enzyme-linked immunosorbent assay for detection of respiratory syncytial virus infection. J Clin Microbiol 16:329–33, 1982.
6. Smith, David W., Frankel, Lorry R., Mather, Larry H., Tang, Allen T.S., Ariagno, Ronald L., Prober, Charles G. A Controlled Trial of Aerosolized Ribavirin in Infants Receiving Mechanical Ventilation for Severe Respiratory Syncytial Virus Infection. The New England Journal of Medicine 1991; 325:24–29.
7. Decker, John, Shultz, Ruth A., Health Hazard Evaluation Report: Florida Hospital, Orlando, Florida, Cincinnati OH: U.S. Department of Health and Human Services, Public Health Service, Centers for NIOSH Report No. HETA 91-104-2229.*
8. Barnes, D.J. and Doursew, M. Reference dose: Description and use in health risk assessments. Regul Tox. and Pharm. Vol. 8; p. 471–486, 1988.
9. Federal Register Vol. 53 No. 126 Thurs. June 30, 1988 p. 24834–24847.
10. American Association for Respirtory Care [1991]. Aerosol Consensus Statement-1991. Respiratory Care 36(9):916–921.

*Copies of the Report may be purchased from National Technical Information Service, 5285 Port Royal Road, Springfield, VA 22161; Ask for Publication PB 93119-345.

1957-07 EL
Rev. 4-02
Manufactured for:
VALEANT PHARMACEUTICALS INTERNATIONAL
3300 Hyland Avenue
Costa Mesa, California 92626
714-545-0100

XELODA®   ℞
[zĕ-lō′də]
(capecitabine)
TABLETS
Rx only

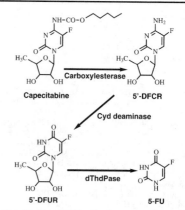

Capecitabine   5′-DFCR

Cyd deaminase

5′-DFUR   5-FU

WARNING

XELODA Warfarin Interaction: Patients receiving concomitant capecitabine and oral coumarin-derivative anticoagulant therapy should have their anticoagulant response (INR or prothrombin time) monitored frequently in order to adjust the anticoagulant dose accordingly. A clinically important XELODA-Warfarin drug interaction was demonstrated in a clinical pharmacology trial (see **CLINICAL PHARMACOLOGY** and **PRECAUTIONS**). Altered coagulation parameters and/or bleeding, including death, have been reported in patients taking XELODA concomitantly with coumarin-derivative anticoagulants such as warfarin and phenprocoumon. Postmarketing reports have shown clinically significant increases in prothrombin time (PT) and INR in patients who were stabilized on anticoagulants at the time XELODA was introduced. These events occurred within several days and up to several months after initiating XELODA therapy and, in a few cases, within 1 month after stopping XELODA. These events occurred in patients with and without liver metastases. Age greater than 60 and a diagnosis of cancer independently predispose patients to an increased risk of coagulopathy.

DESCRIPTION

XELODA (capecitabine) is a fluoropyrimidine carbamate with antineoplastic activity. It is an orally administered systemic prodrug of 5′-deoxy-5-fluorouridine (5′-DFUR) which is converted to 5-fluorouracil.

The chemical name for capecitabine is 5′-deoxy-5-fluoro-N-[(pentyloxy) carbonyl]-cytidine and has a molecular weight of 359.35.

Capecitabine is a white to off-white crystalline powder with an aqueous solubility of 26 mg/mL at 20°C.

XELODA is supplied as biconvex, oblong film-coated tablets for oral administration. Each light peach-colored tablet contains 150 mg capecitabine and each peach-colored tablet contains 500 mg capecitabine. The inactive ingredients in XELODA include: anhydrous lactose, croscarmellose sodium, hydroxypropyl methylcellulose, microcrystalline cellulose, magnesium stearate and purified water. The peach or light peach film coating contains hydroxypropyl methylcellulose, talc, titanium dioxide, and synthetic yellow and red iron oxides.

CLINICAL PHARMACOLOGY

XELODA is relatively non-cytotoxic in vitro. This drug is enzymatically converted to 5-fluorouracil (5-FU) in vivo.

Bioactivation

Capecitabine is readily absorbed from the gastrointestinal tract. In the liver, a 60 kDa carboxylesterase hydrolyzes much of the compound to 5′-deoxy-5-fluorocytidine (5′-DFCR). Cytidine deaminase, an enzyme found in most tissues, including tumors, subsequently converts 5′-DFCR to 5′-deoxy-5-fluorouridine (5′-DFUR). The enzyme, thymidine phosphorylase (dThdPase), then hydrolyzes 5′-DFUR to the active drug 5-FU. Many tissues throughout the body express thymidine phosphorylase. Some human carcinomas express this enzyme in higher concentrations than surrounding normal tissues.

Metabolic Pathway of capecitabine to 5-FU

[See chemical structure at top of next column]

Mechanism of Action

Both normal and tumor cells metabolize 5-FU to 5-fluoro-2′-deoxyuridine monophosphate (FdUMP) and 5-fluorouridine triphosphate (FUTP). These metabolites cause cell injury by two different mechanisms. First, FdUMP and the folate cofactor, N^{5-10}-methylenetetrahydrofolate, bind to thymidylate synthase (TS) to form a covalently bound ternary complex. This binding inhibits the formation of thymidylate from 2′-deoxyuridylate. Thymidylate is the necessary precursor of thymidine triphosphate, which is essential for the synthesis of DNA, so that a deficiency of this compound can inhibit cell division. Second, nuclear transcriptional enzymes can mistakenly incorporate FUTP in place of uridine triphosphate (UTP) during the synthesis of RNA. This metabolic error can interfere with RNA processing and protein synthesis.

Pharmacokinetics in Colorectal Tumors and Adjacent Healthy Tissue

Following oral administration of XELODA 7 days before surgery in patients with colorectal cancer, the median ratio of 5-FU concentration in colorectal tumors to adjacent tissues was 2.9 (range from 0.9 to 8.0). These ratios have not been evaluated in breast cancer patients or compared to 5-FU infusion.

Human Pharmacokinetics

The pharmacokinetics of XELODA and its metabolites have been evaluated in about 200 cancer patients over a dosage range of 500 to 3500 mg/m²/day. Over this range, the pharmacokinetics of XELODA and its metabolite, 5′-DFCR were dose proportional and did not change over time. The increases in the AUCs of 5′-DFUR and 5-FU, however, were greater than proportional to the increase in dose and the AUC of 5-FU was 34% higher on day 14 than on day 1. The elimination half-life of both parent capecitabine and 5-FU was about ¾ of an hour. The inter-patient variability in the C_{max} and AUC of 5-FU was greater than 85%.

Following oral administration of 825 mg/m² capecitabine twice daily for 14 days, Japanese patients (n=18) had about 36% lower C_{max} and 24% lower AUC for capecitabine than the Caucasian patients (n=22). Japanese patients had also about 25% lower C_{max} and 34% lower AUC for FBAL than the Caucasian patients. The clinical significance of these differences is unknown. No significant differences occurred in the exposure to other metabolites (5′-DFCR, 5′-DFUR, and 5-FU).

Absorption, Distribution, Metabolism and Excretion

Capecitabine reached peak blood levels in about 1.5 hours (T_{max}) with peak 5-FU levels occurring slightly later, at 2 hours. Food reduced both the rate and extent of absorption of capecitabine with mean C_{max} and $AUC_{0-\infty}$ decreased by 60% and 35%, respectively. The C_{max} and $AUC_{0-\infty}$ of 5-FU were also reduced by food by 43% and 21%, respectively. Food delayed T_{max} of both parent and 5-FU by 1.5 hours (see **PRECAUTIONS** and **DOSAGE AND ADMINISTRATION**).

Plasma protein binding of capecitabine and its metabolites is less than 60% and is not concentration-dependent. Capecitabine was primarily bound to human albumin (approximately 35%).

Capecitabine is extensively metabolized enzymatically to 5-FU. The enzyme dihydropyrimidine dehydrogenase hydrogenates 5-FU, the product of capecitabine metabolism, to the much less toxic 5-fluoro-5, 6-dihydro-fluorouracil (FUH_2). Dihydropyrimidinase cleaves the pyrimidine ring o yield 5-fluoro-ureido-propionic acid (FUPA). Finally, -ureido-propionase cleaves FUPA to α-fluoro-β-alanine (FBAL) which is cleared in the urine.

Capecitabine and its metabolites are predominantly excreted in urine; 95.5% of administered capecitabine dose is recovered in urine. Fecal excretion is minimal (2.6%). The major metabolite excreted in urine is FBAL which represents 57% of the administered dose. About 3% of the administered dose is excreted in urine as unchanged drug.

A clinical phase 1 study evaluating the effect of XELODA on the pharmacokinetics of docetaxel (Taxotere®) and the effect of docetaxel on the pharmacokinetics of XELODA was conducted in 26 patients with solid tumors. XELODA was found to have no effect on the pharmacokinetics of docetaxel (C_{max} and AUC) and docetaxel has no effect on the pharmacokinetics of capecitabine and the 5-FU precursor 5'-DFUR.

Special Populations

A population analysis of pooled data from the two large controlled studies in patients with metastatic colorectal cancer (n=505) who were administered XELODA at 1250 mg/m^2 twice a day indicated that gender (202 females and 303 males) and race (455 white/Caucasian patients, 22 black patients, and 28 patients of other race) have no influence on the pharmacokinetics of 5'-DFUR, 5-FU and FBAL. Age has no significant influence on the pharmacokinetics of 5'-DFUR and 5-FU over the range of 27 to 86 years. A 20% increase in age results in a 15% increase in AUC of FBAL (see **WARNINGS** and **DOSAGE AND ADMINISTRATION**).

Hepatic Insufficiency

XELODA has been evaluated in 13 patients with mild to moderate hepatic dysfunction due to liver metastases defined by a composite score including bilirubin, AST/ALT and alkaline phosphatase following a single 1255 mg/m^2 dose of XELODA. Both $AUC_{0-\infty}$ and C_{max} of capecitabine increased by 60% in patients with hepatic dysfunction compared to patients with normal hepatic function (n=14). The $AUC_{0-\infty}$ and C_{max} of 5-FU were not affected. In patients with mild to moderate hepatic dysfunction due to liver metastases, caution should be exercised when XELODA is administered. The effect of severe hepatic dysfunction on XELODA is not known (see **PRECAUTIONS** and **DOSAGE AND ADMINISTRATION**).

Renal Insufficiency

Following oral administration of 1250 mg/m^2 capecitabine twice a day to cancer patients with varying degrees of renal impairment, patients with moderate (creatinine clearance = 30 to 50 mL/min) and severe (creatinine clearance <30 mL/min) renal impairment showed 85% and 258% higher systemic exposure to FBAL on day 1 compared to normal renal function patients (creatinine clearance >80 mL/min). Systemic exposure to 5'-DFUR was 42% and 71% greater in moderately and severely renal impaired patients, respectively, than in normal patients. Systemic exposure to capecitabine was about 25% greater in both moderately and severely renal impaired patients (see **CONTRAINDICATIONS**, **WARNINGS**, and **DOSAGE AND ADMINISTRATION**).

Drug-Drug Interactions

Anticoagulants

In four patients with cancer, chronic administration of capecitabine (1250 mg/m^2 bid) with a single 20 mg dose of warfarin increased the mean AUC of S-warfarin by 57% and decreased its clearance by 37%. Baseline corrected AUC of INR in these 4 patients increased by 2.8-fold, and the maximum observed mean INR value was increased by 91% (see **Boxed WARNING** and **PRECAUTIONS: Drug-Drug Interactions**).

Drugs Metabolized by Cytochrome P450 Enzymes

In vitro enzymatic studies with human liver microsomes indicated that capecitabine and its metabolites (5'-DFUR, 5'-DFCR, 5-FU, and FBAL) had no inhibitory effects on substrates of cytochrome P450 for the major isoenzymes such as 1A2, 2A6, 3A4, 2C9, 2C19, 2D6, and 2E1.

Antacid

When Maalox® (20 mL), an aluminum hydroxide- and magnesium hydroxide-containing antacid, was administered immediately after XELODA (1250 mg/m^2, n=12 cancer pa-

tients), AUC and C_{max} increased by 16% and 35%, respectively, for capecitabine and by 18% and 22%, respectively, for 5'-DFCR. No effect was observed on the other three major metabolites (5'-DFUR, 5-FU, FBAL) of XELODA.

XELODA has a low potential for pharmacokinetic interactions related to plasma protein binding.

CLINICAL STUDIES

General

The recommended dose of XELODA was determined in an open-label, randomized clinical study, exploring the efficacy and safety of continuous therapy with capecitabine (1331 mg/m^2/day in two divided doses, n=39), intermittent therapy with capecitabine (2510 mg/m^2/day in two divided doses, n=34), and intermittent therapy with capecitabine in combination with oral leucovorin (LV) (capecitabine 1657 mg/m^2/day in two divided doses, n=35; leucovorin 60 mg/day) in patients with advanced and/or metastatic colorectal carcinoma in the first-line metastatic setting. There was no apparent advantage in response rate to adding leucovorin to XELODA; however, toxicity was increased. XELODA, 1250 mg/m^2 twice daily for 14 days followed by a 1-week rest, was selected for further clinical development based on the overall safety and efficacy profile of the three schedules studied.

Adjuvant Colon Cancer

A multicenter randomized, controlled phase 3 clinical trial in patients with Dukes' C colon cancer provided data concerning the use of XELODA for the adjuvant treatment of patients with colon cancer. The primary objective of the study was to compare disease-free survival (DFS) in patients receiving XELODA to those receiving IV 5-FU/LV alone. In this trial, 1987 patients were randomized either to treatment with XELODA 1250 mg/m^2 orally twice daily for 2 weeks followed by a 1-week rest period, given as 3-week cycles for a total of 8 cycles (24 weeks) or IV bolus 5-FU 425 mg/m^2 and 20 mg/m^2 IV leucovorin on days 1 to 5, given as 4-week cycles for a total of 6 cycles (24 weeks). Patients in the study were required to be between 18 and 75 years of age with histologically-confirmed Dukes' stage C colon cancer with at least one positive lymph node and to have undergone (within 8 weeks prior to randomization) complete resection of the primary tumor without macroscopic or microscopic evidence of remaining tumor. Patients were also required to have no prior cytotoxic chemotherapy or immunotherapy (except steroids), and have an ECOG performance status of 0 or 1 (KPS ≥70%), ANC ≥1.5x10^9/L, platelets ≥100x10^9/L, serum creatinine ≤1.5 ULN, total bilirubin ≤1.5 ULN, AST/ALT ≤2.5 ULN and CEA within normal limits at time of randomization.

The baseline demographics for XELODA and 5-FU/LV patients are shown in **Table 1**. The baseline characteristics were well-balanced between arms.

Table 1   Baseline Demographics

	XELODA (n=1004)	5-FU/LV (n=983)
Age (median, years)	62	63
Range	(25-80)	(22-82)
Gender		
Male (n, %)	542 (54)	532 (54)
Female (n, %)	461 (46)	451 (46)
ECOG PS		
0 (n, %)	849 (85)	830 (85)
1 (n, %)	152 (15)	147 (15)
Staging – Primary Tumor		
PT1 (n, %)	12 (1)	6 (0.6)
PT2 (n, %)	90 (9)	92 (9)
PT3 (n, %)	763 (76)	746 (76)
PT4 (n, %)	138 (14)	139 (14)
Other (n, %)	1 (0.1)	0 (0)

Staging – Lymph Node		
pN1 (n, %)	695 (69)	694 (71)
pN2 (n, %)	305 (30)	288 (29)
Other (n, %)	4 (0.4)	1 (0.1)

All patients with normal renal function or mild renal impairment began treatment at the full starting dose of 1250 mg/m^2 orally twice daily. The starting dose was reduced in patients with moderate renal impairment (calculated creatinine clearance 30 to 50 mL/min) at baseline (see **DOSAGE AND ADMINISTRATION**). Subsequently, for all patients, doses were adjusted when needed according to toxicity. Dose management for XELODA included dose reductions, cycle delays and treatment interruptions (see Table 2).

Table 2   **Summary of Dose Modifications in X-ACT Study**

	XELODA N = 995	5-FU/LV N = 974
Median relative dose intensity (%)	93	92
Patients completing full course of treatment (%)	83	87
Patients with treatment interruption (%)	15	5
Patients with cycle delay (%)	46	29
Patients with dose reduction (%)	42	44
Patients with treatment interruption, cycle delay, or dose reduction (%)	57	52

The median follow-up at the time of the analysis was 53 months. The hazard ratio for DFS for XELODA compared to 5-FU/LV was 0.87 (95% C.I. 0.76–1.00). Because the upper 2-sided 95% confidence limit of hazard ratio was less than 1.20, XELODA was non-inferior to 5-FU/LV. The choice of the non-inferiority margin of 1.20 corresponds to the retention of approximately 75% of the 5-FU/LV effect on DFS. Survival data were not mature at the time of the analysis with a median follow-up of 53 months. The comparison of overall survival did not reach statistical significance for the test of difference (HR 0.88, 95% C.I. 0.74–1.05; p = 0.169).

Table 3   **Efficacy of XELODA vs 5-FU/LV in Adjuvant Treatment of Colon Cancer[a]**

All Randomized Population	XELODA (n=1004)	5-FU/LV (n=983)
Median follow-up (months)	53	53
3-year Disease-free Survival Rates	66.0	62.9
Hazard Ratio (XELODA/5-FU/LV) (95% C.I. for Hazard Ratio), p-value[b]	0.87 (0.76–1.00) p = 0.055	

[a] Approximately 85% had 3-year DFS information
[b] Log-rank test for differences of XELODA vs 5-FU/LV

Figure 1   **Kaplan-Meier Estimates of Disease-Free Survival (All Randomized Population)[a]**

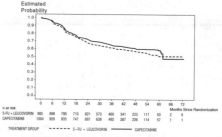

[a]XELODA has been demonstrated to be non-inferior to 5-FU/LV.

Metastatic Colorectal Cancer

Data from two open-label, multicenter, randomized, controlled clinical trials involving 1207 patients support the use of XELODA in the first-line treatment of patients with metastatic colorectal carcinoma. The two clinical studies were identical in design and were conducted in 120 centers in different countries. Study 1 was conducted in the US, Canada, Mexico, and Brazil; Study 2 was conducted in Europe, Israel, Australia, New Zealand, and Taiwan. Altogether, in both trials, 603 patients were randomized to treatment with XELODA at a dose of 1250 mg/m^2 twice daily for 2 weeks followed by a 1-week rest period and given as 3-week cycles; 604 patients were randomized to treat-

Table 4   **Baseline Demographics of Controlled Colorectal Trials**

	Study 1		Study 2	
	XELODA (n=302)	5-FU/LV (n=303)	XELODA (n=301)	5-FU/LV (n=301)
Age (median, years) Range	64 (23-86)	63 (24-87)	64 (29-84)	64 (36-86)
Gender Male (%) Female (%)	181 (60) 121 (40)	197 (65) 106 (35)	172 (57) 129 (43)	173 (57) 128 (43)
Karnofsky PS (median) Range	90 (70-100)	90 (70-100)	90 (70-100)	90 (70-100)
Colon (%) Rectum (%)	222 (74) 79 (26)	232 (77) 70 (23)	199 (66) 101 (34)	196 (65) 105 (35)
Prior radiation therapy (%)	52 (17)	62 (21)	42 (14)	42 (14)
Prior adjuvant 5-FU (%)	84 (28)	110 (36)	56 (19)	41 (14)

Table 5 Efficacy of XELODA vs 5-FU/LV in Colorectal Cancer (Study 1)

	XELODA (n=302)	5-FU/LV (n=303)
Overall Response Rate (%, 95% C.I.)	21 (16-26)	11 (8-15)
(*p*-value)	0.0014	
Time to Progression (Median, days, 95% C.I.)	128 (120-136)	131 (105-153)
Hazard Ratio (XELODA/5-FU/LV) 95% C.I. for Hazard Ratio	0.99 (0.84-1.17)	
Survival (Median, days, 95% C.I.)	380 (321-434)	407 (366-446)
Hazard Ratio (XELODA/5-FU/LV) 95% C.I. for Hazard Ratio	1.00 (0.84-1.18)	

Table 6 Efficacy of XELODA vs 5-FU/LV in Colorectal Cancer (Study 2)

	XELODA (n=301)	5-FU/LV (n=301)
Overall Response Rate (%, 95% C.I.)	21 (16-26)	14 (10-18)
(*p*-value)	0.027	
Time to Progression (Median, days, 95% C.I.)	137 (128-165)	131 (102-156)
Hazard Ratio (XELODA/5-FU/LV) 95% C.I. for Hazard Ratio	0.97 (0.82-1.14)	
Survival (Median, days, 95% C.I.)	404 (367-452)	369 (338-430)
Hazard Ratio (XELODA/5-FU/LV) 95% C.I. for Hazard Ratio	0.92 (0.78-1.09)	

ment with 5-FU and leucovorin (20 mg/m² leucovorin IV followed by 425 mg/m² IV bolus 5-FU, on days 1 to 5, every 28 days).

In both trials, overall survival, time to progression and response rate (complete plus partial responses) were assessed. Responses were defined by the World Health Organization criteria and submitted to a blinded independent review committee (IRC). Differences in assessments between the investigator and IRC were reconciled by the sponsor, blinded to treatment arm, according to a specified algorithm. Survival was assessed based on a non-inferiority analysis.

The baseline demographics for XELODA and 5-FU/LV patients are shown in **Table 4**.
[See table 4 at bottom of previous page]
The efficacy endpoints for the two phase 3 trials are shown in **Table 5** and **Table 6**.
[See table 5 above]
[See table 6 above]
[See figure 2 at right]
XELODA was superior to 5-FU/LV for objective response rate in Study 1 and Study 2. The similarity of XELODA and 5-FU/LV in these studies was assessed by examining the potential difference between the two treatments. In order to assure that XELODA has a clinically meaningful survival effect, statistical analyses were performed to determine the percent of the survival effect of 5-FU/LV that was retained by XELODA. The estimate of the survival effect of 5-FU/LV was derived from a meta-analysis of ten randomized studies from the published literature comparing 5-FU to regimens of 5-FU/LV that were similar to the control arms used in these Studies 1 and 2. The method for comparing the treatments was to examine the worst case (95% confidence upper bound) for the difference between 5-FU/LV and XELODA, and to show that loss of more than 50% of the 5-FU/LV sur-

Figure 2 Kaplan-Meier Curve for Overall Survival of Pooled Data (Studies 1 and 2)

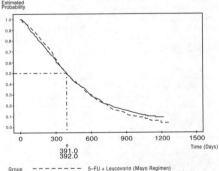

vival effect was ruled out. It was demonstrated that the percent of the survival effect of 5-FU/LV maintained was at least 61% for Study 2 and 10% for Study 1. The pooled result is consistent with a retention of at least 50% of the effect of 5-FU/LV. It should be noted that these values for preserved effect are based on the upper bound of the 5-FU/LV vs XELODA difference. These results do not exclude the possibility of true equivalence of XELODA to 5-FU/LV (see **Table 5, Table 6,** and **Figure 2**).

Breast Cancer
XELODA has been evaluated in clinical trials in combination with docetaxel (Taxotere®) and as monotherapy.

Table 7 Baseline Demographics and Clinical Characteristics XELODA and Docetaxel Combination vs Docetaxel in Breast Cancer Trial

	XELODA + Docetaxel (n=255)	Docetaxel (n=256)
Age (median, years)	52	51
Karnofsky PS (median)	90	90
Site of Disease		
Lymph nodes	121 (47%)	125 (49%)
Liver	116 (45%)	122 (48%)
Bone	107 (42%)	119 (46%)
Lung	95 (37%)	99 (39%)
Skin	73 (29%)	73 (29%)
Prior Chemotherapy		
Anthracycline[1]	255 (100%)	256 (100%)
5-FU	196 (77%)	189 (74%)
Paclitaxel	25 (10%)	22 (9%)
Resistance to an Anthracycline		
No resistance	19 (7%)	19 (7%)
Progression on anthracycline therapy	65 (26%)	73 (29%)
Stable disease after 4 cycles of anthracycline therapy	41 (16%)	40 (16%)
Relapsed within 2 years of completion of anthracycline-adjuvant therapy	78 (31%)	74 (29%)
Experienced a brief response to anthracycline therapy, with subsequent progression while on therapy or within 12 months after last dose	51 (20%)	50 (20%)
No. of Prior Chemotherapy Regimens for Treatment of Metastatic Disease		
0	89 (35%)	80 (31%)
1	123 (48%)	135 (53%)
2	43 (17%)	39 (15%)
3	0 (0%)	2 (1%)

[1]Includes 10 patients in combination and 18 patients in monotherapy arms treated with an anthracenedione

Table 8 Efficacy of XELODA and Docetaxel Combination vs Docetaxel Monotherapy

Efficacy Parameter	Combination Therapy	Monotherapy	p-value	Hazard Ratio
Time to Disease Progression				
Median Days	186	128	0.0001	0.643
95% C.I.	(165-198)	(105-136)		
Overall Survival				
Median Days	442	352	0.0126	0.775
95% C.I.	(375-497)	(298-387)		
Response Rate[1]	32%	22%	0.009	NA[2]

[1] The response rate reported represents a reconciliation of the investigator and IRC assessments performed by the sponsor according to a predefined algorithm.
[2] NA = Not Applicable

Breast Cancer Combination Therapy

The dose of XELODA used in the phase 3 clinical trial in combination with docetaxel was based on the results of a phase 1 study, where a range of doses of docetaxel administered in 3-week cycles in combination with an intermittent regimen of XELODA (14 days of treatment, followed by a 7-day rest period) were evaluated. The combination dose regimen was selected based on the tolerability profile of the 75 mg/m^2 administered in 3-week cycles of docetaxel in combination with 1250 mg/m^2 twice daily for 14 days of XELODA administered in 3-week cycles. The approved dose of 100 mg/m^2 of docetaxel administered in 3-week cycles was the control arm of the phase 3 study.

XELODA in combination with docetaxel was assessed in an open-label, multicenter, randomized trial in 75 centers in Europe, North America, South America, Asia, and Austra-

lia. A total of 511 patients with metastatic breast cancer resistant to, or recurring during or after an anthracycline-containing therapy, or relapsing during or recurring within 2 years of completing an anthracycline-containing adjuvant therapy were enrolled. Two hundred and fifty-five (255) patients were randomized to receive XELODA 1250 mg/m^2 twice daily for 14 days followed by 1 week without treatment and docetaxel 75 mg/m^2 as a 1-hour intravenous infusion administered in 3-week cycles. In the monotherapy arm, 256 patients received docetaxel 100 mg/m^2 as a 1-hour intravenous infusion administered in 3-week cycles. Patient demographics are provided in **Table 7**.

[See table 7 above]

XELODA in combination with docetaxel resulted in statistically significant improvement in time to disease progres-

Table 9   Baseline Demographics and Clinical Characteristics Single-Arm Breast Cancer Trial

	Patients With Measurable Disease (n=135)	All Patients (n=162)
Age (median, years)	55	56
Karnofsky PS	90	90
No. Disease Sites		
1-2	43 (32%)	60 (37%)
3-4	63 (46%)	69 (43%)
>5	29 (22%)	34 (21%)
Dominant Site of Disease		
Visceral[1]	101 (75%)	110 (68%)
Soft Tissue	30 (22%)	35 (22%)
Bone	4 (3%)	17 (10%)
Prior Chemotherapy		
Paclitaxel	135 (100%)	162 (100%)
Anthracycline[2]	122 (90%)	147 (91%)
5-FU	110 (81%)	133 (82%)
Resistance to Paclitaxel	103 (76%)	124 (77%)
Resistance to an Anthracycline[2]	55 (41%)	67 (41%)
Resistance to both Paclitaxel and an Anthracycline[2]	43 (32%)	51 (31%)

[1] Lung, pleura, liver, peritoneum
[2] Includes 2 patients treated with an anthracenedione

---

tion, overall survival and objective response rate compared to monotherapy with docetaxel as shown in **Table 8, Figure 3**, and **Figure 4**.
[See table 8 at top of previous page]

Breast Cancer Monotherapy

Figure 3   Kaplan-Meier Estimates for Time to Disease Progression XELODA and Docetaxel vs Docetaxel

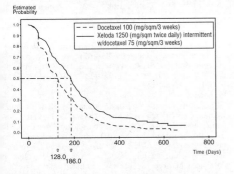

Figure 4   Kaplan-Meier Estimates of Survival XELODA and Docetaxel vs Docetaxel

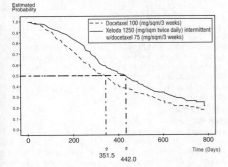

The antitumor activity of XELODA as a monotherapy was evaluated in an open-label single-arm trial conducted in 24 centers in the US and Canada. A total of 162 patients with stage IV breast cancer were enrolled. The primary endpoint was tumor response rate in patients with measurable disease, with response defined as a ≥50% decrease in sum of the products of the perpendicular diameters of bidimensionally measurable disease for at least 1 month. XELODA was administered at a dose of 1255 mg/m^2 twice daily for 2 weeks followed by a 1-week rest period and given as 3-week cycles. The baseline demographics and clinical characteristics for all patients (n=162) and those with measurable disease (n=135) are shown in **Table 9**. Resistance was defined as progressive disease while on treatment, with or without an initial response, or relapse within 6 months of completing treatment with an anthracycline-containing adjuvant chemotherapy regimen.
[See table 9 above]
Antitumor responses for patients with disease resistant to both paclitaxel and an anthracycline are shown in **Table 10**.

Table 10   Response Rates in Doubly-Resistant Patients Single-Arm Breast Cancer Trial

	Resistance to Both Paclitaxel and an Anthracycline (n=43)
CR	0
PR[1]	11
CR + PR[1]	11
Response Rate[1] (95% C.I.)	25.6% (13.5, 41.2)
Duration of Response,[1] Median in days[2] (Range)	154 (63-233)

[1] Includes 2 patients treated with an anthracenedione
[2] From date of first response

For the subgroup of 43 patients who were doubly resistant, the median time to progression was 102 days and the median survival was 255 days. The objective response rate in this population was supported by a response rate of 18.5% (1 CR, 24 PRs) in the overall population of 135 patients with measurable disease, who were less resistant to chemotherapy (see **Table 9**). The median time to progression was 90 days and the median survival was 306 days.

INDICATIONS AND USAGE

Colorectal Cancer

- XELODA is indicated as a single agent for adjuvant treatment in patients with Dukes' C colon cancer who have undergone complete resection of the primary tumor when treatment with fluoropyrimidine therapy alone is preferred. XELODA was non-inferior to 5-fluorouracil and leucovorin (5-FU/LV) for disease-free survival (DFS). Although neither XELODA nor combination chemotherapy prolongs overall survival (OS), combination chemotherapy has been demonstrated to improve disease-free survival compared to 5-FU/LV. Physicians should consider these results when prescribing single-agent XELODA in the adjuvant treatment of Dukes' C colon cancer.
- XELODA is indicated as first-line treatment of patients with metastatic colorectal carcinoma when treatment with fluoropyrimidine therapy alone is preferred. Combination chemotherapy has shown a survival benefit compared to 5-FU/LV alone. A survival benefit over 5-FU/LV has not been demonstrated with XELODA monotherapy. Use of XELODA instead of 5-FU/LV in combinations has not been adequately studied to assure safety or preservation of the survival advantage.

Breast Cancer

- XELODA in combination with docetaxel is indicated for the treatment of patients with metastatic breast cancer after failure of prior anthracycline-containing chemotherapy.
- XELODA monotherapy is also indicated for the treatment of patients with metastatic breast cancer resistant to both paclitaxel and an anthracycline-containing chemotherapy regimen or resistant to paclitaxel and for whom further anthracycline therapy is not indicated, eg, patients who have received cumulative doses of 400 mg/m^2 of doxorubicin or doxorubicin equivalents. Resistance is defined as progressive disease while on treatment, with or without an initial response, or relapse within 6 months of completing treatment with an anthracycline-containing adjuvant regimen.

CONTRAINDICATIONS

XELODA is contraindicated in patients with known hypersensitivity to capecitabine or to any of its components. XELODA is contraindicated in patients who have a known hypersensitivity to 5-fluorouracil. XELODA is contraindicated in patients with known dihydropyrimidine dehydrogenase (DPD) deficiency. XELODA is also contraindicated in patients with severe renal impairment (creatinine clearance below 30 mL/min [Cockroft and Gault]) (see **CLINICAL PHARMACOLOGY: Special Populations**).

WARNINGS

Renal Insufficiency

Patients with moderate renal impairment at baseline require dose reduction (see **DOSAGE AND ADMINISTRATION**). Patients with mild and moderate renal impairment at baseline should be carefully monitored for adverse events. Prompt interruption of therapy with subsequent dose adjustments is recommended if a patient develops a grade 2 to 4 adverse event as outlined in **Table 18** in **DOSAGE AND ADMINISTRATION**.

Coagulopathy

See **Boxed WARNING**.

Diarrhea

XELODA can induce diarrhea, sometimes severe. Patients with severe diarrhea should be carefully monitored and given fluid and electrolyte replacement if they become dehydrated. In 875 patients with either metastatic breast or colorectal cancer who received XELODA monotherapy, the median time to first occurrence of grade 2 to 4 diarrhea was 34 days (range from 1 to 369 days). The median duration of grade 3 to 4 diarrhea was 5 days. National Cancer Institute of Canada (NCIC) grade 2 diarrhea is defined as an increase

of 4 to 6 stools/day or nocturnal stools, grade 3 diarrhea as an increase of 7 to 9 stools/day or incontinence and malabsorption, and grade 4 diarrhea as an increase of ≥10 stools/day or grossly bloody diarrhea or the need for parenteral support. If grade 2, 3 or 4 diarrhea occurs, administration of XELODA should be immediately interrupted until the diarrhea resolves or decreases in intensity to grade 1. Following a reoccurrence of grade 2 diarrhea or occurrence of any grade 3 or 4 diarrhea, subsequent doses of XELODA should be decreased (see **DOSAGE AND ADMINISTRATION**). Standard antidiarrheal treatments (eg, loperamide) are recommended.

Necrotizing enterocolitis (typhlitis) has been reported.

Geriatric Patients

Patients ≥80 years old may experience a greater incidence of grade 3 or 4 adverse events (see **PRECAUTIONS: Geriatric Use**). In 875 patients with either metastatic breast or colorectal cancer who received XELODA monotherapy, 62% of the 21 patients ≥80 years of age treated with XELODA experienced a treatment-related grade 3 or 4 adverse event: diarrhea in 6 (28.6%), nausea in 3 (14.3%), hand-and-foot syndrome in 3 (14.3%), and vomiting in 2 (9.5%) patients. Among the 10 patients 70 years of age and greater (no patients were >80 years of age) treated with XELODA in combination with docetaxel, 30% (3 out of 10) of patients experienced grade 3 or 4 diarrhea and stomatitis, and 40% (4 out of 10) experienced grade 3 hand-and-foot syndrome.

Among the 67 patients ≥60 years of age receiving XELODA in combination with docetaxel, the incidence of grade 3 or 4 treatment-related adverse events, treatment-related serious adverse events, withdrawals due to adverse events, treatment discontinuations due to adverse events and treatment discontinuations within the first two treatment cycles was higher than in the <60 years of age patient group.

In 995 patients receiving XELODA as adjuvant therapy for Dukes' C colon cancer after resection of the primary tumor, 41% of the 398 patients ≥65 years of age treated with XELODA experienced a treatment-related grade 3 or 4 adverse event: hand-and-foot syndrome in 75 (18.8%), diarrhea in 52 (13.1%), stomatitis in 12 (3.0%), neutropenia/granulocytopenia in 11 (2.8%), vomiting in 6 (1.5%), and nausea in 5 (1.3%) patients. In patients ≥65 years of age (all randomized population; capecitabine 188 patients, 5-FU/LV 208 patients) treated for Dukes' C colon cancer after resection of the primary tumor, the hazard ratios for disease-free survival and overall survival for XELODA compared to 5-FU/LV were 1.01 (95% C.I. 0.80–1.27) and 1.04 (95% C.I. 0.79–1.37), respectively.

Pregnancy

XELODA may cause fetal harm when given to a pregnant woman. Capecitabine at doses of 198 mg/kg/day during organogenesis caused malformations and embryo death in mice. In separate pharmacokinetic studies, this dose in mice produced 5′-DFUR AUC values about 0.2 times the corresponding values in patients administered the recommended daily dose. Malformations in mice included cleft palate, anophthalmia, microphthalmia, oligodactyly, polydactyly, syndactyly, kinky tail and dilation of cerebral ventricles. At doses of 90 mg/kg/day, capecitabine given to pregnant monkeys during organogenesis caused fetal death. This dose produced 5′-DFUR AUC values about 0.6 times the corresponding values in patients administered the recommended daily dose. There are no adequate and well-controlled studies in pregnant women using XELODA. If the drug is used during pregnancy, or if the patient becomes pregnant while receiving this drug, the patient should be apprised of the potential hazard to the fetus. Women of childbearing potential should be advised to avoid becoming pregnant while receiving treatment with XELODA.

PRECAUTIONS

General

Patients receiving therapy with XELODA should be monitored by a physician experienced in the use of cancer chemotherapeutic agents. Most adverse events are reversible and do not need to result in discontinuation, although doses may need to be withheld or reduced (see **DOSAGE AND ADMINISTRATION**).

ombination With Other Drugs

se of XELODA in combination with irinotecan has not
en adequately studied.

and-and-Foot Syndrome

and-and-foot syndrome (palmar-plantar erythrodysesthe-
a or chemotherapy-induced acral erythema) is a cutaneous
xicity. Median time to onset was 79 days (range from 11 to
0 days) with a severity range of grades 1 to 3 for patients
ceiving XELODA monotherapy in the metastatic setting.
rade 1 is characterized by any of the following: numbness,
ysesthesia/paresthesia, tingling, painless swelling or ery-
ema of the hands and/or feet and/or discomfort which does
ot disrupt normal activities. Grade 2 hand-and-foot syn-
ome is defined as painful erythema and swelling of the
ands and/or feet and/or discomfort affecting the patient's
ctivities of daily living. Grade 3 hand-and-foot syndrome is
efined as moist desquamation, ulceration, blistering or se-
ere pain of the hands and/or feet and/or severe discomfort
at causes the patient to be unable to work or perform ac-
vities of daily living. If grade 2 or 3 hand-and-foot syn-
ome occurs, administration of XELODA should be inter-
apted until the event resolves or decreases in intensity to
rade 1. Following grade 3 hand-and-foot syndrome, subse-
uent doses of XELODA should be decreased (see **DOSAGE
ND ADMINISTRATION**).

ardiotoxicity

he cardiotoxicity observed with XELODA includes myocar-
ial infarction/ischemia, angina, dysrhythmias, cardiac ar-
est, cardiac failure, sudden death, electrocardiographic
hanges, and cardiomyopathy. These adverse events may be
ore common in patients with a prior history of coronary
rtery disease.

Dihydropyrimidine Dehydrogenase Deficiency

Rarely, unexpected, severe toxicity (eg, stomatitis, diarrhea,
eutropenia and neurotoxicity) associated with 5-fluoroura-
il has been attributed to a deficiency of dihydropyrimidine
ehydrogenase (DPD) activity. A link between decreased
evels of DPD and increased, potentially fatal toxic effects of
-fluorouracil therefore cannot be excluded.

Hepatic Insufficiency

Patients with mild to moderate hepatic dysfunction due to
iver metastases should be carefully monitored when
XELODA is administered. The effect of severe hepatic dys-
unction on the disposition of XELODA is not known (see
CLINICAL PHARMACOLOGY and DOSAGE AND
ADMINISTRATION).

Hyperbilirubinemia

In 875 patients with either metastatic breast or colorectal
ancer who received at least one dose of XELODA
1250 mg/m^2 twice daily as monotherapy for 2 weeks fol-
owed by a 1-week rest period, grade 3 (1.5-3 × ULN) hyperbilirubinemia occurred in 15.2% (n=133) of patients and
grade 4 (>3 × ULN) hyperbilirubinemia occurred in 3.9%
n=34) of patients. Of 566 patients who had prebase-
line at baseline and 309 patients without hepatic metastases at baseline, grade 3 or 4 hyperbilirubinemia occurred in
22.8% and 12.3%, respectively. Of the 167 patients with
grade 3 or 4 hyperbilirubinemia, 18.6% (n=31) also had
postbaseline elevations (grades 1 to 4, without elevations at
baseline) in alkaline phosphatase and 27.5% (n=46) had
postbaseline elevations in transaminases at any time (not
necessarily concurrent). The majority of these patients,
64.5% (n=20) and 71.7% (n=33), had liver metastases at
baseline. In addition, 57.5% (n=96) and 35.3% (n=59) of the
167 patients had elevations (grades 1 to 4) at both prebase-
line and postbaseline in alkaline phosphatase or transaminases, respectively. Only 7.8% (n=13) and 3.0% (n=5)
had grade 3 or 4 elevations in alkaline phosphatase or
transaminases.

In the 596 patients treated with XELODA as first-line therapy for metastatic colorectal cancer, the incidence of grade 3
or 4 hyperbilirubinemia was similar to the overall clinical
trial safety database of XELODA monotherapy. The median
time to onset for grade 3 or 4 hyperbilirubinemia in the colorectal cancer population was 64 days and median total bilirubin increased from 8 μm/L at baseline to 13 μm/L during
treatment with XELODA. Of the 136 colorectal cancer pa-

tients with grade 3 or 4 hyperbilirubinemia, 49 patients had
grade 3 or 4 hyperbilirubinemia as their last measured
value, of which 46 had liver metastases at baseline.

In 251 patients with metastatic breast cancer who received
a combination of XELODA and docetaxel, grade 3 (1.5 to 3 ×
ULN) hyperbilirubinemia occurred in 7% (n=17) and grade
4 (>3 × ULN) hyperbilirubinemia occurred in 2% (n=5).

If drug-related grade 2 to 4 elevations in bilirubin occur, administration of XELODA should be immediately interrupted until the hyperbilirubinemia resolves or decreases in
intensity to grade 1. NCIC grade 2 hyperbilirubinemia is
defined as 1.5 × normal, grade 3 hyperbilirubinemia as 1.5
to 3 x normal and grade 4 hyperbilirubinemia as >3 × normal. (See recommended dose modifications under **DOSAGE
AND ADMINISTRATION**.)

Hematologic

In 875 patients with either metastatic breast or colorectal
cancer who received a dose of 1250 mg/m^2 administered
twice daily as monotherapy for 2 weeks followed by a
1-week rest period, 3.2%, 1.7%, and 2.4% of patients had
grade 3 or 4 neutropenia, thrombocytopenia or decreases in
hemoglobin, respectively. In 251 patients with metastatic
breast cancer who received a dose of XELODA in combination with docetaxel, 68% had grade 3 or 4 neutropenia, 2.8%
had grade 3 or 4 thrombocytopenia, and 9.6% had grade 3 or
4 anemia.

Carcinogenesis, Mutagenesis and Impairment of Fertility

Adequate studies investigating the carcinogenic potential of
XELODA have not been conducted. Capecitabine was not
mutagenic in vitro to bacteria (Ames test) or mammalian
cells (Chinese hamster V79/HPRT gene mutation assay).
Capecitabine was clastogenic in vitro to human peripheral
blood lymphocytes but not clastogenic in vivo to mouse bone
marrow (micronucleus test). Fluorouracil causes mutations
in bacteria and yeast. Fluorouracil also causes chromosomal
abnormalities in the mouse micronucleus test in vivo.

Impairment of Fertility

In studies of fertility and general reproductive performance
in mice, oral capecitabine doses of 760 mg/kg/day disturbed
estrus and consequently caused a decrease in fertility. In
mice that became pregnant, no fetuses survived this dose.
The disturbance in estrus was reversible. In males, this
dose caused degenerative changes in the testes, including
decreases in the number of spermatocytes and spermatids.
In separate pharmacokinetic studies, this dose in mice produced 5'-DFUR AUC values about 0.7 times the corresponding values in patients administered the recommended daily
dose.

Information for Patients (see Patient Package Insert)

Patients and patients' caregivers should be informed of the
expected adverse effects of XELODA, particularly nausea,
vomiting, diarrhea, and hand-and-foot syndrome, and
should be made aware that patient-specific dose adapta-
tions during therapy are expected and necessary (see **DOS-
AGE AND ADMINISTRATION**). Patients should be encouraged to recognize the common grade 2 toxicities
associated with XELODA treatment.

Diarrhea

Patients experiencing grade 2 diarrhea (an increase of 4 to 6
stools/day or nocturnal stools) or greater should be instructed to stop taking XELODA immediately. Standard antidiarrheal treatments (eg, loperamide) are recommended.

Nausea

Patients experiencing grade 2 nausea (food intake significantly decreased but able to eat intermittently) or greater
should be instructed to stop taking XELODA immediately.
Initiation of symptomatic treatment is recommended.

Vomiting

Patients experiencing grade 2 vomiting (2 to 5 episodes in a
24-hour period) or greater should be instructed to stop taking XELODA immediately. Initiation of symptomatic treatment is recommended.

Hand-and-Foot Syndrome

Patients experiencing grade 2 hand-and-foot syndrome
(painful erythema and swelling of the hands and/or feet

Table 11 Percent Incidence of Adverse Events Reported in ≥5% of Patients Treated With XELODA or 5-FU/LV for Colon Cancer in the Adjuvant Setting (Safety Population)

Body System/Adverse Event	Adjuvant Treatment for Colon Cancer (N=1969)			
	XELODA (N=995)		5-FU/LV (N=974)	
	All Grades	Grade 3/4	All Grades	Grade 3/4
Gastrointestinal Disorders				
Diarrhea	47	12	65	14
Nausea	34	2	47	2
Stomatitis	22	2	60	14
Vomiting	15	2	21	2
Abdominal Pain	14	3	16	2
Constipation	9	–	11	<1
Upper Abdominal Pain	7	<1	7	<1
Dyspepsia	6	<1	5	–
Skin and Subcutaneous Tissue Disorders				
Hand-and-Foot Syndrome	60	17	9	<1
Alopecia	6	–	22	<1
Rash	7	–	8	–
Erythema	6	1	5	<1
General Disorders and Administration Site Conditions				
Fatigue	16	<1	16	1
Pyrexia	7	<1	9	<1
Asthenia	10	<1	10	1
Lethargy	10	<1	9	<1
Nervous System Disorders				
Dizziness	6	<1	6	–
Headache	5	<1	6	<1
Dysgeusia	6	–	9	–
Metabolism and Nutrition Disorders				
Anorexia	9	<1	11	<1
Eye Disorders				
Conjunctivitis	5	<1	6	<1
Blood and Lymphatic System Disorders				
Neutropenia	2	<1	8	5
Respiratory Thoracic and Mediastinal Disorders				
Epistaxis	2	–	5	–

and/or discomfort affecting the patients' activities of daily living) or greater should be instructed to stop taking XELODA immediately.

Stomatitis
Patients experiencing grade 2 stomatitis (painful erythema, edema or ulcers of the mouth or tongue, but able to eat) or greater should be instructed to stop taking XELODA immediately. Initiation of symptomatic treatment is recommended (see **DOSAGE AND ADMINISTRATION**).

Fever and Neutropenia
Patients who develop a fever of 100.5°F or greater or other evidence of potential infection should be instructed to call their physician.

Drug-Food Interaction
In all clinical trials, patients were instructed to administer XELODA within 30 minutes after a meal. Since current safety and efficacy data are based upon administration with food, it is recommended that XELODA be administered with food (see **DOSAGE AND ADMINISTRATION**).

Drug-Drug Interactions
Antacid
The effect of an aluminum hydroxide- and magnesium hydroxide-containing antacid (Maalox) on the pharmacokinetics of XELODA was investigated in 12 cancer patients. There was a small increase in plasma concentrations of XELODA and one metabolite (5'-DFCR); there was no effect on the 3 major metabolites (5'-DFUR, 5-FU and FBAL).

Anticoagulants
Patients receiving concomitant capecitabine and oral coumarin-derivative anticoagulant therapy should have their anticoagulant response (INR or prothrombin time) monitored closely with great frequency and the anticoagulant dose should be adjusted accordingly (see **Boxed WARNING** and **CLINICAL PHARMACOLOGY**). Altered coagulation parameters and/or bleeding have been reported in patients taking XELODA concomitantly with coumarin-derivative anticoagulants such as warfarin and phenprocoumon. These events occurred within several days and up to several months after initiating XELODA therapy and, in a few cases, within 1 month after stopping XELODA. These events occurred in patients with and without liver metastases. In a drug interaction study with single-dose warfarin administration, there was a significant increase in the mean AUC of S-warfarin. The maximum observed INR value increased by 91%. This interaction is probably due to an inhibition of cytochrome P450 2C9 by capecitabine and/or its metabolites (see **CLINICAL PHARMACOLOGY**).

CYP2C9 substrates
Other than warfarin, no formal drug-drug interaction studies between XELODA and other CYP2C9 substrates have been conducted. Care should be exercised when XELODA is coadministered with CYP2C9 substrates.

Phenytoin
The level of phenytoin should be carefully monitored in patients taking XELODA and phenytoin dose may need to be

educed (see **DOSAGE AND ADMINISTRATION: Dose Management Guidelines**). Postmarketing reports indicate that some patients receiving XELODA and phenytoin had toxicity associated with elevated phenytoin levels. Formal drug-drug interaction studies with phenytoin have not been conducted, but the mechanism of interaction is presumed to be inhibition of the CYP2C9 isoenzyme by capecitabine and/or its metabolites (see **PRECAUTIONS: Drug-Drug Interactions: Anticoagulants**).

Leucovorin
The concentration of 5-fluorouracil is increased and its toxicity may be enhanced by leucovorin. Deaths from severe enterocolitis, diarrhea, and dehydration have been reported in elderly patients receiving weekly leucovorin and fluorouracil.

Pregnancy
Teratogenic Effects
Category D (see **WARNINGS**). Women of childbearing potential should be advised to avoid becoming pregnant while receiving treatment with XELODA.

Nursing Women
Lactating mice given a single oral dose of capecitabine excreted significant amounts of capecitabine metabolites into the milk. Because of the potential for serious adverse reactions in nursing infants from capecitabine, it is recommended that nursing be discontinued when receiving XELODA therapy.

Pediatric Use
The safety and effectiveness of XELODA in persons <18 years of age have not been established.

Geriatric Use
Physicians should pay particular attention to monitoring the adverse effects of XELODA in the elderly (see **WARNINGS: Geriatric Patients**).

ADVERSE REACTIONS
Adjuvant Colon Cancer
Table 11 shows the adverse events occurring in ≥5% of patients from one phase 3 trial in patients with Dukes' C colon cancer who received at least one dose of study medication and had at least one safety assessment. A total of 995 patients were treated with 1250 mg/m² twice a day of XELODA administered for 2 weeks followed by a 1-week rest period, and 974 patients were administered 5-FU and

leucovorin (20 mg/m² leucovorin IV followed by 425 mg/m² IV bolus 5-FU, on days 1-5, every 28 days). The median duration of treatment was 164 days for capecitabine-treated patients and 145 days for 5-FU/LV-treated patients. A total of 112 (11%) and 73 (7%) capecitabine and 5-FU/LV-treated patients, respectively, discontinued treatment because of adverse events. A total of 18 deaths due to all causes occurred either on study or within 28 days of receiving study drug: 8 (0.8%) patients randomized to XELODA and 10 (1.0%) randomized to 5-FU/LV.
Table 12 shows grade 3/4 laboratory abnormalities occurring in ≥1% of patients from one phase 3 trial in patients with Dukes' C colon cancer who received at least one dose of study medication and had at least one safety assessment. [See table 11 at top of previous page]

Table 12 Percent Incidence of Grade 3/4 Laboratory Abnormalities Reported in ≥1% of Patients Receiving XELODA Monotherapy for Adjuvant Treatment of Colon Cancer (Safety Population)

Adverse Event	XELODA (n=995) Grade 3/4 %	IV 5-FU/LV (n=974) Grade 3/4 %
Increased ALAT (SGPT)	1.6	0.6
Increased calcium	1.1	0.7
Decreased calcium	2.3	2.2
Decreased hemoglobin	1.0	1.2
Decreased lymphocytes	13.0	13.0
Decreased neutrophils*	2.2	26.2
Decreased neutrophils/ granulocytes	2.4	26.4
Decreased platelets	1.0	0.7
Increased bilirubin**	20	6.3

* The incidence of grade 3/4 white blood cell abnormalities was 1.3% in the XELODA arm and 4.9% in the IV 5-FU/LV arm.
**It should be noted that grading was according to NCIC CTC Version 1 (May, 1994). In the NCIC-CTC Version 1, hyperbilirubinemia grade 3 indicates a bilirubin value of

Table 13 Pooled Phase 3 Colorectal Trials: Percent Incidence of Adverse Events in ≥5% of Patients

Adverse Event	XELODA (n=596)			5-FU/LV (n=593)		
	Total %	Grade 3 %	Grade 4 %	Total %	Grade 3 %	Grade 4 %
Number of Patients With > One Adverse Event	96	52	9	94	45	9
Body System/Adverse Event						
GI						
Diarrhea	55	13	2	61	10	2
Nausea	43	4	–	51	3	<1
Vomiting	27	4	<1	30	4	<1
Stomatitis	25	2	<1	62	14	1
Abdominal Pain	35	9	<1	31	5	–
Gastrointestinal Motility Disorder	10	<1	–	7	<1	–
Constipation	14	1	<1	17	1	–
Oral Discomfort	10	–	–	10	–	–
Upper GI Inflammatory Disorders	8	<1	–	10	1	–
Gastrointestinal Hemorrhage	6	1	<1	3	1	–
Ileus	6	4	1	5	2	1
Skin and Subcutaneous						
Hand-and-Foot Syndrome	54	17	NA	6	1	NA
Dermatitis	27	1	–	26	1	–
Skin Discoloration	7	<1	–	5	–	–
Alopecia	6	–	–	21	<1	–

(Table continued on next page)

Table 13 *(cont.)*   Pooled Phase 3 Colorectal Trials:
Percent Incidence of Adverse Events in ≥5% of Patients

Adverse Event	XELODA (n=596)			5-FU/LV (n=593)		
	Total %	Grade 3 %	Grade 4 %	Total %	Grade 3 %	Grade 4 %
Number of Patients With > One Adverse Event	96	52	9	94	45	9
Body System/Adverse Event						
General						
Fatigue/Weakness	42	4	–	46	4	–
Pyrexia	18	1	–	21	2	–
Edema	15	1	–	9	1	–
Pain	12	1	–	10	1	–
Chest Pain	6	1	–	6	1	<1
Neurological						
Peripheral Sensory Neuropathy	10	–	–	4	–	–
Headache	10	1	–	7	–	–
Dizziness*	8	<1	–	8	<1	–
Insomnia	7	–	–	7	–	–
Taste Disturbance	6	1	–	11	<1	1
Metabolism						
Appetite Decreased	26	3	<1	31	2	<1
Dehydration	7	2	<1	8	3	1
Eye						
Eye Irritation	13	–	–	10	<1	–
Vision Abnormal	5	–	–	2	–	–
Respiratory						
Dyspnea	14	1	–	10	<1	1
Cough	7	<1	1	8	–	–
Pharyngeal Disorder	5	–	–	5	–	–
Epistaxis	3	<1	–	6	–	–
Sore Throat	2	–	–	6	–	–
Musculoskeletal						
Back Pain	10	2	–	9	<1	–
Arthralgia	8	1	–	6	1	–
Vascular						
Venous Thrombosis	8	3	<1	6	2	–
Psychiatric						
Mood Alteration	5	–	–	6	<1	–
Depression	5	–	–	4	<1	–
Infections						
Viral	5	<1	–	5	<1	–
Blood and Lymphatic						
Anemia	80	2	<1	79	1	<1
Neutropenia	13	1	2	46	8	13
Hepatobiliary						
Hyperbilirubinemia	48	18	5	17	3	3

– Not observed
* Excluding vertigo
NA = Not Applicable

1.5 to 3.0 × upper limit of normal (ULN) range, and grade 4 a value of > 3.0 × ULN. The NCI CTC Version 2 and above define a grade 3 bilirubin value of >3.0 to 10.0 × ULN, and grade 4 values >10.0 × ULN.

Metastatic Colorectal Cancer

Table 13 shows the adverse events occurring in ≥5% of patients from pooling the two phase 3 trials in first line metastatic colorectal cancer. A total of 596 patients with metastatic colorectal cancer were treated with 1250 mg/m² twice a day of XELODA administered for 2 weeks followed by a 1-week rest period, and 593 patients were administered 5-FU and leucovorin in the Mayo regimen (20 mg/m² leucovorin IV followed by 425 mg/m² IV bolus 5-FU, on days 1–5, every 28 days). In the pooled colorectal database the median duration of treatment was 139 days for capecitabine-treated patients and 140 days for 5-FU/LV-treated patients. A total of 78 (13%) and 63 (11%) capecitabine and 5-FU/LV-treated patients, respectively, discontinued treatment because of adverse events/intercurrent illness. A total of 82 deaths due to all causes occurred either on study or within 28 days of receiving study drug: 50 (8.4%) patients randomized to XELODA and 32 (5.4%) randomized to 5-FU/LV.

Table 14   Percent Incidence of Adverse Events Considered Related or Unrelated to Treatment in ≥5% of Patients Participating in the XELODA and Docetaxel Combination vs Docetaxel Monotherapy Study

Adverse Event	XELODA 1250 mg/m²/bid With Docetaxel 75 mg/m²/3 weeks (n=251)			Docetaxel 100 mg/m²/3 weeks (n=255)		
	Total %	Grade 3 %	Grade 4 %	Total %	Grade 3 %	Grade 4 %
Number of Patients With at Least One Adverse Event	99	76.5	29.1	97	57.6	31.8
Body System/Adverse Event						
GI						
Diarrhea	67	14	<1	48	5	<1
Stomatitis	67	17	<1	43	5	–
Nausea	45	7	–	36	2	–
Vomiting	35	4	1	24	2	–
Constipation	20	2	–	18	–	–
Abdominal Pain	30	<3	<1	24	2	–
Dyspepsia	14	–	–	8	1	–
Dry Mouth	6	<1	–	5	–	–
Skin and Subcutaneous						
Hand-and-Foot Syndrome	63	24	NA	8	1	NA
Alopecia	41	6	–	42	7	–
Nail Disorder	14	2	–	15	–	–
Dermatitis	8	–	–	11	1	–
Rash Erythematous	9	<1	–	5	–	–
Nail Discoloration	6	–	–	4	<1	–
Onycholysis	5	1	–	5	1	–
Pruritus	4	–	–	5	–	–
General						
Pyrexia	28	2	–	34	2	–
Asthenia	26	4	<1	25	6	–
Fatigue	22	4	–	27	6	–
Weakness	16	2	–	11	2	–
Pain in Limb	13	<1	–	13	2	–
Lethargy	7	–	–	6	2	–
Pain	7	<1	–	5	1	–
Chest Pain (non-cardiac)	4	<1	–	6	2	–
Influenza-like Illness	5	–	–	5	–	–
Neurological						
Taste Disturbance	16	<1	–	14	<1	–
Headache	15	3	–	15	2	–
Paresthesia	12	<1	–	16	1	–
Dizziness	12	–	–	8	<1	–
Insomnia	8	–	–	10	<1	–
Peripheral Neuropathy	6	–	–	10	1	–
Hypoaesthesia	4	<1	–	8	<1	–
Metabolism						
Anorexia	13	1	–	11	<1	–
Appetite Decreased	10	–	–	5	–	–
Weight Decreased	7	–	–	5	–	–
Dehydration	10	2	–	7	<1	<1
Eye						
Lacrimation Increased	12	–	–	7	<1	–
Conjunctivitis	5	–	–	4	–	–
Eye Irritation	5	–	–	1	–	–

(Table continued on next page)

[See table 13 on pages 375 and 376]

Breast Cancer Combination

The following data are shown for the combination study with XELODA and docetaxel in patients with metastatic breast cancer in **Table 14** and **Table 15**. In the XELODA and docetaxel combination arm the treatment was XELODA administered orally 1250 mg/m² twice daily as intermittent therapy (2 weeks of treatment followed by 1 week without treatment) for at least 6 weeks and docetaxel administered as a 1-hour intravenous infusion at a dose of 75 mg/m² on the first day of each 3-week cycle for at least 6 weeks. In the monotherapy arm docetaxel was administered as a 1-hour intravenous infusion at a dose of 100 mg/m² on the first day of each 3-week cycle for at least 6 weeks. The mean duration of treatment was 129 days in the combination arm and 98 days in the monotherapy arm. A total of 66 patients (26%) in the combination arm and 49 (19%) in the monotherapy arm withdrew from the study because of adverse events. The

Table 14 *(cont.)*   Percent Incidence of Adverse Events Considered Related or Unrelated to Treatment in ≥5% of Patients Participating in the XELODA and Docetaxel Combination vs Docetaxel Monotherapy Study

Adverse Event	XELODA 1250 mg/m²/bid With Docetaxel 75 mg/m²/3 weeks (n=251)			Docetaxel 100 mg/m²/3 weeks (n=255)		
	Total %	Grade 3 %	Grade 4 %	Total %	Grade 3 %	Grade 4 %
Number of Patients With at Least One Adverse Event	99	76.5	29.1	97	57.6	31.8
Body System/Adverse Event						
Musculoskeletal						
Arthralgia	15	2	–	24	3	–
Myalgia	15	2	–	25	2	–
Back Pain	12	<1	–	11	3	–
Bone Pain	8	<1	–	10	2	–
Cardiac						
Edema	33	<2	–	34	<3	1
Blood						
Neutropenic Fever	16	3	13	21	5	16
Respiratory						
Dyspnea	14	2	<1	16	2	–
Cough	13	1	–	22	<1	–
Sore Throat	12	2	–	11	<1	–
Epistaxis	7	<1	–	6	–	–
Rhinorrhea	5	–	–	3	–	–
Pleural Effusion	2	1	–	7	4	–
Infection						
Oral Candidiasis	7	<1	–	8	<1	–
Urinary Tract Infection	6	<1	–	4	–	–
Upper Respiratory Tract	4	–	–	5	1	–
Vascular						
Flushing	5	–	–	5	–	–
Lymphoedema	3	<1	–	5	1	–
Psychiatric						
Depression	5	–	–	5	1	–

– Not observed
NA = Not Applicable

percentage of patients requiring dose reductions due to adverse events was 65% in the combination arm and 36% in the monotherapy arm. The percentage of patients requiring treatment interruptions due to adverse events in the combination arm was 79%. Treatment interruptions were part of the dose modification scheme for the combination therapy arm but not for the docetaxel monotherapy-treated patients. [See table 14 on previous page and above]

[See table 15 below]

Breast Cancer XELODA Monotherapy
The following data are shown for the study in stage IV breast cancer patients who received a dose of 1250 mg/m² administered twice daily for 2 weeks followed by a 1-week rest period. The mean duration of treatment was 114 days. A total of 13 out of 162 patients (8%) discontinued treatment because of adverse events/intercurrent illness.

Table 15   Percent of Patients With Laboratory Abnormalities Participating in the XELODA and Docetaxel Combination vs Docetaxel Monotherapy Study

Adverse Event	XELODA 1250 mg/m²/bid With Docetaxel 75 mg/m²/3 weeks (n=251)			Docetaxel 100 mg/m²/3 weeks (n=255)		
Body System/Adverse Event	Total %	Grade 3 %	Grade 4 %	Total %	Grade 3 %	Grade 4 %
Hematologic						
Leukopenia	91	37	24	88	42	33
Neutropenia/Granulocytopenia	86	20	49	87	10	66
Thrombocytopenia	41	2	1	23	1	2
Anemia	80	7	3	83	5	<1
Lymphocytopenia	99	48	41	98	44	40
Hepatobiliary						
Hyperbilirubinemia	20	7	2	6	2	2

Table 16 Percent Incidence of Adverse Events Considered Remotely, Possibly or Probably Related to Treatment in ≥5% of Patients Participating in the Single Arm Trial in Stage IV Breast Cancer

Adverse Event	Phase 2 Trial in Stage IV Breast Cancer (n=162)		
Body System/Adverse Event	Total %	Grade 3 %	Grade 4 %
GI			
Diarrhea	57	12	3
Nausea	53	4	–
Vomiting	37	4	–
Stomatitis	24	7	–
Abdominal Pain	20	4	–
Constipation	15	1	–
Dyspepsia	8	–	–
Skin and Subcutaneous			
Hand-and-Foot Syndrome	57	11	N/A
Dermatitis	37	1	–
Nail Disorder	7	–	–
General			
Fatigue	41	8	–
Pyrexia	12	1	–
Pain in Limb	6	1	–
Neurological			
Paresthesia	21	1	–
Headache	9	1	–
Dizziness	8	–	–
Insomnia	8	–	–
Metabolism			
Anorexia	23	3	–
Dehydration	7	4	1
Eye			
Eye Irritation	15	–	–
Musculoskeletal			
Myalgia	9	–	–
Cardiac			
Edema	9	1	–
Blood			
Neutropenia	26	2	2
Thrombocytopenia	24	3	1
Anemia	72	3	1
Lymphopenia	94	44	15
Hepatobiliary			
Hyperbilirubinemia	22	9	2

– Not observed
NA = Not Applicable

[See table 16 above]

XELODA and Docetaxel in Combination

Shown below by body system are the clinically relevant adverse events in <5% of patients in the overall clinical trial safety database of 251 patients (Study Details) reported as related to the administration of XELODA in combination with docetaxel and that were clinically at least remotely relevant. In parentheses is the incidence of grade 3 and 4 occurrences of each adverse event.

It is anticipated that the same types of adverse events observed in the XELODA monotherapy studies may be observed in patients treated with the combination of XELODA plus docetaxel.

Gastrointestinal: ileus (0.39), necrotizing enterocolitis (0.39), esophageal ulcer (0.39), hemorrhagic diarrhea (0.80)

Neurological: ataxia (0.39), syncope (1.20), taste loss (0.80), polyneuropathy (0.39), migraine (0.39)

Cardiac: supraventricular tachycardia (0.39)

Infection: neutropenic sepsis (2.39), sepsis (0.39), bronchopneumonia (0.39)

Blood and Lymphatic: agranulocytosis (0.39), prothrombin decreased (0.39)

Vascular: hypotension (1.20), venous phlebitis and thrombophlebitis (0.39), postural hypotension (0.80)

Renal: renal failure (0.39)

Hepatobiliary: jaundice (0.39), abnormal liver function tests (0.39), hepatic failure (0.39), hepatic coma (0.39), hepatotoxicity (0.39)

Immune System: hypersensitivity (1.20)

XELODA Monotherapy Metastatic Breast and Colorectal Cancer

Shown below by body system are the clinically relevant adverse events in <5% of patients in the overall clinical trial safety database of 875 patients (phase 3 colorectal studies — 596 patients, phase 2 colorectal study — 34 patients,

Table 17 XELODA Dose Calculation According to Body Surface Area

Dose Level 1250 mg/m² Twice a Day		Number of Tablets to be Taken at Each Dose (Morning and Evening)	
Surface Area (m²)	Total Daily* Dose (mg)	150 mg	500 mg
≤ 1.25	3000	0	3
1.26-1.37	3300	1	3
1.38-1.51	3600	2	3
1.52-1.65	4000	0	4
1.66-1.77	4300	1	4
1.78-1.91	4600	2	4
1.92-2.05	5000	0	5
2.06-2.17	5300	1	5
≥ 2.18	5600	2	5

*Total Daily Dose divided by 2 to allow equal morning and evening doses

Table 18 XELODA in Combination With Docetaxel Dose Reduction Schedule

Toxicity NCIC Grades*	Grade 2	Grade 3	Grade 4
1st appearance	Grade 2 occurring during the 14 days of XELODA treatment: interrupt XELODA treatment until resolved to grade 0-1. Treatment may be resumed during the cycle at the same dose of XELODA. Doses of XELODA missed during a treatment cycle are not to be replaced. Prophylaxis for toxicities should be implemented where possible. Grade 2 persisting at the time the next XELODA/docetaxel treatment is due: delay treatment until resolved to grade 0-1, then continue at 100% of the original XELODA and docetaxel dose. Prophylaxis for toxicities should be implemented where possible.	Grade 3 occurring during the 14 days of XELODA treatment: interrupt the XELODA treatment until resolved to grade 0-1. Treatment may be resumed during the cycle at 75% of the XELODA dose. Doses of XELODA missed during a treatment cycle are not to be replaced. Prophylaxis for toxicities should be implemented where possible. Grade 3 persisting at the time the next XELODA/docetaxel treatment is due: delay treatment until resolved to grade 0-1. For patients developing grade 3 toxicity at any time during the treatment cycle, upon resolution to grade 0-1, subsequent treatment cycles should be continued at 75% of the original XELODA dose and at 55 mg/m² of docetaxel. Prophylaxis for toxicities should be implemented where possible.	Discontinue treatment unless treating physician considers it to be in the best interest of the patient to continue with XELODA at 50% of original dose.

(Table continued on next page)

phase 2 breast cancer studies — 245 patients) reported as related to the administration of XELODA and that were clinically at least remotely relevant. In parentheses is the incidence of grade 3 or 4 occurrences of each adverse event.
Gastrointestinal: abdominal distension, dysphagia, proctalgia, ascites (0.1), gastric ulcer (0.1), ileus (0.3), toxic dilation of intestine, gastroenteritis (0.1)
Skin and Subcutaneous: nail disorder (0.1), sweating increased (0.1), photosensitivity reaction (0.1), skin ulceration, pruritus, radiation recall syndrome (0.2)
General: chest pain (0.2), influenza-like illness, hot flushes, pain (0.1), hoarseness, irritability, difficulty with walking, thirst, chest mass, collapse, fibrosis (0.1), hemorrhage, edema, sedation

Neurological: insomnia, ataxia (0.5), tremor, dysphasia, encephalopathy (0.1), abnormal coordination, dysarthria, loss of consciousness (0.2), impaired balance
Metabolism: increased weight, cachexia (0.4), hypertriglyceridemia (0.1), hypokalemia, hypomagnesemia
Eye: conjunctivitis
Respiratory: cough (0.1), epistaxis (0.1), asthma (0.2), hemoptysis, respiratory distress (0.1), dyspnea
Cardiac: tachycardia (0.1), bradycardia, atrial fibrillation, ventricular extrasystoles, extrasystoles, myocarditis (0.1), pericardial effusion
Infections: laryngitis (1.0), bronchitis (0.2), pneumonia (0.2), bronchopneumonia (0.2), keratoconjunctivitis, sepsis (0.3), fungal infections (including candidiasis) (0.2)

Table 18 (cont.)   XELODA in Combination With Docetaxel Dose Reduction Schedule

Toxicity NCIC Grades*	Grade 2	Grade 3	Grade 4
2nd appearance of same toxicity	Grade 2 occurring during the 14 days of XELODA treatment: interrupt XELODA treatment until resolved to grade 0-1. Treatment may be resumed during the cycle at 75% of original XELODA dose. Doses of XELODA missed during a treatment cycle are not to be replaced. Prophylaxis for toxicities should be implemented where possible. Grade 2 persisting at the time the next XELODA/docetaxel treatment is due: delay treatment until resolved to grade 0-1. For patients developing 2nd occurrence of grade 2 toxicity at any time during the treatment cycle, upon resolution to grade 0-1, subsequent treatment cycles should be continued at 75% of the original XELODA dose and at 55 mg/m^2 of docetaxel. Prophylaxis for toxicities should be implemented where possible.	Grade 3 occurring during the 14 days of XELODA treatment: interrupt the XELODA treatment until resolved to grade 0-1. Treatment may be resumed during the cycle at 50% of the XELODA dose. Doses of XELODA missed during a treatment cycle are not to be replaced. Prophylaxis for toxicities should be implemented where possible. Grade 3 persisting at the time the next XELODA/docetaxel treatment is due: delay treatment until resolved to grade 0-1. For patients developing grade 3 toxicity at any time during the treatment cycle, upon resolution to grade 0-1, subsequent treatment cycles should be continued at 50% of the original XELODA dose and the docetaxel discontinued. Prophylaxis for toxicities should be implemented where possible.	Discontinue treatment.
3rd appearance of same toxicity	Grade 2 occurring during the 14 days of XELODA treatment: interrupt XELODA treatment until resolved to grade 0-1. Treatment may be resumed during the cycle at 50% of the original XELODA dose. Doses of XELODA missed during a treatment cycle are not to be replaced. Prophylaxis for toxicities should be implemented where possible. Grade 2 persisting at the time the next XELODA/docetaxel treatment is due: delay treatment until resolved to grade 0-1. For patients developing 3rd occurrence of grade 2 toxicity at any time during the treatment cycle, upon resolution to grade 0-1, subsequent treatment cycles should be continued at 50% of the original XELODA dose and the docetaxel discontinued. Prophylaxis for toxicities should be implemented where possible.	Discontinue treatment.	
4th appearance of same toxicity	Discontinue treatment.		

*National Cancer Institute of Canada Common Toxicity Criteria were used except for hand-and-foot syndrome (see **PRECAUTIONS**).

Musculoskeletal: myalgia, bone pain (0.1), arthritis (0.1), muscle weakness
Blood and Lymphatic: leukopenia (0.2), coagulation disorder (0.1), bone marrow depression (0.1), idiopathic thrombocytopenia purpura (1.0), pancytopenia (0.1)
Vascular: hypotension (0.2), hypertension (0.1), lymphoedema (0.1), pulmonary embolism (0.2), cerebrovascular accident (0.1)

Psychiatric: depression, confusion (0.1)
Renal: renal impairment (0.6)
Ear: vertigo
Hepatobiliary: hepatic fibrosis (0.1), hepatitis (0.1), cholestatic hepatitis (0.1), abnormal liver function tests
Immune System: drug hypersensitivity (0.1)
Postmarketing: hepatic failure, lacrimal duct stenosis

OVERDOSAGE

The manifestations of acute overdose would include nausea, vomiting, diarrhea, gastrointestinal irritation and bleeding, and bone marrow depression. Medical management of overdose should include customary supportive medical interventions aimed at correcting the presenting clinical manifestations. Although no clinical experience using dialysis as a treatment for XELODA overdose has been reported, dialysis may be of benefit in reducing circulating concentrations of 5'-DFUR, a low–molecular-weight metabolite of the parent compound.

Single doses of XELODA were not lethal to mice, rats, and monkeys at doses up to 2000 mg/kg (2.4, 4.8, and 9.6 times the recommended human daily dose on a mg/m^2 basis).

DOSAGE AND ADMINISTRATION

The recommended dose of XELODA is 1250 mg/m^2 administered orally twice daily (morning and evening; equivalent to 2500 mg/m^2 total daily dose) for 2 weeks followed by a 1-week rest period given as 3-week cycles. XELODA tablets should be swallowed with water within 30 minutes after a meal. In combination with docetaxel, the recommended dose of XELODA is 1250 mg/m^2 twice daily for 2 weeks followed by a 1-week rest period, combined with docetaxel at 75 mg/m^2 as a 1-hour intravenous infusion every 3 weeks. Pre-medication, according to the docetaxel labeling, should be started prior to docetaxel administration for patients receiving the XELODA plus docetaxel combination. **Table 17** displays the total daily dose by body surface area and the number of tablets to be taken at each dose.

Adjuvant treatment in patients with Dukes' C colon cancer is recommended for a total of 6 months, ie, XELODA 1250 mg/m^2 orally twice daily for 2 weeks followed by a 1-week rest period, given as 3-week cycles for a total of 8 cycles (24 weeks).

[See table 17 at top of page 380]

Dose Management Guidelines

XELODA dosage may need to be individualized to optimize patient management. Patients should be carefully monitored for toxicity and doses of XELODA should be modified as necessary to accommodate individual patient tolerance to treatment (see **CLINICAL STUDIES**). Toxicity due to XELODA administration may be managed by symptomatic treatment, dose interruptions and adjustment of XELODA dose. Once the dose has been reduced it should not be increased at a later time.

The dose of phenytoin and the dose of coumarin-derivative anticoagulants may need to be reduced when either drug is administered concomitantly with XELODA (see **PRECAUTIONS: Drug-Drug Interactions**).

XELODA dose modification scheme as described below (see **Table 18** and **Table 19**) is recommended for the management of adverse events.

[See table 18 on pages 380 and 381]

Dose modification for the use of XELODA as monotherapy is shown in **Table 19**.

[See table 19 below]

Dosage modifications are not recommended for grade 1 events. Therapy with XELODA should be interrupted upon the occurrence of a grade 2 or 3 adverse experience. Once the adverse event has resolved or decreased in intensity to grade 1, then XELODA therapy may be restarted at full dose or as adjusted according to **Table 18** and **Table 19**. If a grade 4 experience occurs, therapy should be discontinued or interrupted until resolved or decreased to grade 1, and therapy should be restarted at 50% of the original dose. Doses of XELODA omitted for toxicity are not replaced or restored; instead the patient should resume the planned treatment cycles.

Adjustment of Starting Dose in Special Populations

Hepatic Impairment

In patients with mild to moderate hepatic dysfunction due to liver metastases, no starting dose adjustment is necessary; however, patients should be carefully monitored. Patients with severe hepatic dysfunction have not been studied.

Renal Impairment

No adjustment to the starting dose of XELODA is recommended in patients with mild renal impairment (creatinine clearance = 51 to 80 mL/min [Cockroft and Gault, as shown below]). In patients with moderate renal impairment (base-

Table 19   Recommended Dose Modifications With XELODA Monotherapy

Toxicity NCIC Grades*	During a Course of Therapy	Dose Adjustment for Next Treatment (% of starting dose)
• *Grade 1*	Maintain dose level	Maintain dose level
• *Grade 2*		
-1st appearance	Interrupt until resolved to grade 0-1	100%
-2nd appearance	Interrupt until resolved to grade 0-1	75%
-3rd appearance	Interrupt until resolved to grade 0-1	50%
-4th appearance	Discontinue treatment permanently	
• *Grade 3*		
-1st appearance	Interrupt until resolved to grade 0-1	75%
-2nd appearance	Interrupt until resolved to grade 0-1	50%
-3rd appearance	Discontinue treatment permanently	
• *Grade 4*		
-1st appearance	Discontinue permanently *OR* If physician deems it to be in the patient's best interest to continue, interrupt until resolved to grade 0-1	50%

*National Cancer Institute of Canada Common Toxicity Criteria were used except for the hand-and-foot syndrome (see **PRECAUTIONS**).

Cockroft and Gault Equation:

$$\text{Creatinine clearance for males} = \frac{(140 - \text{age [yrs]}) (\text{body wt [kg]})}{(72) (\text{serum creatinine [mg/dL]})}$$

Creatinine clearance for females = $0.85 \times$ male value

ine creatinine clearance = 30 to 50 mL/min), a dose reduction to 75% of the XELODA starting dose when used as monotherapy or in combination with docetaxel (from 1250 mg/m^2 to 950 mg/m^2 twice daily) is recommended (see **CLINICAL PHARMACOLOGY: Special Populations**). Subsequent dose adjustment is recommended as outlined in **Table 18** and **Table 19** if a patient develops a grade 2 to 4 adverse event (see **WARNINGS**). The starting dose adjustment recommendations for patients with moderate renal impairment apply both to XELODA monotherapy and XELODA in combination use with docetaxel.
[See table above]

Geriatrics
Physicians should exercise caution in monitoring the effects of XELODA in the elderly. Insufficient data are available to provide a dosage recommendation.

HOW SUPPLIED
XELODA is supplied as biconvex, oblong film-coated tablets, available in bottles as follows:

150 mg
color: light peach
engraving: XELODA on one side, 150 on the other
150 mg tablets are packaged in bottles of 60 (NDC 0004-1100-20).

500 mg
color: peach
engraving: XELODA on one side, 500 on the other
500 mg tablets are packaged in bottles of 120 (NDC 0004-1101-50).

Storage Conditions
Store at 25°C (77°F); excursions permitted to 15° to 30°C (59° to 86°F). [See USP Controlled Room Temperature].
KEEP TIGHTLY CLOSED.
Maalox is a registered trademark of Novartis Consumer Health.
Taxotere is a registered trademark of Aventis Pharmaceuticals Inc.
For full Taxotere prescribing information, please refer to Taxotere Package Insert.

PATIENT INFORMATION (TEXT ONLY)
Read this leaflet before you start taking XELODA® [zeh-LOE-duh] and each time you refill your prescription in case the information has changed. This leaflet contains important information about XELODA. However, this information does not take the place of talking with your doctor. This information cannot cover all possible risks and benefits of XELODA. Your doctor should always be your first choice for discussing your medical condition and this medicine.

What is XELODA?
XELODA is a medicine you take by mouth (orally). XELODA is changed in the body to 5-fluorouracil (5-FU). In some patients with colon, rectum or breast cancer, 5-FU stops cancer cells from growing and decreases the size of the tumor.
XELODA is used to treat:
— cancer of the colon after surgery
— cancer of the colon or rectum (colorectal cancer) that has spread to other parts of the body (metastatic colorectal cancer). You should know that in studies, other medicines showed improved survival when they were taken together with 5-FU and leucovorin. In studies, XELODA was no worse than 5-FU and leucovorin taken together but did not improve survival compared to these two medicines.
— breast cancer that has spread to other parts of the body (metastatic breast cancer) together with another medicine called docetaxel (Taxotere®)
— breast cancer that has spread to other parts of the body and has not improved after treatment with other medi-

cines such as paclitaxel (Taxol®) and anthracycline-containing medicine such as Adriamycin® and doxorubicin

What is the most important information about XELODA?
XELODA may increase the effect of other medicines used to thin your blood such as warfarin (Coumadin®). It is very important that your doctor knows if you are taking a blood thinner such as warfarin because XELODA may increase the effect of this medicine and could lead to serious side effects. If you are taking blood thinners and XELODA, your doctor needs to check more often how fast your blood clots and change the dose of the blood thinner, if needed.

Who should not take XELODA?
1. DO NOT TAKE XELODA IF YOU
— are nursing a baby. Tell your doctor if you are nursing. XELODA may pass to the baby in your milk and harm the baby.
— are allergic to 5-fluorouracil
— are allergic to capecitabine or to any of the ingredients in XELODA
— have been told that you lack the enzyme DPD (dihydropyrimidine dehydrogenase)

2. TELL YOUR DOCTOR IF YOU
— take a blood thinner such as warfarin (Coumadin). This is very important because XELODA may increase the effect of the blood thinner. If you are taking blood thinners and XELODA, your doctor needs to check more often how fast your blood clots and change the dose of the blood thinner, if needed.
— take phenytoin (Dilantin®). Your doctor needs to test the levels of phenytoin in your blood more often or change your dose of phenytoin.
— are pregnant or think you may be pregnant. XELODA may harm your unborn child.
— have kidney problems. Your doctor may prescribe a different medicine or lower the XELODA dose.
— have liver problems. You may need to be checked for liver problems while you take XELODA.
— have heart problems because you could have more side effects related to your heart.
— take the vitamin folic acid. It may affect how XELODA works.

How should I take XELODA?
Take XELODA exactly as your doctor tells you to. Your doctor will prescribe a dose and treatment plan that is right for you. Your doctor may want you to take both 150 mg and 500 mg tablets together for each dose. If so, you must be able to identify the tablets. Taking the wrong tablets could cause an overdose (too much medicine) or underdose (too little medicine). The 150 mg tablets are light peach in color with 150 on one side. The 500 mg tablets are peach in color with 500 on one side. Your doctor may change the amount of medicine you take during your treatment. Your doctor may prescribe XELODA Tablets with Taxotere or docetaxel injection.
— XELODA is taken in 2 daily doses, a morning dose and an evening dose
— Take XELODA tablets **within 30 minutes after the end of a meal** (breakfast and dinner)
— **Swallow XELODA tablets with water**
— If you miss a dose of XELODA, do not take the missed dose at all and do not double the next dose. Instead, continue your regular dosing schedule and check with your doctor.
— XELODA is usually taken for 14 days followed by a 7-day rest period (no drug), for a 21-day cycle. Your doctor will tell you how many cycles of treatment you will need.
— If you take too much XELODA, contact your doctor or local poison control center or emergency room **right away**.

What should I avoid while taking XELODA?
— Women should not become pregnant while taking XELODA. XELODA may harm your unborn child. Use effective birth control while taking XELODA. Tell your doctor if you become pregnant.
— Do not breast-feed. XELODA may pass through your milk and harm your baby.
— Men should use birth control while taking XELODA

What are the most common side effects of XELODA?
The most common side effects of XELODA are:
— diarrhea, nausea, vomiting, sores in the mouth and throat (stomatitis), stomach area pain (abdominal pain), upset stomach, constipation, loss of appetite, and too much water loss from the body (dehydration). These side effects are more common in patients age 80 and older.
— hand-and-foot syndrome (palms of the hands or soles of the feet tingle, become numb, painful, swollen or red), rash, dry, itchy or discolored skin, nail problems, and hair loss
— tiredness, weakness, dizziness, headache, fever, pain (including chest, back, joint, and muscle pain), trouble sleeping, and taste problems

These side effects may differ when taking XELODA with Taxotere. Please consult your doctor for possible side effects that may be caused by taking XELODA with Taxotere.

If you are concerned about these or any other side effects while taking XELODA, talk to your doctor.

Stop taking XELODA immediately and contact your doctor right away if you have the side effects listed below, or other side effects that concern you. Your doctor can then adjust XELODA to a dose that is right for you or stop your XELODA treatment for a while. This should help to reduce the side effects and stop them from getting worse.
— *Diarrhea:* if you have an additional 4 bowel movements each day beyond what is normal or any diarrhea at night
— *Vomiting:* if you vomit more than once in a 24-hour time period
— *Nausea:* if you lose your appetite, and the amount of food you eat each day is much less than usual
— *Stomatitis:* if you have pain, redness, swelling or sores in your mouth
— *Hand-and-Foot Syndrome:* if you have pain, swelling or redness of your hands or feet that prevents normal activity

— *Fever or Infection:* if you have a temperature of 100.5°F or greater, or other signs of infection

Your doctor may tell you to lower the dose or to stop XELODA treatment for a while. If caught early, most of these side effects usually improve after you stop taking XELODA. If they do not improve within 2 to 3 days, call your doctor again. After your side effects have improved, your doctor will tell you whether to start taking XELODA again and what dose to take. Adjusting the dose of XELODA to be right for each patient is an important part of treatment.

How should I store and use XELODA?
— Never share XELODA with anyone
— Store XELODA at normal room temperature (about 65 to 85°F)
— Keep XELODA and all other medicines out of the reach of children
— If you take too much XELODA by mistake, contact your doctor or local poison control center or emergency room right away

General advice about prescription medicines:
Medicines are sometimes prescribed for conditions that are not mentioned in patient information leaflets. Do not use XELODA for a condition for which it was not prescribed. Do not give XELODA to other people, even if they have the same symptoms you have. It may harm them.

This leaflet summarizes the most important information about XELODA. If you would like more information, talk with your doctor. You can ask your pharmacist or doctor for information about XELODA that is written for health professionals.

Adriamycin is a registered trademark of Bristol-Myers Squibb Company.

Coumadin is a registered trademark of Bristol-Myers Squibb Company.

Dilantin is a registered trademark of Parke-Davis.

Taxol is a registered trademark of Bristol-Myers Squibb Company.

Taxotere is a registered trademark of Aventis Pharmaceuticals Inc.

Revised: June 2005

Section IV
Professional Resources

Advances in Colon Cancer Chemotherapy— Nursing Implications

Teri Vega-Stromberg, MSN, RN, AOCN
Clinical Nurse Specialist, Oncology
St. Joseph Regional Medical Center
Milwaukee, WI

Adjuvant chemotherapy for colon cancer has changed significantly during the past five years. The traditional agent fluorouracil has been joined by new drugs, including capecitabine, irinotecan, oxaliplatin, and targeted agents such as bevacizumab and cetuximab. These new agents bring different mechanisms of action, different side effects, and new home care nursing implications. Significant improvements in disease-free remissions and survival rates are among the many benefits of these therapies to persons with colon cancer. This article covers these newer agents, targeted therapies for colon cancer, and associated nursing and patient implications, including detailed drug information.

Colon cancer has held the post of the third highest incidence and the third highest cause of death from cancer among both men and women.[1] Patients with stage III colorectal cancer are dependent on adjuvant chemotherapy for control of their disease.[2]

For more than 40 years, systemic therapy combining fluorouracil, more commonly called 5-FU, and leucovorin had been the main chemotherapy agents for persons with stage III colon cancer. This chemotherapy regimen had afforded, at best, a five-year cure rate of 35%.[3] During the past decade, several new agents have shown efficacy in the treatment of colorectal cancer, improving the median survival of patients with metastatic disease from approximately eight months to 20 months.[4] Infusions of 5-FU and leucovorin form the basis of current combinations with newer drugs, including irinotecan and oxaliplatin (**Table 1**).

In home care, chemotherapy and especially infusion regimens have unique considerations for clinicians. Priorities are planning for the initiation of the infusion, medications given prior to the chemotherapy to prevent side effects, follow-up visits, safety precautions, and patient education. This article covers these newer agents, targeted therapies for colon cancer, and associated nursing and patient implications. Detailed drug information appears in **Table 2**.

Table 1. Examples of Chemotherapy Combinations for Colorectal Cancer

Name	Regimen	Dosing and Schedule
5-FU/LV (Mayo)	Fluorouracil Leucovorin	Leucovorin 20 mg/m^2 IV: days 1–5; 5-FU bolus 370 mg/m^2 IV over 2–4 min: 1 hr after start of leucovorin: days 1–5 Repeat at 4 and 8 wk and q 5 wk after
IFL	Irinotecan Fluorouracil Leucovorin	Irinotecan 125 mg/m^2 IV over 90 min: days 1, 8, 15, 22 Bolus 5-FU 500 mg/m^2 IV: days 1, 8, 15, 22 Leucovorin 20 mg/m^2 IV: days 1, 8, 15, 22 Repeat q 6 wk
FOLFIRI	Fluorouracil Leucovorin Irinotecan	Irinotecan 180 mg/m^2 IV over 90 min: day 1; Leucovorin 200 mg/m^2 IV over 2-hr infusion during irinotecan: day 1; 5-FU bolus 400 mg/m^2 IV: day 1 ...followed by: 5-FU 2.4—3.0 g/m^2 continuous infusion IV over 46 hr: days 1 and 2 Repeat q 2 wk
FOLFOX 4	Fluorouracil Leucovorin Oxaliplatin	Leucovorin 200 mg/m^2 IV over 2 hr: days 1 and 2; Oxaliplatin 85 mg/m^2 IV over 2 hr: day 1 5-FU bolus of 400 mg/m^2 IV over 2–4 min and 5-FU infusion of 600 mg/m^2 IV over 22 hr: days 1 and 2 Repeat q 2 wk
FOLFOX 6	Fluorouracil Leucovorin Oxaliplatin	Oxaliplatin 100 mg/m^2 IV over 2 hr: day 1 Leucovorin 200 mg/m^2 IV over 2 hr: day 1 5-FU 400 mg/m^2 IV bolus, then 5-FU 2.4—3.0 g/m^2 IV over 46-hr continuous infusion Repeat q 2 wk
XELIRI or CAPIRI	Xeloda Irinotecan	Xeloda/capecitabine 1000 mg/m^2 PO, BID: days 1–14 then 1 wk of rest for a 3-wk cycle Irinotecan 250 mg/m^2 IV: day 1 Repeat q 3 wk
XELOX or CAPOX	Xeloda Oxaliplatin	Xeloda/capecitabine 1000 mg/m^2 PO, BID: days 1–14 Oxaliplatin 130 mg/m^2 IV over 2 hr: day 1 Repeat every 3 wk

Note. IV = intravenously; PO = by mouth; BID = twice a day

Table 2. New Chemotherapy and Targeted Agents for Colorectal Cancer

Drug Names and Manufacturer	Class and Action	Dose and Administration	Side Effects and Toxicity	Patient Education
Bevacizumab (Avastin); Genetech	• Monoclonal antibody • Anti-angiogenesis • Binds to VEGF • Inhibits VEGF-induced angiogenesis • Half-life, 20 days	• 5 mg/kg q 14 days • IV infusion • First dose over 90 min, if tolerated well, 2nd dose over 60 min, reduce to 30 min for further doses. • Mix with normal saline only; dilute in 100 mL normal saline. • Dilute drug stable for 8 hr if refrigerated. Contraindications: • Pediatric patients • Patients with tumors with high likelihood of hemorrhage	Infusion reaction • Chills, fever, rigors, myalgias, allergic reaction GI perforation Cardiovascular • Hypertension • Thromboemboli • Bleeding Proteinuria Delays wound healing	Safety • Refrigerate • Protect from light • Do not shake or freeze Cardiovascular • Monitor blood pressure prior to every dose and weekly • Assess for edema, pain in abdomen, leg or thigh, chest or shoulder pain, shortness of breath, hemoptysis, visual changes, lightheadedness • Caution in head/neck cancer. • Proteinuria • Monitor serial urine analysis

Capecitabine (Xeloda); Roche Laboratories	• Antimetabolite
	• Inhibits DNA and RNA synthesis
	• Converted to 5-FU at tumor site
	• Absorbed through GI tract
		• 1000–1250 mg/m²
		• PO: swallow whole
		• BID: 12 hr apart
		• Days 1–14 followed by 7 days of rest
		Repeat q 3 wk.
		Give in am and pm with glass of water and 30 min after a meal.
		Increases warfarin levels, phenytoin, folic acid.
		Antacids decrease absorption of drug.
			GI: diarrhea, stomatitis, mild nausea
			Hand-and-foot syndrome
			Hyperbilirubin
			Paraesthesia
			Fatigue
			Bone marrow: anemia
				Safety
				• Store at room temperature
				• Handle pills with gloves
				• Use excretion precautions for 5–7 days throughout treatment cycle
				GI
				• Track number of diarrhea episodes and amount
				• Report diarrhea >5 per day to MD
				• Increase fluid intake
				• Check nausea, especially in elderly; if nausea/vomiting > 3 per day, call MD
				• Eat small meals, bland foods
				• Oral care
				Hand-and-foot syndrome
				• Baseline skin assessment, prior to each cycle and every visit
				• Report tingling, redness, tenderness, numbness or pain on palms of hand or feet
				  • Protect skin from hot/cold weather
				  • Tepid or cool shower
				  • Avoid constrictive clothing, gloves, socks, and so forth
				  • Caution with sharp utensils, tools, and so forth; reduce friction
				• Use mild soap
				• Keep hands moist
				• Consider use of pyridoxine (vitamin B_6)
				• Bag balm

continued on following page

Table 2. (continued from previous page)

Drug Names and Manufacturer	Class and Action	Dose and Administration	Side Effects and Toxicity	Patient Education
Cetuximab (Erbitux); Imclone Systems, Bristol-Myers Squibb	• Monoclonal antibody • Binds to EGFR, blocks ability of EGFR to initiate receptor activation and signal tumor growth, invasions, or cell repair	• Initial dose 400 mg/m² (IV) over 2 hr • Subsequent doses 250 mg/m² (IV) over 1 hr q wk until disease progression • Maximum rate of 5 mL/min • Requires in-line filter, non-PVC bag and tubing • Premedication: diphenhydramine 50 mg IV • Observe patient for 1 hr postinfusion	Hypersensitivity reactions • Grade 1–2: reduce infusion rate by 50% • Grade 3–4: stop drug immediately and permanently Integument • Acne-like rash during first 3 wk of treatment • Rash resolves in 1–2 mo after drug stopped	Safety • Refrigerate • Do not freeze or shake Integument • Assess skin frequently during beginning of treatment • Assess need for pain medication • Assess need for topical or PO antibiotic; clindamycin
Irinotecan (Camptosar); Pfizer	Inhibits topoisomerase to cause double-strand DNA changes	• 125 mg/m² IV over 90 min • Given weekly X 4 wk, followed by 2-wk rest period. • Very acidic: dilute in 500 mL of D5W. • Contraindicated in patients with bone marrow depression, decreased hepatic function, existing infection, pulmonary disease.	Myelosuppression: neutropenia, alopecia, moderate nausea, strong irritant • Early diarrhea occurs in 1st 24 hr of administration: cholinergic; precipitated by abdominal cramping or diaphoresis. • Treated with IV atropine: 0.25–1.0 mg • Late-onset diarrhea (after 24 hr–12 days) occurs in 80% of patients; dose-limiting toxicity; may be life-threatening. • Treat with loperamide; 4 mg at onset, then 2 mg q 2 hr until diarrhea subsides for 12 hr.	Safety: Store at room temperature; protect from light Diarrhea • Reinforce need for patient to report and record diarrhea immediately • Increase fluids • Recommend bland, lowfat diet Patient should have prescription for loperamide for diarrhea prophylactically.

FAMILIAR CHEMOTHERAPY AGENTS

Fluorouracil (5-FU)

Fluorouracil remains the consistent ingredient within old and new colon cancer chemotherapy combinations. Although 5-FU is well known, a word of caution follows. When given alone, fluorouracil has a mild side effect profile with mild gastrointestinal effects, mild myelosuppression, and no alopecia. Generally, 5-FU is well tolerated by patients. However, 5-FU commonly is given with leucovorin.

Leucovorin is a potent biologic modulator that increases the entry of 5-FU into both cancer cells and normal cells, producing an increase in the frequency and severity of side effects of 5-FU. The patient and family require education about the potential for nausea, stomatitis, loose stools and/or diarrhea, and the risk for infection. Hand-and-foot syndrome is an additional side effect of 5-FU when the drug is given via infusion, and special precautions are necessary. The knowledge and experience of working with 5-FU remains applicable to many of the newer chemotherapy regimens containing the 5-FU and leucovorin combination.

Table 2. *(continued from previous page)*

Drug Names and Manufacturer	Class and Action	Dose and Administration	Side Effects and Toxicity	Patient Education
Oxaliplatin (Eloxatin); Sanofi-Synthelabo	• Third-generation platin • Inhibits DNA synthesis and repair; promotes cellular apoptosis • Excretion through kidneys • Binds to protein	• 85–100 mg/m^2 • Two-week cycle • IV bolus for 1–2 days or 2- to 6-hr infusion in 250–500 mL of dextrose only • Give prior to 5-FU • Can give simultaneously with leucovorin in dextrose • Vesicant? • Avoid aluminum products • Incompatible with diazepam Premedication • 5HT3 anti-emetic • Dexamethasone, 10–20 mg Sequence of Administration 1. Premedications 2. Flush with D5W 3. Oxaliplatin 4. Flush with D5W 5. 5-FU Rate adjustment • If infusion reaction (including erythematic) of hands and face, hives, chest tightness, dyspnea...slow rate to 6-hr infusion • Next administrations include antihistamine and corticosteroid with premedications; administer over 6 hr.	Neurotoxicity • Acute onset: pain, burning in arm or throat, tongue numbness, tightness in throat, inability to get air (usually cold induced) • Acute onset: occurs during infusion or as late as 5–7 days after drug is administered • Calcium or magnesium infusion during infusion may decrease neurotoxicity • Late onset: cumulative peripheral sensory neuropathy, especially with total dose >800 mg/m^2; appears as dysesthesia of hands and feet • Late onset: occurs after 10–12 cycles, presents as stocking glove distribution • Recovery from neurotoxicity in 3–4 mo after drug is stopped GI • Mild nausea • Diarrhea • Mucositis Bone marrow: • Mild thrombocytopenia • Mild neutropenia	Neurotoxicity • Assess baseline functional and neurocheck, especially fine motor dexterity of hands: writing, holding objects, buttoning clothing, picking up coins, and so forth. Reassess every cycle or visit. • Acute onset: teach patient to avoid cold objects and cold beverages or food for 2–4 days after drug; drink warm beverages; dress warmly; use pot holders or gloves. • Late onset: reassess neuro/functional status; protect hands and feet from weather extremes and sharp objects or tools; dress warmly.

Note. VEGF = vascular endothelial growth factor; EGFR = epidermal growth factor receptor; IV = intravenously; 5-FU = 5-fluorouracil; GI = gastrointestinal; PO = by mouth; BID = twice a day; MD = doctor; PVC = polyvinylchloride; D5W = dextrose 5% in water; 5HT3 = serotonin receptor. Full prescribing information is available at: http://www.xeloda.com; http://www.eloxatin.com/hcp/pi/asp; http://www.fda.gov.cder/foi/label/2004/1250841bl.pdf; and http://www.pfizer.com/download/uspi_camptosar.pdf.

NEW CHEMOTHERAPY AGENTS FOR COLON CANCER

Irinotecan (Camptosar, CPT-11)

Irinotecan is an agent that inhibits the enzyme topoisomerase to stop DNA synthesis. It has indications for use in metastatic colon cancer.[5] Nausea/vomiting, anorexia, mucositis, and grade 3 or 4 diarrhea are the main untoward effects on the gastrointestinal tract. The drug causes early- and late-onset diarrhea, which can be dose limiting.

Early-onset diarrhea occurs within the first 24 hours of administration and is generally cholinergic.

Late-onset diarrhea has symptoms of watery or poorly formed stool, increase in bowel movements, and late abdominal cramping.

A thorough nursing assessment of the patient's baseline bowel status is followed by thorough patient education regarding the management of diarrhea. A proactive pharmaceutical plan to control diarrhea typically is needed.

Table 3. Summary of Safe Drug-Handling Guidelines for the Home Setting

	Oral Route	Parenteral Route
Drug handling	• Wear gloves • Do not crush tablets or open capsules • Unit dose package sealed in plastic bag	• Wear gloves and gown • Face shield or goggles as needed for splashing • Four x four gauze for use around injection port • Disposable plastic-backed wrapper
Drug disposal	Sealable hazardous drug waste container	Puncture-resistant sharps container labeled for hazardous waste only
Drug spills	Wear gloves, place in sealable plastic bag	• Spill kit in home • Wear gown, double glove • Wear mask if aerosol spill • Wear face shield if liquid spill • Use absorbent pad to absorb spill • Dispose of all contaminated equipment in drug disposal or hazardous waste container
Body fluids	• Standard precautions for 48 hr following drug administration: wear gloves, wash hands when handling body wastes • Double flush toilets with lids down • Use of toilets rather than urinals or bedpan	Same
Skin exposure	• Wash hands with soap and water	• Wash skin immediately with soap and water • Flush eyes for 15 min with water or isotonic solution
Soiled linens	• Wear gloves • Double wash soiled linens separately	Same

Note. Data from *Safe Handling of Hazardous Drugs,* by B. Povolich, C. Lecher, E. Glynn-Tucker, M. McDiamid, & S. Newton, 2003, Pittsburgh: Oncology Nursing Society. Copyright 2003 by the Oncology Nursing Society.

Capecitabine (Xeloda)

Capecitabine is a prodrug of fluorouracil. It is an oral fluoropyrimidine and converts to the drug fluorouracil after it is absorbed through the gastrointestinal tract. Capecitabine is considered tumor selective in that one enzyme needed for the conversion to fluorouracil is found in higher concentrations among tumors. It permits a sustained exposure to fluorouracil, creating a steady state or drug level similar to that produced by infu-sional fluorouracil.[6] Capecitabine currently is indicated as single-agent therapy in the first-line treatment of metastatic colon cancer when fluorouracil alone is needed.[7,8]

Capecitabine is an oral agent that eliminates the need for a central line catheter and ambulatory infusion pump needed for the traditional infusion of 5-FU. Capecitabine is a cytotoxic drug that requires the safe handling precautions outlined by the Oncology Nursing Society (**Table 3**).

The capecitabine side effect profile mimics that seen with infusional fluorouracil, including diarrhea, stomatitis, anorexia, and hand-and-foot syndrome or palmar plantar erythrodysesthesia. Anemia and fatigue also are common, but neutropenia and thrombocytopenia are uncommon. Irinotecan also produces a cholinergic syndrome, characterized by rhinor

Table 4. Example of Oxaliplatin Scheduling: FOLFOX 4

Day 1		Day 2	
Leucovorin, 200 mg/m²	*5-FU bolus:* 400 mg/m² followed by *5-FU infusion:* 600 mg/m²	Leucovorin, 200 mg/m²	*5-FU bolus:* 400 mg/m² followed by *5-FU infusion:* 600 mg/m²
Oxaliplatin, 85 mg/m²	22-hr infusion →	2-hr infusion →	22-hr infusion →
2-hr infusion →			

Note. 5-FU = 5-fluorouracil.

rhea, lacrimation, increased salivation, nausea and vomiting, diaphoresis, flushing, and nasal congestion occurring shortly after infusion.

Oxaliplatin (Eloxatin)

Oxaliplatin is a third-generation platinum agent, following cisplatin and carboplatin. Oxaliplatin:
- inhibits DNA synthesis
- is indicated in first- and second-line treatment of metastatic colon cancer[9]
- is part of multiple chemotherapy combinations used for metastatic colon cancer, and is administered into the largest peripheral vein possible during a period of two to six hours. A warm compress above the insertion site may help reduce vein irritation during the infusion.

Dextrose is the only solvent permitted with oxaliplatin because normal saline will degrade oxaliplatin.[10] Thus, adequate flushing with a dextrose-based solution is required before and between drugs. A particular challenge to the home care nurse is the timing of home visits because of the administration schedule for oxaliplatin. **Table 4** lists examples of combinations using oxaliplatin and the timed sequence of administration. Home visits must be arranged accordingly.

Advantages of oxaliplatin include
- a milder side effect profile with only mild emetogenicity
- no delayed nausea or vomiting
- no myelosuppression, nephrotoxicity, ototoxicity, or alopecia.

Neurotoxicity is the main dose-limiting toxicity. The acute form of neurotoxicity occurs in as many as 85% to 95% of patients[11] and more frequently after approximately 10 to 12 cycles. It presents as a cold-induced dysesthesia of the hands, feet, or throat.[12] Chronic or late-onset neurotoxicity occurs as a sensory peripheral neuropathy when total doses of oxaliplatin approach 800 mg/m².[13] Several pharmacologic agents are used to manage neurotoxicity, such as antiepileptic drugs, calcium-magnesium, amifostine, alpha-lipoic acid, and glutathione.

NOVEL AGENTS: TARGETED THERAPY FOR COLON CANCER

Targeted therapies are systemic biologic agents with a specific molecular target in cancer cells. Monoclonal antibodies that target specific antigens are the new hope in the fight against cancer.[14]

In colon cancer, two monoclonal antibodies are reported to be effective: bevacizumab and cetuximab. These drugs are designed to focus on a specific antigen or receptor or growth factor on the surface of the cell. By directing the action to the cancer cell alone, the new drug will affect cancer cells without harming normal cells.

Angiogenesis or the formation of new blood vessels is a second destination for targeted therapies. A tumor's ability to perform angiogenesis directly impacts its growth and metastasis. Specific growth factors, such as vascular endothelial growth factor (VEGF), are found to begin the angiogenesis process. New chemotherapy agents that block angiogenesis are thought to be the fifth cancer treatment modality.[15]

Bevacizumab (Avastin)

Bevacizumab is a monoclonal antibody with action directed at VEGF. VEGF is responsible for embryogenesis, wound healing, and follicular development, and it promotes blood vessel formation. It is an important factor in tumor growth and in the tumor's ability to metastasize via the newly formed blood vessels.

Bevacizumab is an antiangiogenic agent that binds to VEGF to reduce microvascular growth and inhibit progress of metastatic disease.[16] It has shown promising first-line clinical activity in the treatment of metastatic colon cancer with 5-FU-based regimens, resulting in statistically significant improvements in overall progression-free survival and response rates.[17]

Various combinations of bevacizumab pose complex administration issues, such as compatibility of agents, diluents, sequencing, and duration of infusion. For example, bevacizumab must be diluted only with normal saline, never dextrose. Yet oxaliplatin requires use of only dextrose, never saline. Thus, adequate flushing between drugs or the use of multiple lines must be considered.

Patients need to be prepared for the length of clinic visits. The administration of the initial dose of bevacizumab requires 90 minutes to avoid a hypersensitivity reaction. If the patient tolerates the first dose, subsequent infusion times are 60 minutes and eventually 30 minutes.

Gastrointestinal perforation and wound healing complications, hypertension, and bleeding are the most important safety considerations in the use of bevacizumab. Other adverse effects are thrombosis, proteinuria, asthenia, pain, diarrhea, leukopenia, and stomatitis.

Cetuximab (Erbitux)

Cetuximab is the first monoclonal antibody that binds specifically to the epidermal growth factor (EGFR) on both normal and cancer cells. EGFR is responsible for tumor growth and metastasis. It promotes cell growth and replication and enhances angiogenesis.[18,19] Cetuximab inhibits these proliferation signals and enhances the sensitivity of tumors to chemotherapy.

Cetuximab is indicated for the treatment of EGFR-positive metastatic colorectal carcinoma for patients who have experienced relapse or are intolerant to irinotecan-based chemotherapy. The effectiveness of cetuximab is based solely on objective response rates. Currently, no data are available that demonstrate an improvement in disease-related symptoms or increased survival rates.

Cetuximab is given as a single agent or in combination with irinotecan. Common side effects include asthenia/malaise, diarrhea, nausea, abdominal pain, and vomiting. The most serious adverse reactions associated with cetuximab are infusion reaction; pulmonary toxicity, such as interstitial lung disease or pulmonary emboli; dermatologic toxicity; dehydration; fever; sepsis; and kidney failure. Fever and headache usually occur within the first 24 hours but resolve with acetaminophen use. Nausea is mild or non-existent.

Cetuximab carries the possibility of an infusion reaction. Grade 3 to 4 infusion reactions occur in about 3% of patients requiring premedication with an H1 antagonist such as diphenhydramine. These infusion reactions are characterized by rapid onset of bronchospasm, stridor, hoarseness, urticaria, and hypotension. Severe infusion reactions require immediate and permanent discontinuation of cetuximab therapy. Direct observation for a minimum of one hour is recommended for each infusion.

Appropriate medical therapy, including epinephrine, corticosteroids, IV antihistamines, bronchodilators, and oxygen should be available when the drug is given. The possibility of infusion reactions, especially with the first infusion, contraindicates the use of the home as an appropriate setting for use of this drug.

Cetuximab is known for causing an acne-form rash in almost all patients within the first three weeks of treatment. The rash consists of macular pustules most commonly found on the face, upper chest, and back.

Grade 1 rash is considered mild and is characterized by eruptions or erythema without symptoms. There is no change in treatment.

Grade 2 rash consisting of eruptions with pruritus covering less than 50% of the body surface is also well tolerated without a change in treatment. In both grades 1 and 2, the rash resolves without scarring one to two months after the treatment is complete.

Grade 3 rash, which covers more than 50% of the body surface area with pain or erosion of the skin, often causes a treatment delay of two consecutive weeks. No change in the dose is needed if the rash returns to a status of grade 2 or less.

Grade 4 rash involves exfoliation, dermatitis, or ulceration, requiring that use of the drug be stopped. The rash is treated with topical and/or oral antibiotics. Topical corticosteroids are not recommended.

RECENT INQUIRIES: CHEMOTHERAPY IN THE ELDERLY AND MANAGEMENT OF HEPATIC METASTASES

The treatment of colon cancer in the elderly (those older than 70 years of age) is an area of attention. Aging can affect the pharmacokinetics of chemotherapy, including drug absorption, distribution, elimination, and metabolism.[20] The option of administering chemotherapy in the elderly is determined after weighing the degree of comorbid conditions and the patient's performance status.

In general, recent literature suggests that there is no evidence of increased rates of nausea/vomiting, stomatitis, or diarrhea in patients 70 to 80 years of age who are treated with fluorouracil and leucovorin.[21,22] Thus, age itself, without the presence of

Two Specific Syndromes Associated with Capecitabine

- **Hand-and-foot syndrome.** Symptoms to assess for hand-and-foot syndrome (palmar-plantar erythrodysesthesia) include redness, pain, numbness and tingling, scaling, and swelling in the palms of the hands or soles of the feet. Patient instructions include:
  - protect the hands and feet from extreme weather temperatures, hot showers, and hot/cold utensils
  - keep hands and feet moist; use mild soap, bag balm
  - consider using pyridoxine.

- **Cholinergic syndrome** is noted by runny nose (rhinorrhea), excess tearing (lacrimation), excess salivation, and diaphoresis.

- *Monitoring for bone marrow suppression consists of awareness of decreased blood counts, such as:*
  - Neutropenia: decreased white blood cell count and specifically neutrophils, which fight infection. An absolute neutrophil count of less than 1,000/mm³ places a patient at high risk for infection. Patient instructions need to emphasize good hand washing and hygiene, avoiding crowds or persons with upper respiratory tract infections, and safe cooking practices. Patients are to report fevers (temperature greater than 100.5 degrees), signs of upper respiratory tract infection, open wounds, headaches, and redness, pain, or tenderness around central line catheters.
  - Thrombocytopenia: decreased platelet count of less than 150,000 cells/mm³. Patients are at high risk for bleeding and need to report bleeding from any orifice, petechiae, headaches, shortness of breath, abdominal pain, dizziness, and blurred vision.

comorbid conditions, does not preclude the use of chemotherapy in patients with colon cancer.

The liver is a site of life-threatening colorectal cancer metastasis. The delivery of chemotherapy directly to the liver, called hepatic arterial infusion, is being explored again in clinical trials.[23] Hepatic arterial infusion exposes cancer cells to high concentrations of chemotherapy while sparing normal liver cells. Chemotherapy agents administered by this route include cisplatin, 5-FU, oxaliplatin, irinotecan, and others.

Early data show significantly improved rates of overall, median, and progression-free survival.[24] Patient and caregiver education centers on the use of a pump, access device, and assessing complications such as infection, bleeding, and thrombosis. Hepatic arterial infusion does affect quality-of-life components with activity restrictions, changes in sleep patterns, and body image disturbances.

Drug Administration Highlights

- **Bevacizumab** is mixed with normal saline only, never dextrose! The first infusion is given slowly during a period of 90 minutes.
- **Capecitabine** is taken orally with full glass of water 30 minutes after a meal.
- **Cetuximab** requires an in-line filter and non-PVC tubing and bag. Administer diphenhydramine before administration of cetuximab and observe for infusion reaction.
- **Irinotecan** will cause early onset diarrhea requiring use of atropine to avoid dehydration.
- **Oxaliplatin** is mixed only with dextrose, never saline!

NURSING IMPLICATIONS: A SUMMARY

With the use of newer agents to fight colon cancer, particular attention must be given to drug administration, scheduling of drugs, home visits, follow-up assessments, caregiver instructions, and physician communications. Key points for drug administration include the following:

- Close attention must be given to the necessary solvents, tubing required, flushing sequence, and risk for infusion reactions.
- The flow of the sequencing of drugs within any given combination will dictate timing of nursing visits, length of nursing visit, and appropriate timing for follow-up calls.
- Key differences in patient and family education regarding expected side effects and signs of toxicity should be noted between conventional chemotherapy agents and targeted therapies.
- Newer agents are associated with less familiar side effects, and additional education for the patient and caregiver is needed.
- Communication with patients, care-givers, and physicians is vital. Patients and caregivers may not consider a rash or other less common reaction to be abnormal, but drug doses may need to be delayed or altered, depending on the severity of reaction.
- The follow-through of patients in taking oral medications such as capecitabine is another area for home care assessment. Research has suggested that as many as 43% of patients are not compliant with prescribed medications.[25] Medication knowledge, cost, polypharmacy, and resulting side effects are among the factors to evaluate.
- Finally, although not cytotoxic, newer agents are classified as bio-hazardous drugs. Therefore, safety principles regarding drug storage, handling, and precautions with patient excretions are still necessary (**Table 3**).

Patients with colon cancer now have a wide selection of chemotherapy regimens. These new regimens bring new hope for increases in survival rates. For home care clinicians, expansion of our knowledge of these new drugs will assist patients to complete the recommended therapy and maintain their quality of life throughout the process.

REFERENCES

1. American Cancer Society. Cancer facts & figures 2004. Retrieved September 10, 2004 from *http://www.cancer.org*.
2. Jemal A, Tiwari RC, Murray T, et al. Cancer statistics, 2004. *CA Cancer J Clin*. 2004;54:8-29.
3. Abbruzzese J. An annual review of gastrointestinal cancers. *Oncol News Int*. 2004;13 (3), Suppl 1.
4. Gill S, Goldberg RM. First-line treatment strategies to improve survival in patients with advanced colorectal cancer. *Drugs*. 2004;64:27-44.
5. Grothey A, Sargent D, Goldberg RM, et al. Survival of patients with advanced colorectal cancer improves with the availability of fluorouracil-leucovorin, irinotecan, and oxaliplatin in the course of treatment. *J Clin Oncol*. 2004; 22:1209-1214.
6. Birner A. Pharmacology of oral chemotherapy agents. *Clin J Oncol Nurs*. 2003;7 (6) Suppl:11-20.
7. Cassidy J, Tabernero J, Twelves C, et al. XELOX: Active first line therapy for patients with metastatic colorectal cancer. *J Clin Oncol*. 2004;22:2084-2091.
8. Simpson D, Dunn C, Curran M, et al. Oxaliplatin: A review of its use in combination therapy for advanced metastatic colorectal cancer. *Drugs*. 2003;63:2127-2156.
9. Pelley RJ. Oxaliplatin: A new agent for colorectal cancer. *Curr Oncol Rep*. 2001;3:147-155.
10. Sorich J, Taubes B, Wagner A, et al. Oxaliplatin: Practical guidelines for administration. *Clin J Oncol Nurs*. 2004; 18:251-255.
11. Armand JP, Boige V, Raymond E, et al. Oxaliplatin in colorectal cancer: an overview. *Semin Oncol*. 2000;27:96-104.
12. Barhamand B. Management of pharyngolaryngeal dysesthesia associated with oxaliplatin therapy. *Clin J Oncol Nurs*. 2003;7:452-453.
13. Berg D. Oxaliplatin: A novel platinum analog with activity in colorectal cancer. *Oncol Nurs Forum*. 2003;30:957-966.
14. National Cancer Institute, NCI. Cancer dictionary. Accessed September 10, 2004 at *http://www.cancer.gov/dictionary*.
15. Camp-Sorrell D. Antiangiogenesis: The fifth cancer treatment modality. *Oncol Nurs Forum*. 2003;30:934-944.
16. Kerbel R, Fulkman J. Clinical translation of angiogenesis inhibitors. *Natl Rev Cancer*. 2002;26:727-739.
17. Hurwitz H, Fehrenbacher L, Novotny W, et al. Bevacizumab plus irinotecan, fluorouracil and leucovorin for metastatic colon cancer. *N Engl J Med*. 2004;350:2335-2342.
18. Ellis LM, Hoff PM. Targeting the epidermal growth factor receptor: An important incremental step in the battle against colorectal cancer. *J Clin Oncol*. 2004;22:1177-1179.
19. Krozely P. Epidermal growth factor receptor tyrosine kinase inhibitors: Evolving role in treatment of solid tumors. *Clin J Oncol Nurs*. 2004;8:163-168.
20. Veena J, Mashru S, Lichtman S. Pharmacologic factors influencing anticancer drug selection in the elderly. *Drugs & Aging*. 2003;20:737-759.
21. Arora A, Potter J. Older patients with colon cancer: Is adjuvant chemotherapy safe and effective? *J Am Geriatr Soc*. 2003; 51:567-569.
22. Sargent D, Goldberg R, Jacobsen S, et al. A polled analysis of adjuvant chemotherapy for resectable colon cancer in elderly patients. *N Engl J Med*. 2001;345:1091-1097.
23. Barber FD, Fabugais-Nazario LE. What's old is new again: Patients receiving hepatic arterial infusion chemotherapy. *Clin J Oncol Nurs*. 2003;7:647-652.
24. Blair SL, Grant M, Chu DZ, et al. Quality of life in patients with colorectal metastasis and intrahepatic chemotherapy. *Ann Surg Oncol*. 2003;10:144-149.
25. Hartigan K. Patient education: The cornerstone of successful oral chemotherapy treatment. *Clin J Oncol Nurs*. 2003;7 (6) Suppl:21-24.

SECTION V
PATIENT EDUCATION

COLON CANCER (PDQ®): TREATMENT PATIENT VERSION

GENERAL INFORMATION ABOUT COLON CANCER

Colon cancer is a disease in which malignant (cancer) cells form in the tissues of the colon.

The colon is part of the body's digestive system. The digestive system removes and processes nutrients (vitamins, minerals, carbohydrates, fats, proteins, and water) from foods and helps pass waste material out of the body. The digestive system is made up of the esophagus, stomach, and the small and large intestines. The first six feet of the large intestine are called the large bowel or colon. The last six inches are the rectum and the anal canal. The anal canal ends at the anus (the opening of the large intestine to the outside of the body).

Age and health history can affect the risk of developing colon cancer.

Risk factors include the following:
- Age 50 or older.
- A family history of cancer of the colon or rectum.
- A personal history of cancer of the colon, rectum, ovary, endometrium, or breast.
- A history of polyps in the colon.
- A history of ulcerative colitis (ulcers in the lining of the large intestine) or Crohn's disease.
- Certain hereditary conditions, such as familial adenomatous polyposis and hereditary nonpolyposis colon cancer (HNPCC; Lynch Syndrome).

Possible signs of colon cancer include a change in bowel habits or blood in the stool.

These and other symptoms may be caused by colon cancer. Other conditions may cause the same symptoms. A doctor should be consulted if any of the following problems occur:
- A change in bowel habits.
- Blood (either bright red or very dark) in the stool.
- Diarrhea, constipation, or feeling that the bowel does not empty completely.
- Stools that are narrower than usual.
- Frequent gas pains, bloating, fullness, or cramps.
- Weight loss for no known reason.
- Feeling very tired.
- Vomiting.

Tests that examine the rectum, rectal tissue, and blood are used to detect (find) and diagnose colon cancer.

The following tests and procedures may be used:

- Physical exam and history: An exam of the body to check general signs of health, including checking for signs of disease, such as lumps or anything else that seems unusual. A history of the patient's health habits and past illnesses and treatments will also be taken.
- Fecal occult blood test: A test to check stool (solid waste) for blood that can only be seen with a microscope. Small samples of stool are placed on special cards and returned to the doctor or laboratory for testing.
- Digital rectal exam: An exam of the rectum. The doctor or nurse inserts a lubricated, gloved finger into the rectum to feel for lumps or anything else that seems unusual.
- Barium enema: A series of x-rays of the lower gastrointestinal tract. A liquid that contains barium (a silver-white metallic compound) is put into the rectum. The barium coats the lower gastrointestinal tract and x-rays are taken. This procedure is also called a lower GI series.
- Sigmoidoscopy: A procedure to look inside the rectum and sigmoid (lower) colon for polyps, abnormal areas, or cancer. A sigmoidoscope (a thin, lighted tube) is inserted through the rectum into the sigmoid colon. Polyps or tissue samples may be taken for biopsy.
- Colonoscopy: A procedure to look inside the rectum and colon for polyps, abnormal areas, or cancer.

A colonoscope (a thin, lighted tube) is inserted through the rectum into the colon. Polyps or tissue samples may be taken for biopsy.

- Biopsy: The removal of cells or tissues so they can be viewed under a microscope to check for signs of cancer.
- Virtual colonoscopy: A procedure that uses a series of x-rays called computed tomography to make a series of pictures of the colon. A computer puts the pictures together to create detailed images that may show polyps and anything else that seems unusual on the inside surface of the colon. This test is also called colonography or CT colonography.

Certain factors affect prognosis (chance of recovery) and treatment options.

The prognosis (chance of recovery) depends on the following:

- The stage of the cancer (whether the cancer is in the inner lining of the colon only, involves the whole colon, or has spread to other places in the body).
- Whether the cancer has blocked or created a hole in the colon.
- The blood levels of carcinoembryonic antigen (CEA; a substance in the blood that may be increased when cancer is present) before treatment begins.
- Whether the cancer has recurred.
- The patient's general health.

Treatment options depend on the following:

- The stage of the cancer.
- Whether the cancer has recurred.
- The patient's general health.

TAGES OF COLON CANCER

After colon cancer has been diagnosed, tests are done to find out if cancer cells have spread within the colon or to other parts of the body.

The process used to find out if cancer has spread within the colon or to other parts of the body is called staging. The information gathered from the staging process determines the stage of the disease. It is important to know the stage in order to plan treatment. The following tests and procedures may be used in the staging process:

CT scan (CAT scan): A procedure that makes a series of detailed pictures of areas inside the body, taken from different angles. The pictures are made by a computer linked to an x-ray machine. A dye may be injected into a vein or swallowed to help the organs or tissues show up more clearly. This procedure is also called computed tomography, computerized tomography, or computerized axial tomography.

• Lymph node biopsy: The removal of all or part of a lymph node. A pathologist views the tissue under a microscope to look for cancer cells.

• Complete blood count (CBC): A procedure in which a sample of blood is drawn and checked for the following:
  – the number of red blood cells, white blood cells, and platelets.
  – the amount of hemoglobin (the protein that carries oxygen) in the red blood cells.
  – the portion of the blood sample made up of red blood cells.

• Carcinoembryonic antigen (CEA) assay: A test that measures the level of CEA in the blood. CEA is released into the bloodstream from both cancer cells and normal cells. When found in higher than normal amounts, it can be a sign of colon cancer or other conditions.

• MRI (magnetic resonance imaging): A procedure that uses a magnet, radio waves, and a computer to make a series of detailed pictures of areas inside the colon. A substance called gadolinium is injected into the patient through a vein. The gadolinium collects around the cancer cells so they show up brighter in the picture. This procedure is also called nuclear magnetic resonance imaging (NMRI).

• Chest x-ray: An x-ray of the organs and bones inside the chest. An x-ray is a type of energy beam that can go through the body and onto film, making a picture of areas inside the body.

• Surgery: A procedure to remove the tumor and see how far it has spread through the colon.

The following stages are used for colon cancer:

Stage 0 (carcinoma in situ)

In stage 0, the cancer is found only in the innermost lining of the colon. Stage 0 cancer is also called carcinoma in situ.

Stage I

In stage I, the cancer has spread beyond the innermost tissue layer of the colon wall to the middle layers. Stage I colon cancer is sometimes called Dukes' A colon cancer.

Stage II

Stage II colon cancer is divided into stage IIA and stage IIB.

- Stage IIA: Cancer has spread beyond the middle tissue layers of the colon wall or has spread to nearby tissues around the colon or rectum.
- Stage IIB: Cancer has spread beyond the colon wall into nearby organs and/or through the peritoneum.

Stage II colon cancer is sometimes called Dukes' B colon cancer.

Stage III

Stage III colon cancer is divided into stage IIIA, stage IIIB, and stage IIIC.

- Stage IIIA: Cancer has spread from the innermost tissue layer of the colon wall to the middle layers and has spread to as many as three lymph nodes.
- Stage IIIB: Cancer has spread to as many as three nearby lymph nodes and has spread:
  - beyond the middle tissue layers of the colon wall; or
  - to nearby tissues around the colon or rectum; or
  - beyond the colon wall into nearby organs and/or through the peritoneum.
- Stage IIIC: Cancer has spread to four or more nearby lymph nodes and has spread:
  - to or beyond the middle tissue layers of the colon wall; or
  - to nearby tissues around the colon or rectum; or
  - to nearby organs and/or through the peritoneum.

Stage III colon cancer is sometimes called Dukes' C colon cancer.

Stage IV

In stage IV, cancer may have spread to nearby lymph nodes and has spread to other parts of the body, such as the liver or lungs. Stage IV colon cancer is sometimes called Dukes' D colon cancer.

RECURRENT COLON CANCER

Recurrent colon cancer is cancer that has recurred (come back) after it has been treated. The cancer may come back in the colon or in other parts of the body, such as the liver, lungs, or both.

TREATMENT OPTION OVERVIEW

There are different types of treatment for patients with colon cancer.

Different types of treatment are available for patients with colon cancer. Some treatments are standard (the currently used treatment), and some are being tested in clinical trials. Before starting treatment, patients may want to think about taking part in a clinical trial. A treatment clinical trial is a research study meant to help improve current treatments or obtain information on new treatments for patients with cancer. When clinical trials show that a new treatment is better than the standard treatment, the new treatment may become the standard treatment.

Three types of standard treatment are used. These include the following:

Surgery

Surgery (removing the cancer in an operation) is the most common reatment for all stages of colon cancer. doctor may remove the cancer using ne of the following types of surgery:

Local excision: If the cancer is found at a very early stage, the doctor may remove it without cutting through the abdominal wall. Instead, the doctor may put a tube through the rectum into the colon and cut the cancer out. This is called a local excision. If the cancer is found in a polyp (a small bulging piece of tissue), the operation is called a polypectomy.

Resection: If the cancer is larger, the doctor will perform a partial colectomy (removing the cancer and a small amount of healthy tissue around it). The doctor may then perform an anastomosis (sewing the healthy parts of the colon together). The doctor will also usually remove lymph nodes near the colon and examine them under a microscope to see whether they contain cancer.

- Resection and colostomy: If the doctor is not able to sew the two ends of the colon back together, a stoma (an opening) is made on the outside of the body for waste to pass through. This procedure is called a colostomy. A bag is placed around the stoma to collect the waste. Sometimes the colostomy is needed only until the lower colon has healed, and then it can be reversed. If the doctor needs to remove the entire lower colon, however, the colostomy may be permanent.

- Radiofrequency ablation: The use of a special probe with tiny electrodes that kill cancer cells. Sometimes the probe is inserted directly through the skin and only local anesthesia is needed. In other cases, the probe is inserted through an incision in the abdomen. This is done in the hospital with general anesthesia.

- Cryosurgery: A treatment that uses an instrument to freeze and destroy abnormal tissue, such as carcinoma in situ. This type of treatment is also called cryotherapy.

Even if the doctor removes all the cancer that can be seen at the time of the operation, some patients may be given chemotherapy or radiation therapy after surgery to kill any cancer cells that are left. Treatment given after the surgery, to increase the chances of a cure, is called adjuvant therapy.

Chemotherapy

Chemotherapy is a cancer treatment that uses drugs to stop the growth of cancer cells, either by killing the cells or by stopping the cells from dividing. When chemotherapy is taken by mouth or injected into a vein or muscle, the drugs enter the bloodstream and can reach cancer cells throughout the body (systemic chemotherapy). When chemotherapy is placed directly into the spinal column, an organ, or a body cavity such as the abdomen, the drugs mainly affect cancer cells in those areas (regional chemotherapy).

Chemoembolization of the hepatic artery may be used to treat cancer that has spread to the liver. This involves blocking the hepatic artery (the main artery that supplies blood to the liver) and injecting anticancer drugs between the blockage and the liver. The liver's arteries then deliver the drugs throughout the liver. Only a small amount of the drug reaches other parts of the body. The blockage may be temporary or permanent, depending on what is used to block the artery. The liver continues to receive some blood from the hepatic portal vein, which carries blood from the stomach and intestine.

The way the chemotherapy is given depends on the type and stage of the cancer being treated.

Radiation therapy

Radiation therapy is a cancer treatment that uses high-energy x-rays or other types of radiation to kill cancer cells. There are two types of radiation therapy. External radiation therapy uses a machine outside the body to send radiation toward the cancer. Internal radiation therapy uses a radioactive substance sealed in needles, seeds, wires, or catheters that are placed directly into or near the cancer. The way the radiation therapy is given depends on the type and stage of the cancer being treated.

Other types of treatment are being tested in clinical trials. These include the following:

Biologic therapy

Biologic therapy is a treatment that uses the patient's immune system to fight cancer. Substances made by the body or made in a laboratory are used to boost, direct, or restore the body's natural defenses against cancer. This type of cancer treatment is also called biotherapy or immunotherapy.

Follow-up exams may help find recurrent colon cancer earlier.

After treatment, a blood test to measure carcinoembryonic antigen (CEA; a substance in the blood that may be increased when colon cancer is present) may be done along with other tests to see if the cancer has come back.

TREATMENT OPTIONS FOR COLON CANCER

Stage 0 Colon Cancer (Carcinoma in Situ)

Treatment of stage 0 (carcinoma in situ) may include the following types of surgery:
- Local excision or simple polypectomy.
- Resection/anastomosis. This is done when the cancerous tissue is too large to remove by local excision.

Stage I Colon Cancer

Treatment of stage I colon cancer is usually resection/anastomosis.

Stage II Colon Cancer

Treatment of stage II colon cancer may include the following:
- Resection/anastomosis.
- Clinical trials of chemotherapy, radiation therapy, or biologic therapy after surgery.

Stage III Colon Cancer

Treatment of stage III colon cancer may include the following:
- Resection/anastomosis with chemotherapy.
- Clinical trials of chemotherapy, radiation therapy, and/or biologic therapy after surgery.

Stage IV and Recurrent Colon Cancer

Treatment of stage IV and recurrent colon cancer may include the following:

- Resection/anastomosis (surgery to remove the cancer or bypass the tumor and join the cut ends of the colon).
- Surgery to remove parts of other organs, such as the liver, lungs, and ovaries, where the cancer may have recurred or spread.
- Radiation therapy or chemotherapy may be offered to some patients as palliative therapy to relieve symptoms and improve quality of life.
- Clinical trials of chemotherapy and/or biologic therapy.

Treatment of locally recurrent colon cancer may be local excision.

Special treatments of cancer that has spread to or recurred in the liver may include the following:

- Radiofrequency ablation or cryosurgery.
- Clinical trials of hepatic chemoembolization with radiation therapy.

Patients whose colon cancer spreads or recurs after initial treatment with chemotherapy may be offered further chemotherapy with a different drug or combination of drugs.

A NOTE ABOUT CLINICAL TRIALS

Clinical trials are taking place in many parts of the country. Information about ongoing clinical trials is available from the NCI Web site. Choosing the most appropriate cancer treatment is a decision that ideally involves the patient, family, and healthcare team.

RECTAL CANCER (PDQ®): TREATMENT PATIENT VERSION

GENERAL INFORMATION ABOUT RECTAL CANCER

Rectal cancer is a disease in which malignant (cancer) cells form in the tissues of the rectum.

The rectum is part of the body's digestive system. The digestive system removes and processes nutrients (vitamins, minerals, carbohydrates, fats, proteins, and water) from foods and helps pass waste material out of the body. The digestive system is made up of the esophagus, stomach, and the small and large intestines. The first six feet of the large intestine are called the large bowel or colon. The last six inches are the rectum and the anal canal. The anal canal ends at the anus (the opening of the large intestine to the outside of the body).

Age and family history can affect the risk of developing rectal cancer.

The following are possible risk factors for rectal cancer:
Age 50 or older.
- A family history of cancer of the colon or rectum.
- A personal history of cancer of the colon, rectum, ovary, endometrium,

or breast.
- A personal history of ulcerative colitis (ulcers in the lining of the large intestine) or Crohn's disease.
- Certain hereditary conditions, such as familial adenomatous polyposis and hereditary nonpolyposis colon cancer (HNPCC; Lynch syndrome).

Possible signs of rectal cancer include a change in bowel habits or blood in the stool.

These and other symptoms may be caused by rectal cancer. Other conditions may cause the same symptoms. A doctor should be consulted if any of the following problems occur:
- A change in bowel habits.
- Blood (either bright red or very dark) in the stool.
- Diarrhea, constipation, or feeling that the bowel does not empty completely.
- Stools that are narrower than usual.
- General abdominal discomfort (frequent gas pains, bloating, fullness, or cramps).
- Weight loss for no known reason.
- Feeling very tired.
- Vomiting.

Tests that examine the rectum and colon are used to detect (find) and diagnose rectal cancer.

Tests used in diagnosing rectal cancer include the following:

- Fecal occult blood test: A test to check stool (solid waste) for blood that can only be seen with a microscope. Small samples of stool are placed on special cards and returned to the doctor or laboratory for testing.
- Digital rectal exam: An exam of the rectum. The doctor or nurse inserts a lubricated, gloved finger into the lower part of the rectum to feel for lumps or anything else that seems unusual.
- Barium enema: A series of x-rays of the lower gastrointestinal tract. A liquid that contains barium (a silver-white metallic compound) is put into the rectum. The barium coats the lower gastrointestinal tract and x-rays are taken. This procedure is also called a lower GI series.
- Sigmoidoscopy: A procedure to look inside the rectum and sigmoid (lower) colon for polyps, abnormal areas, or cancer. A sigmoidoscope (a thin, lighted tube) is inserted through the rectum into the sigmoid colon. Polyps or tissue samples may be taken for biopsy.
- Colonoscopy: A procedure to look inside the rectum and colon for polyps, abnormal areas, or cancer. A colonoscope (a thin, lighted tube) is inserted through the rectum into the colon. Polyps or tissue samples may be taken for biopsy.
- Biopsy: The removal of cells or tissues so they can be viewed under a microscope to check for signs of cancer.

Certain factors affect prognosis (chance of recovery) and treatment options.

The prognosis (chance of recovery) and treatment options depend on the following:

- The stage of the cancer (whether it affects the inner lining of the rectum only, involves the whole rectum, or has spread to other places in the body).
- The patient's general health.
- Whether the cancer has just been diagnosed or has recurred (come back).

STAGES OF RECTAL CANCER

After rectal cancer has been diagnosed, tests are done to find out if cancer cells have spread within the rectum or to other parts of the body.

The process used to find out whether cancer has spread within the rectum or to other parts of the body is called staging. The information gathered from the staging process determines the stage of the disease. It is important to know the stage in order to plan treatment. The following tests and procedures may be used in the staging process:

- Digital rectal exam: An exam of the rectum. The doctor or nurse inserts a lubricated, gloved finger into the lower part of the rectum to feel for lumps or anything else that seems unusual.
- CT scan (CAT scan): A procedure that makes a series of detailed pictures of areas inside the body, taken from different angles. The pictures are made by a computer

linked to an x-ray machine. A dye may be injected into a vein or swallowed to help the organs or tissues show up more clearly. This procedure is also called computed tomography, computerized tomography, or computerized axial tomography.

- MRI (magnetic resonance imaging): A procedure that uses a magnet, radio waves, and a computer to make a series of detailed pictures of areas inside the body. This procedure is also called nuclear magnetic resonance imaging (NMRI).

- Sigmoidoscopy or colonoscopy and biopsy: A procedure to look inside the rectum and colon for polyps, abnormal areas, or cancer. A sigmoidoscope or colonoscope is inserted through the rectum into the colon. Polyps or tissue samples may be taken for biopsy.

- Endoscopic ultrasound (EUS): A procedure in which an endoscope (a thin, lighted tube) is inserted into the body. The endoscope is used to bounce high-energy sound waves (ultrasound) off internal tissues or organs and make echoes. The echoes form a picture of body tissues called a sonogram. This procedure is also called endosonography.

The following stages are used for rectal cancer:

Stage 0 (carcinoma in situ)

In stage 0, cancer is found only in the innermost lining of the rectum. Stage 0 cancer is also called carcinoma in situ.

Stage I

In stage I, cancer has spread beyond the innermost lining of the rectum to the second and third layers and involves the inside wall of the rectum but it has not spread to the outer wall of the rectum or outside the rectum. Stage I rectal cancer is sometimes called Dukes' A rectal cancer.

Stage II

In stage II, cancer has spread outside the rectum to nearby tissue, but it has not gone into the lymph nodes (small bean-shaped structures found throughout the body that filter substances in a fluid called lymph and help fight infection and disease). Stage II rectal cancer is sometimes called Dukes' B rectal cancer.

Stage III

In stage III, cancer has spread to nearby lymph nodes, but it has not spread to other parts of the body. Stage III rectal cancer is sometimes called Dukes' C rectal cancer.

Stage IV

In stage IV, cancer has spread to other parts of the body, such as the liver, lungs, or ovaries. Stage IV rectal cancer is sometimes called Dukes' D rectal cancer.

RECURRENT RECTAL CANCER

Recurrent rectal cancer is cancer that has recurred (come back) after it has been treated. The cancer may come back in the rectum or in other parts of the body, such as the colon, pelvis, liver, or lungs.

TREATMENT OPTION OVERVIEW

There are different types of treatment for patients with rectal cancer.

Different types of treatment are available for patients with rectal cancer. Some treatments are standard (the currently used treatment), and some are being tested in clinical trials. Before starting treatment, patients may want to think about taking part in a clinical trial. A treatment clinical trial is a research study meant to help improve current treatments or obtain information on new treatments for patients with cancer. When clinical trials show that a new treatment is better than the standard treatment, the new treatment may become the standard treatment.

Three types of standard treatment are used:

Surgery

Surgery is the most common treatment for all stages of rectal cancer. A doctor may remove the cancer using one of the following types of surgery:

- Local excision: If the cancer is found at a very early stage, the doctor may remove it without cutting into the abdomen. If the cancer is found in a polyp (a growth that protrudes from the rectal mucous membrane), the operation is called a polypectomy.
- Resection: If the cancer is larger, the doctor will perform a resection of the rectum (removing the cancer and a small amount of healthy tissue around it). The doctor will then perform an anastomosis (sewing the healthy parts of the rectum together, sewing the remaining rectum to the colon, or sewing the colon to the anus). The doctor will also take out lymph nodes near the rectum and examine them under a microscope to see if they contain cancer.
- Resection and colostomy: If the doctor is not able to sew the rectum back together, a stoma (an opening) is made on the outside of the body for waste to pass through. This procedure is called a colostomy. A bag is placed around the stoma to collect the waste. Sometimes the colostomy is needed only until the rectum has healed, and then it can be reversed. If the doctor needs to remove the entire rectum, however, the colostomy may be permanent.

Even if the doctor removes all the cancer that can be seen at the time of the operation, some patients may be given chemotherapy or radiation therapy after surgery to kill any cancer cells that are left. Treatment given after surgery to increase the chances of a cure is called adjuvant therapy.

Radiation therapy

Radiation therapy is a cancer treatment that uses high-energy x-rays or other types of radiation to kill cancer cells. There are two types of radiation therapy. External radiation therapy uses a machine outside the body to send radiation toward the cancer. Internal radiation therapy uses a radioactive substance sealed in needles, seeds, wires, or catheters that are placed directly into or near the cancer. The way the radiation therapy is given depends on the type and stage of the cancer being treated.

Chemotherapy

Chemotherapy is a cancer treatment that uses drugs to stop the growth of cancer cells, either by killing the cells or by stopping the cells from dividing. When chemotherapy is taken by mouth or injected into a vein or muscle, the drugs enter the bloodstream and can reach cancer cells throughout the body (systemic chemotherapy). When chemotherapy is placed directly in the spinal column, an organ, or a body cavity such as the abdomen, the drugs mainly affect cancer cells in those areas (regional chemotherapy). The way the chemotherapy is given depends on the type and stage of the cancer being treated.

After treatment, a blood test to measure amounts of carcinoembryonic antigen (a substance in the blood that may be increased when cancer is present) may be done to see if the cancer has come back.

New types of treatment are being tested in clinical trials. These include the following:

Biologic therapy

Biologic therapy is a treatment that uses the patient's immune system to fight cancer. Substances made by the body or made in a laboratory are used to boost, direct, or restore the body's natural defenses against cancer. This type of cancer treatment is also called biotherapy or immunotherapy.

Treatment Options by Stage

Stage 0 rectal cancer

Treatment of stage 0 (carcinoma in situ) rectal cancer may include the following:

- Local excision (surgery to remove the tumor without cutting into the abdomen) or simple polypectomy (surgery to remove a growth that protrudes from the rectal mucous membrane).
- Resection (surgery to remove the cancer). This is done when the cancerous tissue is too large to remove by local excision.
- Internal or external radiation therapy.

Stage I rectal cancer

Treatment of stage I rectal cancer may include the following:
- Surgery to remove the tumor with or without anastomosis (joining the cut ends of the rectum).
- Surgery to remove the tumor with or without radiation therapy and chemotherapy.
- Internal and/or external radiation therapy.

Stage II rectal cancer

Treatment of stage II rectal cancer may include the following:
- Resection with or without anastomosis (joining the cut ends of the rectum and colon, or the colon and anus) followed by chemotherapy and radiation therapy.
- Partial or total pelvic exenteration (surgery to remove the organs and nearby structures of the pelvis), depending on where the cancer has spread. Surgery is followed by radiation therapy and chemotherapy.
- Radiation therapy with or without chemotherapy followed by surgery and chemotherapy.
- Radiation therapy during surgery followed by external-beam radiation therapy and chemotherapy.

- A clinical trial evaluating new treatment options.

Stage III rectal cancer

Treatment of stage III rectal cancer may include the following:
- Resection with or without anastomosis (joining the cut ends of the rectum and colon, or the colon and anus) followed by chemotherapy and radiation therapy.
- Partial or total pelvic exenteration (surgery to remove the organs and nearby structures of the pelvis), depending on where the cancer has spread. Surgery is followed by radiation therapy and chemotherapy.
- Radiation therapy with or without chemotherapy followed by surgery and chemotherapy.
- Radiation therapy during surgery followed by external-beam radiation therapy and chemotherapy.
- Chemotherapy and radiation therapy to relieve symptoms caused by advanced cancer.
- A clinical trial evaluating new treatment options.

Stage IV rectal cancer

Treatment of stage IV rectal cancer may include the following:
- Resection/anastomosis (surgery to remove the cancer and join the cut ends of the rectum and colon, or colon and anus) to relieve symptoms caused by advanced cancer.

- Surgery to remove parts of other organs, such as the liver, lung, and ovaries, where the cancer may have spread.
- Chemotherapy and radiation therapy to relieve symptoms caused by advanced cancer.
- Chemotherapy following surgery.
- Clinical trials of chemotherapy and biological therapy.

Treatment Options for Recurrent Rectal Cancer

Treatment of recurrent rectal cancer may include the following:
- Surgery to remove the tumor or as palliative therapy to relieve symptoms caused by advanced cancer.
- Surgery to remove parts of other organs, such as the liver, lungs, and ovaries, where the cancer may have spread.
- Radiation therapy and/or chemotherapy as palliative therapy to reduce the size of the tumor and relieve symptoms caused by advanced cancer.

A NOTE ABOUT CLINICAL TRIALS

Clinical trials are taking place in many parts of the country. Information about ongoing clinical trials is available from the NCI website (*www.nci.nih.gov*). Choosing the most appropriate cancer treatment is a decision that ideally involves the patient, family, and healthcare team.

SECTION VI
INTERNET RESOURCES

INTERNET RESOURCES

The Internet offers practically limitless information relating to every conceivable health condition. The danger is that not all health-related websites are reliable. While no one—whether patient or healthcare professional—should take action based on something learned from even a reliable website without first consulting a physician, the following sites are believed to be reputable and home to solid, potentially helpful information about colorectal cancer or related issues.

For the sake of convenience, they have been separated according to the type of content they offer.

GENERAL INFORMATION

American Cancer Society: Learn About Colon and Rectum Cancer

The American Cancer Society provides a comprehensive online information resource on colon and rectal cancer. The visitor can find everything from an overview of both cancers to treatment options, as well as other information on cancer. Personal anecdotes, a handy glossary of terms, and tips on how to speak to others about this condition are also provided as links. Free brochures, alternate websites, and specific books are offered for those seeking further information on the subject.

Website: http://www.cancer.org/docroot/lrn/lrn_0.asp

Cancer Education: Colorectal Cancer

Intended as a resource for both patients and professionals, Cancer Education's information on colorectal cancer goes above and beyond typical reporting. Text links on numerous topics such as risk factors and prevention, signs and symptoms, screening, diagnosis, and treatment options are all present. The patient is also able to connect to audio and video information on numerous subjects, from dealing with fatigue to risk factors, prevention, and early detection. From the main screen at the address below, click on the "Choose a Topc" box under Patient and Family Center", then select "colorectal cancer" from the menu.

Website: http://www.cancereducation.com

CancerHealthOnline: Colorectal Cancer

A division of HealthCentersOnline, this site provides comprehensive informa
tion pertaining to the types of colorectal cancer, risk factors, signs and symp
toms, diagnosis and treatment, staging, and even ongoing research. Clinica
terms that may be new to the user are defined. A video about colorectal cancer
is provided within the summary heading on the first page. Registration, which
is free of charge, is required.
Website: http://cancer.healthcentersonline.com/gastrointestinalsystemcancer/
colorectalcancer.cfm

Centers for Disease Control: Colorectal Cancer Prevention and Control Initiatives

Awareness is thoroughly promoted throughout CDC's website. Statements and
statistics pertaining to the number cases and diagnoses to-date, and projected
throughout the United States are included. A fact sheet and information about
screening promote immediate medical evaluation.
Website: http://www.cdc.gov/cancer/colorctl/index.htm

Cooper: Colorectal Cancer

The Cancer Institute of New Jersey, at Cooper University Hospital, briefly
defines colorectal cancer. Reading the bullet points on the side of the page, the
visitor may learn about the colon's anatomy (ascending, transverse, descending
and sigmoid sections) followed by the symptoms of colorectal cancer. Clearly
bulleted throughout the remainder of the page are prevention techniques
screening methods, and a practical screening guide for the patient. Also, the
website offers an account of the staging of cancer.
Website: http://www.coopercancer.org/content3/greystone_21488.asp

National Cancer Institute: Colon and Rectal Cancer Homepage

The National Cancer Institute provides a basic overview of colon and rectal can
cer. Separate addresses for each of these diseases, combined with prevention
screening and testing, treatments, clinical trials, and a literature review allow
the patient to view the facts and to understand treatment strategy. Links to
equivalent pages and databases, like the National Institute of Health, are also
presented. At the top of the page, a link to a dictionary of cancer terms is offered
accompanied by a version translated into Spanish.
Website: http://www.cancer.gov/cancertopics/types/colon-and-rectal

Oncolink: Colorectal Cancer

Though listed under the same heading, both colon and rectal cancer are defined
and expressed independently in this source. It describes the anatomical feature
specifically, but also explains the stages, diagnosis, and therapeutic options
General information such as risk, prevention, and screening has been subdivided

for quick location. Additional features of the page allow visitors to browse clinical trials and upcoming conferences.
Website: http://www.oncolink.com/types/article.cfm?c=5&s=11&ss=81&id=7336

RISKS, SCREENING & PREVENTION

American Cancer Society: Can Colorectal Cancer Be Prevented?

Concerns on how to prevent this type of cancer are thoroughly addressed by the American Cancer Society in this webpage. Screening, diet and exercise, and the use of nonsteroidal anti-inflammatory drugs are just a few of the prevention methods explained to the visitor. A general overview of colorectal cancer is available in menu form just opposite the helpful glossary and drug guide. This page is printer-friendly and available for e-mail to others.
Website: http://www.cancer.org/docroot/CRI/content/CRI_2_4_2X_Can_colon_and_rectum_cancer_be_prevented.asp?sitearea=

American Cancer Society: What Are the Risk Factors for Colorectal Cancer?

The text opens with a brief definition of the term "risk factor"; the ACS lists a number of factors that contribute to cancer growth. Family history, ethnic background, age, and diet are among those described. In the margin, there is a list of questions that may frequently be asked; for example, if the cause of the cancer is known and if it may be prevented. There is also a glossary of terms for the vocabulary used throughout the text.
Website: http://www.cancer.org/docroot/CRI/content/CRI_2_4_2X_What_are_the_risk_factors_for_colon_and_rectum_cancer.asp

Cancer Research and Prevention Foundation: Colorectal Screening

This website dives directly into the issue of screening; the text begins with a brief mention of commonly used exams (later discussed in detail), and how often they should be performed. Each of the four assessments is color coded. The basics, before the test, during the test, after the test, and the potential complications, are tended to in this brief description. This site continues to describe the tools and procedure used to remove the polyps if found during the procedure.
Website: http://www.preventcancer.org/colorectal/aboutcolorectal/about_screening.cfm

Dana-Farber Cancer Institute: Screening and Detection

Screening for colorectal cancer is the principal focus of this text. At the top of the page there is a list of topics that will be addressed throughout the website, such as the definition of screening, a brief description of colorectal cancer, and risks of screening. Toward the end of the text there is a catalog offering further data on

this subject. Throughout the entire site, key terms are linked to a glossary to allow quick and easy access to their definition. (From the page at the address below, click on one of the links under "Colorectal Cancer.") From the screen at the address below, click on the "Choose a Diagnosis" bar, then select from the menu.
Website: http://www.dana-farber.org/can/screening/

National Cancer Institute: Colorectal Cancer Screening: Q & A

This site starts with a brief summary of what colorectal cancer is, then goes on to more lengthy explanations. Digital rectal exam (DRE), blood test, and colonoscopy are select tests presented within the text. A tabulated version of the advantages and disadvantages of all five colorectal screenings is presented for easy reading and strategy-planning.
Website: http://www.cancer.gov/cancertopics/factsheet/Detection/colorectal-screening

New York-Presbyterian: Digestive Diseases: Diagnostic Procedures

The University Hospital of Columbia and Cornell offers this page to link the visitor to any of the 19 screening procedures that may diagnose colon or rectal cancer, or other gastrointestinal diseases. By selecting one of the numerous exams, ranging from colonoscopies to sigmoidoscopies, the viewer is privy to a paragraph about the physical process and what it may or may not detect. (From the page at the address below, click on "Diagnostic Procedures" from the menu on the left.)
Website: http://wo-pub2.med.cornell.edu/cgi-bin/WebObjects/PublicA.woa/5/healthindex?website=nyp+digestive

Princeton Longevity Center: Virtual Colonoscopy

This site is devoted to showing the advantages of the three-dimensional virtual colonoscopy in comparison to the typical colonoscopy; for example, there is no need for sedation, or extensive tubing into the rectum. Questions a patient might have on the advanced practice are addressed.
Website: http://www.theplc.net/colonography.shtml

STAGING & TREATMENT

American Cancer Society: After the Tests: Staging

The staging of colorectal cancer is thoroughly detailed by the American Cancer Society. The meaning of the stages is explained, leading up to a description of the three systems which comprise the staging formula. The significance of differences between the various states is explained, as well.
Website: http://www.cancer.org/docroot/CRI/content/CRI_2_2_3X_after_the_tests_staging_10.asp?sitearea=

American Society of Clinical Oncology: Follow-up Care for Colorectal Cancer

This guide aids patients in their quest to remain cancer-free. Recommended frequency of doctor visits and explanations of procedures are provided. A colorful table is given to assist the person in maintaining a healthy lifestyle. A list of questions to ask the doctor during visits, and a collection of alternate sources of data are also made available.

Website: http://www.asco.org/plwc/external_files/Colorectal_Cancer_Patient_Guide.pdf

Eloxatin®: About Eloxatin

The Eloxatin homepage is specific to those who are trying to learn about treatment types. There are multiple links with information for the patient relevant to who should and should not use this drug, how it is administered, the side effects, and management. Prescribing information and brochures are also available.

Website: http://www.eloxatin.com/patient/index.asp

Healthline: Colon Cancer

This Healthline page describes relevant anatomy, incidence, symptoms, and treatment options, as well as complications such as metastasis, recurrence, and development of a second primary colorectal cancer. Diagnostic imaging and color illustrations are used to explain the digestive system, colonoscopy, anatomical structures, and cancer staging in a patient-friendly way.

Website: http://www.healthline.com/article?contentId=000262

National Cancer Institute: Colon and Rectal Cancer: Treatment

Colon and rectal cancer treatments are discussed with emphasis on stages, recurrent cancer, a treatment overview, and treatment options. Large, colorful diagrams, distinctly labeled, help explain general anatomy, where polyps may occur, and what examinations (ie, sigmoidoscopy or colonoscopy) are necessary to find them. A definition will appear in another window to explain the meaning of certain terms. The page is available in both a printable version and a Spanish translation.

Website: http://www.cancer.gov/cancertopics/treatment/colon-and-rectal

NEWS, DATABASES & ARTICLES

Biologics in Cancer Education Initiative: Colorectal Cancer

Access to this site is free, although a quick registration must be completed. By signing in and accessing the link to colorectal cancer, visitors may be educated on therapy combinations and clinical updates through audio/visual tools. Various case studies, specific journal articles, and alternate links, are also provided for further self-education.

Website: http://www.bcei.org/index.asp?/CMEAll.asp%3ftherapy=2

Cancer.com: Colon/Colorectal Cancer

Cancer.com presents a compilation of websites relevant to those affected by cancer. Links relating to therapies, side effects, trials, and research are provided along with a physician locator. Each is defined by the type of knowledge they afford to the patient.
Website: http://www.cancer.com/cancertype?ID=COLCANC

CancerWise: Your Link to Cancer News & Information

Provided by the University of Texas' M.D. Anderson Cancer Center, CancerWise is a free monthly newsletter that discusses cancer of all types. The reader is kept abreast of the latest news, research and treatments. The primary page will display each month's featured article; archived articles cover colon, rectal, or colorectal cancer. This site gives the patients a full background on the foci of their choice, along with a look into the future of cancer research.
Website: http://www.cancerwise.org/

MedicineNet: What's Inside the Colon Cancer Health Center

MedicineNet provides over 100 articles assembled into subheadings for easy access. The site offers a "Good Place to Start"; this gives a full background on the illness. From there, the visitor may move on to more complex questions and answers. At the bottom of the page, there are lists of what is new in colon cancer research, coupled with how to choose a doctor and make the most of the appointment.
Website: http://www.medicinenet.com/colon_cancer/index.htm

People Living with Cancer: About Clinical Trials

A grouping from the American Society of Clinical Oncology, People Living With Cancer takes the visitor through a step-by-step evaluation of a clinical trial. Through distinctive links, this page addresses what a clinical trial actually is, rights and safety, how to make the decision to participate (weighing the risks and benefits), questions to ask the research team, and where to find a trial to participate in. (From the main page below, click on the "Understanding Cancer" button on the left side of the screen, then look for the link to the "Clinical Trials" page.) From the main screen at the address below, type "Clinical Trials" in the search box in the upper left corner
Website: http://www.plwc.org/

FRIENDS & FAMILY

Colon Cancer Alliance: How to Talk About CRC

The Colon Cancer Alliance encourages communication with friends and family. Specific questions to ask a family about history and their personal screenings are

bulleted for simple access. This site supports the idea of being direct, along with expressing needs and feelings. It also offers a link to "conversation starters," providing a perfect introduction to speaking with loved ones about their health.
Website: http://www.ccalliance.org/talk/how_communicating.html

KidsHealth: Dealing with Cancer

Sponsored by the Nemours Foundation, KidsHealth helps children understand what cancer is and how they can help themselves, and others with the disease. The text is written in simple terms for a child or teen, and may be translated to Spanish, as well. The article attempts to define for youngsters exactly what cancer is, and describes how they may better themselves both physically and emotionally, as well as sharing ways to help others who may already be afflicted through volunteer work.
Website: http://kidshealth.org/teen/diseases_conditions/cancer/deal_with_cancer.html

Mayo Clinic: Colon Cancer: Coping Skills

In recognition of the fact that a diagnosis of cancer can be challenging, the Mayo Clinic provides a resource on how to handle it with dignity. The site provides bullet points that explain to the patient what to expect, how to be proactive, why building a support system is important, how to set goals, and the importance of taking time alone. Article sections cover general topics ranging from when to seek medical advice to prevention. Plus, the text is available to print as a whole or in sections, or in larger type. Links to related articles, specialists, centers, a bookstore, and web resources are offered at the bottom of the page. From the screen at the address below, click on "Coping Skills" in the box labeled "Article Sections".
Website: http://www.mayoclinic.com/health/colon-cancer/DS00035/

The University of Texas, M.D. Anderson Cancer Center: Support Programs

M.D. Anderson Cancer Center has dedicated an entire section of its website to support programs for those who are afflicted with cancer, and the individuals close to them. Links lead to group and one-on-one support via telephone, educational resources offering classes for the ill and their loved ones, online and spiritual support, and patient stories. Unless otherwise noted, most of the support groups are free to patients, caregivers, and family/friends. The website is available in Spanish and in a printer-friendly version.
Website: http://www.mdanderson.org/patients_public/support_programs/

University of California: Helping Children Understand Cancer

When cancer strikes a family, children may sense something is wrong even if they're not told. The University of California brings forth a site to help adults talk to children about the disease. Headings such as *Protecting Children Can Make Things Worse* and *How to Tell Them a Loved One Has Cancer* give the adult guidance through the typically tough conversation. Moreover, the text lists numerous ways to answer a child's questions, including suggestions on how to handle the difficult and frightening subject of death.

Website: http://cc.ucsf.edu/crc/hm_talking_with_children.html

WebMD/The Cleveland Clinic: Tips for Family and Friends

Patients with colorectal cancer (or any type of cancer) are not the only ones affected by the diagnosis. WebMD collaborated with The Cleveland Clinic to address how friends and family may cope. The tips are bulleted and deal with topics like what to ask doctors, how the patient might react to the disease physically, mentally, and emotionally, and how to keep a healthy body and mind.

Website: http://www.webmd.com/content/article/45/1811_50431.htm

Section VII
Visual Identification Guide

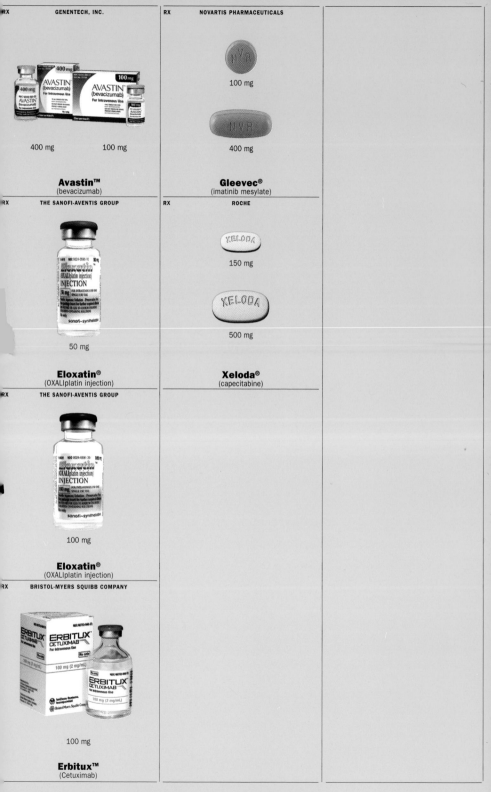

RX GENENTECH, INC.

400 mg   **100 mg**

Avastin™
(bevacizumab)

RX THE SANOFI-AVENTIS GROUP

50 mg

Eloxatin®
(OXALIplatin injection)

RX THE SANOFI-AVENTIS GROUP

100 mg

Eloxatin®
(OXALIplatin injection)

RX BRISTOL-MYERS SQUIBB COMPANY

100 mg

Erbitux™
(Cetuximab)

RX NOVARTIS PHARMACEUTICALS

100 mg

400 mg

Gleevec®
(imatinib mesylate)

RX ROCHE

150 mg

500 mg

Xeloda®
(capecitabine)